Orthopedic
Rehabilitation Science

Orthopedic Rehabilitation Science
Principles for Clinical Management of Bone

Katie Lundon, B.Sc. (P.T.), M.Sc., Ph.D.

Assistant Professor, Department of Physical Therapy and Graduate Department of Rehabilitation Science, Faculty of Medicine, University of Toronto, Toronto, Ontario

With Two Contributing Authors

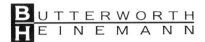

BUTTERWORTH
HEINEMANN

Boston   Oxford   Auckland   Johannesburg   Melbourne   New Delhi

MTHS

 Butterworth–Heinemann supports the efforts of American Forests and the Global ReLeaf program in its campaign for the betterment of trees, forests, and our environment.

Library of Congress Cataloging-in-Publication Data

Lundon, Katie.
   Orthopedic rehabilitation science : principles for clinical management of bone / Katie Lundon.
      p.   cm.
   Includes bibliographical references and index.
   ISBN 0-7506-7155-6
   1. Bones--Diseases--Pathophysiology. 2. Physical therapy.
   3. Connective tissues--Diseases 4. Biomechanics. 5. Orthopedics.
   I. Title.
   [DNLM: 1. Bone Diseases--physiopathology. 2. Biomechanics.
   3. Bone Diseases--rehabilitiation. 4. Bone and Bones--physiology.
   5. Physical Therapy--methods.   WE 225 L962o 2000]
   RC930.L86   2000
   616.7'1--dc21
   DNLM/DLC
   for Library of Congress   99-39419
                                                                     CIP

British Library Cataloguing-in-Publication Data
A catalogue record for this book is available from the British Library.

The publisher offers special discounts on bulk orders of this book.
For information, please contact:

Manager of Special Sales
Butterworth–Heinemann
225 Wildwood Avenue
Woburn, MA 01801-2041
Tel: 781-904-2500
Fax: 781-904-2620

For information on all Butterworth–Heinemann publications available, contact our World Wide Web home page at: http://www.bh.com

10 9 8 7 6 5 4 3 2 1

Printed in the United States of America

7/19/02

In memory of my uncle, Bill Drynan

Contents

Contributing Authors

Aileen M. Davis, B.Sc. (P.T.), M.Sc., Ph.D.
Assistant Professor, Department of Physical Therapy and Graduate Department of Public Health Science, Faculty of Medicine, University of Toronto; Director of Clinical Research, University Musculoskeletal Oncology Unit, Division of Orthopedic Surgery, Mount Sinai Hospital, Toronto, Ontario

Marc D. Grynpas, Ph.D.
Professor, Department of Laboratory Medicine and Pathophysiology, Faculty of Medicine, University of Toronto; Senior Scientist, Samuel Lunenfeld Research Institute, Mount Sinai Hospital, Toronto, Ontario

Katie Lundon, B.Sc. (P.T.), M.Sc., Ph.D.
Assistant Professor, Department of Physical Therapy and Graduate Department of Rehabilitation Science, Faculty of Medicine, University of Toronto, Toronto, Ontario

Preface

This text provides a description of the relationship between the basic and clinical science approaches to the dense mineralized connective tissues as they relate to orthopedic disorders. The book is designed to help clinicians

1. Gain a basic understanding of the biology of dense mineralized connective tissues in terms of normal structure, function, growth, and repair processes in the adult skeleton.
2. Obtain a basic level of knowledge of pathophysiologic processes inherent to dense mineralized connective tissue in response to injury and disease.
3. Understand the rationale for physical intervention in the orthopedic management of bone in health and disease.
4. Be cognizant of the direction for future research studies of mineralized connective tissues that would impact on the field of knowledge in evidence-based orthopedic rehabilitation of bone and bone disorders.

The goals of this book are

1. To effectively present current basic science background underlying mineralized dense connective tissue dynamics in health and selected disease states commonly encountered in physical rehabilitation practice.
2. To serve as a practical reference for undergraduate students and practicing clinicians alike by offering a comprehensive and integrated text on bone metabolism, selected skeletal disorders, and pertinent applications to clinical practice in physical rehabilitation.
3. To facilitate the clinician's understanding of the basic science mechanisms of skeletal pathophysiology that underlie clinical decision making in the physical assessment and treatment of selected mineralized connective tissue disorders and metabolic bone diseases.
4. To enhance clinical practice by providing current rationale as well as potential research directions in the field of physical assessment and treatment of conditions affecting bone.

The book is organized into three parts. Part I is comprised of basic science fundamentals in which structure, composition, and function of bone is presented. Part II encompasses basic bone biomechanics, the impact of physical activity on bone, and bone injury and repair. Part III addresses some pathologic conditions of bone encountered in orthopedic rehabilitation practice. The role of physical rehabilitation management of these common bone disorders is also presented.

The intent of this book is to effectively present the basic science principles underlying mineralized connective tissue pathobiology that are important to evidence-based orthopedic rehabilitation practice. In addition, the current rationale for physical intervention strategies in the management of mineralized connective tissue dynamics in both health and disease are examined.

The need for a concise presentation of the scientific principles underlying the clinical care of dense mineralized connective tissues in physical rehabilitation practice has been recognized. The physical management of bone should reflect, incorporate, and be guided by knowledge of dynamics of bone metabolism in health and disease as well as across the lifespan. This subject is topical, with the increasing demand for evidence-based practice, and serves as a member of the front of specialization in orthopedic physical therapy, which inherently carries an expected fluency between both the basic science and clinical practice disciplines. Hence, this text endeavours to reflect the needs of the contemporary physical rehabilitation practitioner with a keen interest in skeletal metabolism.

K.L.

Acknowledgments

I am indebted to many people for their assistance in creating this work. Specifically, I would like to thank the following people who contributed significant effort to and were extremely supportive of its production: Diane Gasner, Beatrice Poroger, Margaret Furman, Dr. J. Lundon, Alice Lundon, Audrey Li, Harpul (Polly) Gahunia, Dr. Edna Becker, Dr. Marc Grynpas, Dr. Aileen Davis, Sonia Bibershtein, Sarah McCutcheon, and Dr. Lis Mosekilde. I would also like to express my gratitude to both Mary Drabot, Medical Editor, and Leslie Kramer, Assistant Editor, in the medical division of Butterworth–Heinemann for their enthusiasm and guidance. Many thanks go to JoAnn Schambier, Production Editor at Silverchair Science + Communications, for her efficient and thorough handling of this work.

Finally, I wish to thank my husband, Robert L. Gordon, and my *most* wonderful children, Robyn and Sam, for their unfailing love and patience.

K.L.

Part I
Structure and Function of Mineralized Connective Tissue

Chapter 1
Connective Tissues: Structure, Function, and Metabolic Properties

Connective tissues serve to support and connect as well as protect tissues and organs throughout the body. In addition, connective tissues have other specialized functions (Table 1-1). The interstitial tissue of the musculoskeletal system is composed of various forms of specialized connective tissues. Common to all forms of connective tissue found in the musculoskeletal system is the presence of connective tissue cells embedded in an abundant extracellular matrix that the cells produce. This interstitial or extracellular matrix is composed of protein-based structures and complex polysaccharides, the presence and distribution of which determine the metabolic and biomechanical characteristics of each form and contribute to their specialized functions. In health, the connective tissues are not inert structures, but are quite metabolically active and achieve a continuous balance of degradation and replacement of their components.

The term *connective tissue* is often used to describe the extracellular matrix plus resident cells such as fibroblasts, macrophages, and mast cells. The amount of connective tissue in organs varies greatly: Skin and bone are composed mainly of connective tissue, whereas the brain and spinal cord contain minimal amounts. The relative amounts of the different types of matrix macromolecules and the way in which they are organized within the extracellular matrix vary to a great extent, allowing a large diversity of forms, each specific to the functional requirements of the particular tissue. The extracellular matrix can, for example, calcify to

form bone or teeth, or it may assume the ropelike organization of the collagen fibers in tendons, imparting tensile strength. The ligaments, fasciae, tendons, sclera, and cornea of the eye are all examples of "soft" connective tissues. Hard connective tissues, such as the bone tissues of the skeleton, dentine, and cementum, are mineralized through the deposition of calcium phosphate in the form of hydroxyapatite $[Ca_{10}(PO_4)_6OH_2]$ crystals. Cartilage, which can be mineralized but usually is not, is also a hard connective tissue (Table 1-2).

Connective tissue exists diversely and is integral to systems that perform particular functions. For example, the joints that have bone, cartilage, ligaments, and synovial fluid function to allow movement between long bones. Periodontal tissues, gingivae, the periodontal ligament, alveolar bone, and cementum, which together form an organ known as the *periodontium*, cooperatively support the teeth and tooth movement. The heart, blood vessels, and blood cells are all formed from cells that develop in the mesenchyme, the embryonic germ layer responsible for connective tissue development. In this way, the blood circulating in vessels that are confined to connective tissue is considered a specialized connective tissue similar to synovial fluid that is confined to the joint.

Because the properties of ordinary connective tissues can differ markedly, two main groups of connective tissue can be described histologically. Depending on the relative amount of fibers, ordinary connective tissue can be distinguished as being

Table 1-1. Main Types of Connective Tissues and Their Function

Type	Presentation	Function
Ordinary connective tissue	Loose (e.g., areolar tissue)	Tissue/organ protection
	Dense	
	Irregular (e.g., capsule, dermis)	Connecting functions
	Regular	
	Cartilage	Connects, supports, bears weight
	Bone	Connects, protects, supports, bears weight
	Ligament, tendon	Connects, supports, stabilizes, and imparts tensile strength
Specialized connective tissue	Adipose (fat) tissue	Space occupying and has cushioning effects
	Blood cells and blood-forming tissue	

loose or *dense* in nature. Loose connective tissue is also known as *areolar* (*small space*) *tissue*. It is ubiquitous throughout the body and forms a protective covering for many tissues and organs. Loose connective tissue is cellular, compliant, and endowed with many vessels and nerves. Fibers are loosely woven and randomly oriented. Loose connective tissue characteristically has a considerable amount of extracellular matrix containing much the same components as found in dense connective tissues but at lower concentrations. It is also typically high in tissue fluid, which is important for the supply of nutrients and removal of waste products from the dependent tissues.

The dense connective tissues may be further classified as *regular* or *irregular*, depending on their

Table 1-2. Forms of Connective Tissue: Hard versus Soft

Soft
Ligaments
Fasciae
Tendon
Sclera
Cornea of the eye
Hard
Bone[a]
Dentine[a]
Cementum[a]
Cartilage[b]

[a]Mineralized.
[b]Non-mineralized.

internal spatial organization. Dense irregular connective tissue (e.g., dermis, joint capsules) has a three-dimensional framework, often accompanied by elastic fibers. Dense regular connective tissue (e.g., tendon) displays highly ordered fibers arranged parallel to one another, reflecting the mechanical demands of the tissues. Bone is therefore classified as a mineralized, dense, regular connective tissue. The following twelve chapters deal exclusively with the basic and clinical science related to form and function of bone tissue in the human skeleton across the lifespan.

An appreciation of the morphology, cell biology, biochemistry, and biomechanics inherent to the connective tissues is essential to understand the behavior of normal connective tissues, the response of these tissues to injury, and the potential of these tissues to repair themselves once injured. The study of the repair of connective tissues in the musculoskeletal system is fascinating in that the majority of connective tissues have significant regenerative potential, as can be witnessed by the cellular proliferation and biosynthetic events that occur most notably in response to injury. The response of bone tissue to chronic or prolonged abnormal stresses provides the opportunity to study adaptive behavior that differs considerably from acute conditions. Although each tissue has unique intrinsic and extrinsic qualities that influence its response to injury and repair, several common events and processes apply to the musculoskeletal connective tissues. Bone is an excellent example; it continuously adapts to diverse systemic and mechanical environments.

Chapter 2
Anatomy and Biology of Bone Tissue

Composition and Ultrastructure of Bone

Bone is a dynamic form of dense connective tissue consisting of living cells embedded within, or lining the surfaces of, a mineralized organic matrix. Bone provides mechanical support for the body as well as a structure for muscle attachment to allow mobility. The human skeleton is a mechanically optimized biological system whose composition and organization reflect the functional demands made on it. The molecular, cellular, and metabolic changes that occur in bone are directed to maintain its mechanical environment and to adapt to any new loading conditions that it may experience. Failure to do this leads to the development of bone incompetence (fracture) and the skeletal pain associated with a variety of metabolic bone diseases. Under optimal conditions, the human skeleton can fulfill all of its required activities, including locomotion, protection of vital organs, and the ability to participate in metabolic pathways associated with mineral homeostasis.

Bone is a two-phase material composed of a mineral phase deposited in a protein-rich matrix reservoir. By weight, bone consists of approximately 70% mineral, 22% protein, and 8% water. The skeleton serves as a reservoir of calcium, playing an essential role in calcium homeostasis across the body. In fact, the skeleton is a repository for 99% of the calcium, 80% of the phosphate, and a large proportion of the stores of magnesium, sodium, and carbonate found throughout the body. The skeleton provides a response to conditions of systemic acidosis and assists the renal and respiratory systems in the maintenance of acid-base balance. In addition, bone contains the marrow that produces erythrocytes, granular leukocytes, and platelets. Long bone growth and modeling are regulated by complex interactions between an individual's genetic potential, environmental influences, and nutritional status. Functionally appropriate morphology balanced with the skeleton's role in mineral (calcium and phosphorus) homeostasis are the result of these interactions that, in turn, determine bone architecture.

Types of Bone

The human skeleton is comprised of 206 bones. These bones vary in shape and are categorized as long bones, short bones, flat bones, irregular bones, sesamoid bones, and accessory bones. Two basic types of bone exist in the human skeleton, each with a different role and function. In humans, bone consists of dense cortical (compact) bone found on the outer surface of the long bones (e.g., femur, tibia, and humerus) and spongy or cancellous bone present at the ends (epiphyses) of the long bones and in the axial skeleton (e.g., vertebral bodies). The amount, distribution, and representation of compact and cancellous bone varies between bones.

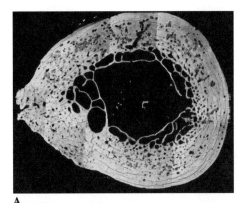

A

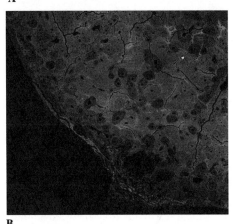

B

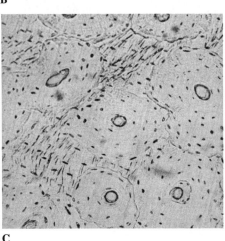

C

Figure 2-1. A. Cross section through the diaphysis of a long bone. Note the periosteal, intracortical (haversian), and endosteal envelopes or surfaces. (Photo courtesy of Dr. Marc Grynpas, Ph.D., Samuel Lunenfeld Research Institute, Mount Sinai Hospital, Toronto.) **B.** Ultrastructural view of a quadrant of a cross section of cortical bone. This backscattered image demonstrates the variation of size and other characteristics of osteons within the intracortical compartment. **C.** Intracortical compartment: secondary osteons as seen under reversed polarized light, 150×.

Cortical Bone

Cortical, or compact bone, is found in the shafts of long bones. Cortical bone comprises approximately 80–85% of the human skeleton and serves significant mechanical and protective functions in that it is densely (80–90%) mineralized. It is therefore a macroscopically dense type of bone tissue. Cortical bone is the most abundant type of bone represented in the long bones of the appendicular skeleton and forms the outer protective shell of all bones. Three main envelopes or remodeling surfaces can be described in cortical bone: endosteal, intracortical or haversian, and periosteal (Figure 2-1). Cortical bone volume is regulated by bone formation or resorption on the endosteal and periosteal surfaces as well as by remodeling within the haversian systems. Cortical bone is removed in metabolic bone disease and across the aging process primarily by endosteal resorption and resorption within the haversian canals (Mundy 1995). Because of the architecture of cortical bone, its metabolic activity is relatively low in comparison to cancellous bone.

The shaft of a long bone is referred to as the *diaphysis*; the flared portion, the *metaphysis*; and the ends of the bone, the *epiphyses* (Figure 2-2). With the exception of regions of the bone covered by articular cartilage, a membrane known as the *periosteum* lines the outer surface of cortical bone. The periosteum consists of an inner layer of loosely arranged, vascular connective tissue that contains osteoblasts, the cells responsible for bone formation. These osteoblasts are referred to as *lining cells*. The *endosteum* is a thin internal membrane that lines the marrow cavity and the internal spaces in the cancellous bone of the epiphysis. The endosteum is considerably thinner than the periosteum and consists of a single layer of flattened cells also with osteogenic potential. Therefore, the periosteum and the endosteum have osteogenic potential that is critical in the maturing skeleton and in fracture-healing processes. Continuing periosteal apposition of lamellar bone in adulthood leads to greater skeletal dimensions in older individuals; however, endosteal resorption also occurs, which has the overall effect of reduced bone volume seen with age (Lazenby 1990).

Haversian canals are longitudinally arranged channels in the bone from which haversian systems or osteons are derived (Figure 2-3). Haversian systems consist of lamellae that may be visualized in cross section as concentric rings surrounding the

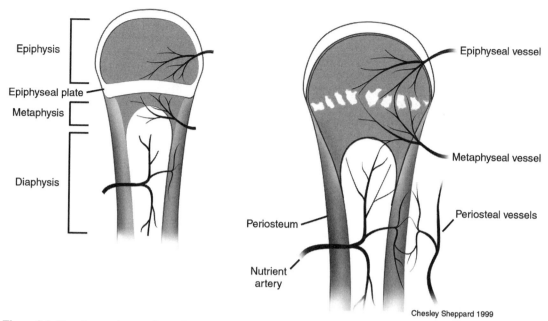

Chesley Sheppard 1999

Figure 2-2. Vascular supply to regions of a long bone.

haversian canals to form an osteon (Figure 2-4). Each channel contains capillaries and some nerve fibers. A second system of vascular channels are known as *Volkmann's canals*. These run perpendicular to the haversian canals and permit communication with the outer (periosteal) and inner (endosteal) envelopes of cortical bone. The outer layer of the periosteum consists of dense connective tissue that contains fewer, but larger, blood vessels that supply branches to the Volkmann's canals. This layer is also the site where bundles of collagenous fibers (Sharpey's fibers) exit from the outer layer into the outer part of the bone.

Cancellous Bone

Cancellous, or trabecular, bone comprises 20% of the skeleton. Cancellous bone is found in structures such as the vertebral bodies, distal radius,

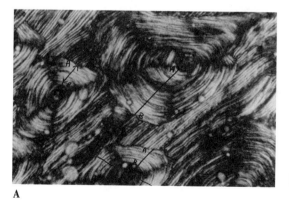

A

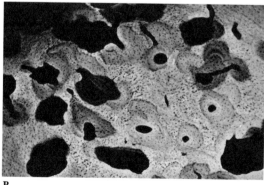

B

Figure 2-3. A. Osteons. Note the different widths for each osteon representing where local changes in bone remodeling have occurred. **B.** Normal bone is heterogeneous in nature. This backscattering image of cortical bone demonstrates the different mineralization phases typical of bone tissue. Lighter areas reflect more mineralized regions, whereas darker ones represent less, or newly mineralized, bone tissue. (Courtesy of Dr. Marc Grynpas, Ph.D., Samuel Lunenfeld Research Institute, Mount Sinai Hospital, Toronto.)

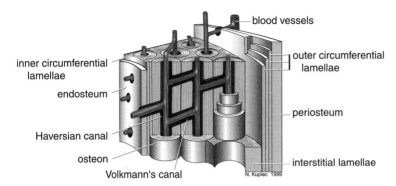

Figure 2-4. Cross section through the diaphysis of a long bone. Note the vascular network.

and proximal femur (Table 2-1). Cancellous bone displays relatively high metabolic activity in comparison to cortical bone. As bone remodeling occurs only on bone surfaces, the large surface area of cancellous bone is conducive to higher metabolic activity than cortical bone. Cancellous bone is less dense than cortical bone; it is only 5–20% mineralized. Cancellous bone has an internal arrangement consisting of bony spicules that branch and intersect in multiple directions to assume a sponge-like network, the cavities of which are filled with bone marrow (Figure 2-5). Like cortical bone, cancellous bone also consists of lamellae, but not arranged in the form of haversian systems. Regions of parallel lamellae often run along the length of a trabecula. The architecture or distribution of trabeculae within different regions of cancellous bone varies. For instance, in vertebral bodies, horizontally and vertically arranged trabeculae 0.12–0.24 mm thick are oriented parallel to lines of stress. In the anterior two-thirds of the vertebral body, vertically oriented trabeculae predominate in comparison to the posterior elements and pedicles where horizontal tra-

beculae predominate (Singh 1978). Within the larger (>200 µm) trabeculae, a central channel containing blood vessels may be found.

Composition of Bone Tissue

The inter- or extracellular bone matrix is comprised of both an inorganic, or mineral, phase and an organic phase consisting of collagen, noncollagenous proteins, lipids, and water (Figure 2-6). Mineralizing bone provides an excellent system for the sequestration and subsequent immobilization of molecules normally soluble in physiologic fluid. These molecules, whether produced locally or exogenously, adsorb to the bone hydroxyapatite or

Table 2-1. Proportion of Cancellous Bone at Various Skeletal Sites

Skeletal Site	Representation (%)
Vertebral body	66–75
Hip (intertrochanteric)	50
Hip (femoral neck)	25
Distal radius	25
Mid-radius	1
Femoral shaft	5

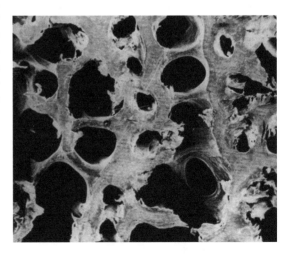

Figure 2-5. Scanning electron microscopic view of intact cancellous bone displaying typical internal architecture of horizontal and vertical trabeculae. Note its honeycomb appearance.

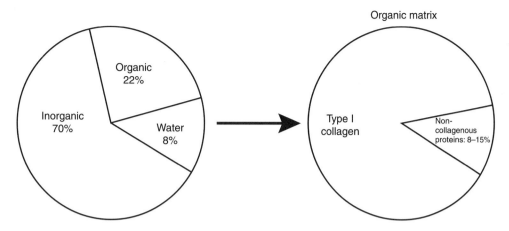

Figure 2-6. Composition of cortical bone by volume.

become entrapped in the bone matrix collagen (Termine 1990).

Inorganic Phase

The inorganic, or mineral, phase makes up approximately two-thirds the weight of mature adult bone. The mineral phase of bone plays a role in mineral homeostasis, maintaining stable systemic acid-base balance (Bushinsky 1989), as well as imparts great mechanical strength to the bone tissue and skeleton at large. The inorganic phase of bone is composed of calcium (99% of the total body calcium is stored in the skeleton) and phosphorus in the form of hydroxyapatite $[Ca_{10}(PO_4)_6(OH)_2]$. In addition, Na^+, K^+, and Mg^{2+} may be present. Bone apatite readily associates with anions other than the hydroxyl group such as CO_3^{2-} and F^-.

Organic Phase

The organic phase of bone consists of collagen fibers and cells embedded within a ground substance. The organic matrix of bone is composed of proteins from both local and exogenous sources. The collagen component of bone is largely made up of type I (92%) and type V (8%) (Bätge et al. 1992) and represents 85–92% of the organic phase by volume in addition to the non-collagenous proteins (NCPs) (8–15%). Type I collagen is a 1.5 × 300-nm rigid rod formed from three polypeptide (alpha) chains that assume a triple helical structure and are linked end to end and side to side to form fibrils. One of the alpha chains has a high proportion of the amino acids proline and hydroxyproline. The covalent intermolecular cross-links between collagen molecules are essential in providing connective tissue matrices with their stability and tensile strength. The collagen fibrils in skeletal tissues such as bone have structures that change in response to imposed forces. Type I collagen serves to impart resilience to bone as well as an organizing template and receptacle for mineral crystals. It is this mineral-collagen composite that ultimately renders bone tissue incompressible (Volpi and Katz 1991).

Although the major constituent of bone organic matrix is collagen, other macromolecules are also present in smaller amounts, and they have important functions as well. The 8–15% NCP component of the organic matrix of bone is unique, with at least 17 different NCPs identified therein. The most largely represented NCP constituents are osteopontin, bone sialoprotein, osteonectin, and osteocalcin (this protein is also referred to as *bone Gla [growth] protein*, or BGP, and is the second most abundant protein in bone), proteoglycans (biglycan and decoran), and matrix Gla protein (Azria 1989; Young et al. 1992). These proteins are considered important to the unique quality of bone as a mineralizing connective tissue. The NCPs of the organic matrix consist of proteins synthesized in situ by osteoblasts and related cells, and of circulating proteins adsorbed or concentrated on bone surfaces at the time of mineralization (Boskey 1989; Fiore et al. 1991). In altered metabolic states, NCP production and incorporation in bone may be affected with the result that the architecture, remodeling, and structural integrity of bone tissue may be compromised (Ingram et al. 1993). The distinct patterns of NCP localization in bone supports the concept that, in addition to their structural and mineral-inducing properties, these proteins may influence the events associated with bone remodeling such as recruitment, attachment, differentiation, and activity of bone cells (Ingram et al. 1993). Many of these proteins are growth factors concentrated in mineralized bone that contribute to the regeneration of injured bone (Termine 1990). As bone Gla protein (osteocalcin) is produced almost exclusively by osteoblasts, its serum values represent new synthesis of BGP, which is primarily an index of bone formation. Osteocalcin constitutes 20% of the NCPs of bone. In addition, osteocalcin may function as a matrix signal in the control of recruitment and differentiation of bone-resorbing cells (Glowacki et al. 1991). Osteopontin is an NCP with cell attachment properties, is a prominent constituent of the bone matrix (Chen et al. 1993), and is important in the mineral turnover of newly formed bone (Hultenby et al. 1991), but is not totally bone specific (Butler 1989; Epstein 1989; Tanaka et al. 1991). Bone sialoprotein is a major NCP of bone and other mineralizing connective tissues and is believed to have a specific role in mediating the initial stages of connective tissue mineralization (Chen et al. 1992). Osteonectin (SPARC) is an NCP that is involved in regulating mineralization processes of collagen and is the most abundant NCP of bone, constituting 2–4% of the total organic matrix of bone (Epstein 1989). Osteonectin is not specific to bone and most of what is found in the circulation is derived from platelets. The major proteoglycans that have been isolated from bone all contain chondroitin sulphate. Known differences in the content of NCPs in cortical compared to cancellous bone suggest functional heterogeneity in these two types of bone tissue (Ninomiya et al. 1990).

Key Players: Osteoblast, Osteoclast, and Osteocyte

Three types of bone cells are involved in bone tissue dynamics: the osteoclast, the osteoblast, and the osteocyte. Of these, the two main cells involved in the bone remodeling sequence are the osteoblast and osteoclast. These two cell types belong to different lineages: The osteoblast is derived from pluripotential mesenchymal stem cells of the bone marrow (Figure 2-7), and the osteoclast originates

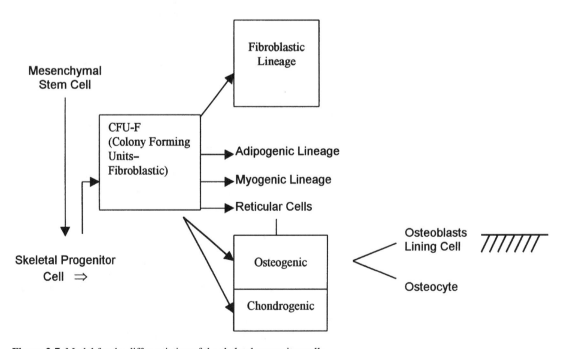

Figure 2-7. Model for the differentiation of the skeletal progenitor cells.

from the hemopoietic granulocyte-macrophage colony-forming unit (CFU) lineage. Stem and progenitor cells present within bone marrow give rise to fibroblastic CFUs (CFU-Fs) that can differentiate into fibroblastic, osteogenic, chondrogenic, myogenic, adipogenic, and reticular cells (Oreffo et al. 1998; Yoo et al. 1998). Mesenchymal progenitor cells have an important role in the repair of musculoskeletal tissues.

Osteoblasts

Osteoblasts are the bone cells responsible for bone formation in that they synthesize and secrete bone matrix. Osteoblasts are derived from fibroblast precursors (mesenchymally derived) and synthesize bone matrix or osteoid (organic component of bone) that subsequently mineralizes. Osteoblasts represent a heterogeneous group of cells that originate from stromal (marrow) tissue. Bone deposition is a primary activity in the maintenance of bone mass and is controlled by the number and activity of osteoblasts available at any one time. Sites for bone formation include those areas recently resorbed by osteoclasts in addition to areas of already established bone. Osteoblasts assume different shapes corresponding to their various tasks associated with bone deposition. For instance, osteoblasts located on the surface of an active bone formation site have a large, rounded shape and are responsible for the synthesis and deposition of bone matrix or osteoid. However, up to 70% of the osteoblasts initially present at a remodeling site may undergo apoptosis (cell death) as regulated by growth factors and cytokines produced in the bone microenvironment (Jilka et al. 1998). Osteoblasts may assume a resting state and present as elongated and flat cells lining bone surfaces. During this stage osteoblasts secrete minimal matrix and may in fact become embedded within the matrix. Once entombed within the matrix, these cells are referred to as *osteocytes*, cells that communicate via long processes by gap junctions. Because of this network, a highly organized communication system exists between surface osteoblasts and osteocytes. The coupling of cell shape and gene expression via the linkage of dynamic skeletal networks provides a molecular framework for sensing and responding to mechanical stimuli, fluid flow,

and diffusion-based chemical signaling pathways (Bidwell et al. 1998).

Osteoblasts have the capacity to synthesize bone matrix proteins including type I collagen and BGP (osteocalcin). In addition, osteoblasts contain alkaline phosphatase, which plays an essential role in bone mineralization. Osteoblasts secrete growth factors that are stored in the bone matrix, such as transforming growth factor β, bone morphogenetic proteins, platelet-derived growth factor, and the insulin-like growth factors (Hauschka et al. 1986). Osteoblasts have receptors for tissue-specific hormones, cytokines, and growth factors that all govern bone growth, differentiation, and metabolism (Rodan and Noda 1991). Proteins in bone synthesized by osteoblasts are believed to be important, not only in the formation of the organic matrix, but also in the formation, growth, and regulated dissolution of the hydroxyapatite crystal.

Osteocytes

Osteocytes are mature descendants of osteoblasts that become entrapped within calcified, mineralized bone in spaces known as *lacunae*. They are the most numerous of the bone cells in mature bone. Osteocytes are interconnected by long dendritic cell processes that run through small channels, known as *canaliculi*, in the bone matrix. This communication network may transmit information about mechanical forces and, in turn, potentially influences bone resorption and formation processes. In addition to their cell-to-cell communication, osteocytes also reside in a labyrinth of extracellular space through which bone tissue may be perfused. Osteocytes communicate with one another via gap junctions. A number of roles have been proposed for osteocytes and the lacunar-canalicular labyrinth they occupy, including the arrest of fatigue cracks, mineral exchange, osteocytic osteolysis, strain detection, and the control of mechanically related bone modeling/remodeling (Lanyon 1993). One hypothesized role of the communication network provided by the team of surface osteoblasts and osteocytes is to respond to dynamic strain within the bone tissue by processing this strain-related information, and subsequently influencing modeling/remodeling activity in a strain-related manner to establish and maintain structurally appropriate bone architecture (Lanyon 1993).

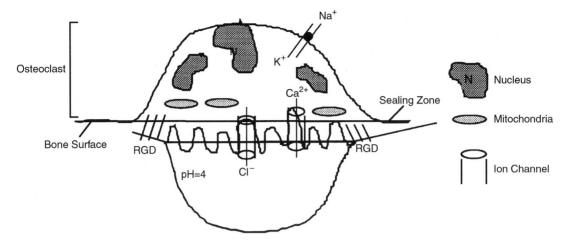

Figure 2-8. Model for the structure and activity of osteoclasts in bone resorption. (RGD = [arginine-glycine-aspartic acid] amino acid sequence.)

Osteoclasts

Osteoclasts are highly motile, multinucleate cells derived from monocyte-macrophage lineage precursors in the bone marrow that act to resorb bone, releasing mineral and removing degraded organic material. In contrast to the osteoblast, the osteoclast is bloodborne. The osteoclast progenitor cells are recruited from the hemopoietic tissues (e.g., bone marrow, splenic tissues) to bone via the blood stream. They proliferate and differentiate into osteoclasts through a mechanism involving cell-to-cell interaction with osteoblastic stromal cells (Suda 1997). The osteoclast participates in bone remodeling, repair, and growth, as well as mobilization of mineral to maintain homeostasis. Osteoclastic bone resorption consists of several complicated processes: (1) osteoclast development, (2) attachment of osteoclasts to calcified tissues, (3) development of a ruffled border and clear zone, and (4) secretion of acids and lysosomal enzymes into the space beneath the ruffled border (Suda et al. 1997). Resorption of bone is accomplished by the dissolution of hydroxyapatite crystals and the disintegration of organic matrix by osteoclastic acid enzymes (Blair 1998). The mechanism of the acidification of the sub-osteoclastic bone-resorbing compartment involves the action of a polarized proton pump located at the level of the ruffled border of the osteoclast (Delaissé and Vaes 1992). A clear zone surrounds the ruffled border and contains actin filaments that

appear to anchor the ruffled border area to the bone surface undergoing resorption. Adhesion molecules on osteoclast cytoplasmic membranes are important for osteoclast function and resorption of bone. These integral membrane proteins (integrins) bind to molecules present in the bone matrix (e.g., osteopontin) through specific RGD (Arg-Gly-Asp) amino acid sequences, an event that leads to osteoclast activation (Mundy 1995). Attachment of osteoclasts to certain proteins containing RGD-sequence, through vitronectin receptors, may be the first step involved in inducing osteoclast polarization (Suda et al. 1997).

Osteoclasts have apical and basolateral poles that differ both morphologically and functionally. The osteoclast's apical pole has a fenestrated membrane oriented in the direction of the bone matrix; the membrane is the region where enzymes and protons are secreted (Figure 2-8). The basolateral pole of the osteoclast is oriented toward the local environment and is involved in physiologic functions involving its receptors for hormones and other substances (Suda et al. 1997). Osteoclasts frequently lie in depressions on the surface of bone known as *Howship's lacunae*. The Howship's lacunae is an eroded region of bone created as a result of an acidic microenvironment.

Although the osteoclast is the principal cell involved in bone resorption, the osteoblast appears to trigger the initial breakdown of bone. For the osteoclast to begin resorption of bone, it must be in contact with the mineralized surface. Studies suggest that osteoblasts may act as helper cells in the process of osteoclastic resorption by preparing the bone surface for later attack by osteoclastic enzymes (Mundy 1995; Suda et al. 1997). The elongated resting state osteoblast releases collagenases and removes the osteoid layer of bone, allowing the osteoclast to reach the underlying mineralized matrix. Therefore, osteoblasts may be involved in osteoclast activation through a cell-to-cell contact mechanism (Suda et al. 1997).

In certain pathologic conditions, such as osteoporosis (a disease endemic in Western society and Asia), enhanced osteoclastic activity causes greater bone resorption than bone formation. Hence, efforts to treat osteoporosis have been most successful when therapies involved the inhibition of osteoclastic bone resorption (Teitelbaum et al. 1997). Regulation of osteoclastic bone resorption is achieved by either altering recruitment of osteoclast precursors into fully differentiated osteoclasts or by regulating the rate at which mature osteoclasts degrade bone. Inhibitors of osteoclast function include the bisphosphonates (carbon-substituted pyrophosphate [P-C-P] compounds) with a high affinity for hydroxyapatite and the ability to inhibit osteoclastic bone resorption, estrogen therapies, and calcitonin (see Chapter 4).

Blood and Nerve Supply of Bones

Vascular supply is one of the most important prerequisites for biological activity; high capillarization is considered a sign of vitality in any body tissue. The vascular network of adult bone supplies the bone tissue, bone marrow, periosteum, and, in part, articular cartilage. Long bones are pierced by the one or two main arteries referred to as *diaphyseal nutrient arteries*. These nutrient arteries run through the nutrient foramen and nutrient canal, located on the shaft of the bone, and branch internally as depicted in Figure 2-2. At the medullary cavity, the nutrient artery divides into two branches known as the *central longitudinal arteries*. The metaphyseal and epiphyseal regions are supplied by ramifications of the nutrient artery. These arteries are quantitatively the most important, and may substitute the diaphyseal

arterial supply (Geneser 1986). The large epiphyseal arteries form a network within the bone tissue and have branches that anastomose near the articular cartilage. In fact, terminal arteries that emerge from the anastomosis form loops that pierce the external portion of compact bone and persevere into the deep calcified zone portion of articular cartilage.

Skeletal blood flow can be measured based on the unidirectional clearance of ^{18}F into bone, permitting evaluation of vascular events in certain conditions (Green et al. 1987). Total bone blood flow was observed to be slightly lower than normal, although skeletal perfusion was normal in crush fractures resulting from osteoporosis (see Chapter 12) which suggests a microvascular defect in the pathogenesis of this condition (Burkhardt et al. 1987). High values of bone blood flow are characteristic in a large number of patients with osteomalacia (see Chapter 12) and very high values are typical in individuals with Paget's disease (Green et al. 1987).

Effects of Vascularity on Bone Cells

Osteoblasts and osteoclasts are metabolically demanding cells with high levels of energy consumption that, therefore, require an adequate blood supply. Specifically, osteoblasts are also thought to be sources of prostaglandins (e.g., prostaglandin E_2), some of which are local regulators of blood flow (Green et al. 1987).

Lymph

Lymph vessels accompany the larger bone blood vessels; however, lymph capillaries have not been identified within the haversian canals.

Nerves

The vertebrae, larger flat bones, and epiphyses of the long bones have an extensive nerve supply. The periosteum houses several branches of these nerves that, in turn, give rise to tiny myelinated and nonmyelinated nerve fibers that accompany the nutrient vessels as they enter the bone. These extend as far as the perivascular spaces of the haversian canals. Whereas bone tissue per se is relatively insensitive to pain, the periosteum is extremely sensitive to pain stimuli. Pain originating from bone may be perceived by unmyelinated (C) afferent nociceptors (defined morphologically and physiologically by their patterns of response to mechanical, thermal, and chemical cutaneous stimuli) that, once activated, conduct impulses via lightly myelinated afferent fibers (A-δ mechanoreceptors), both located in the joint capsule and periosteum (Payne 1997).

Bone and the Hematopoietic and Immune Systems

Observations suggest interaction among bone, marrow, and the immune system in the mature skeleton (Sharrock 1998). Marrow stromal cells include the precursors of the osteochondrogenic lineage, exert important influences on osteoclastogenesis and lymphopoiesis, and mediate the effects of some systemic factors on bone turnover. Evidence exists to support the idea that hematopoietic cells can influence the differentiation of osteogenic cells in that mature lymphocytes can influence osteoclastic and osteoblastic functions (Mundy 1990; Sharrock 1998).

Skeletal Dynamics: Regulation of Bone Remodeling and Modeling

The regulation of bone *remodeling* and its corresponding role in the maintenance of adult bone mass is a separate process from bone *modeling*, which refers to the process controlling skeletal growth in the immature skeleton.

Modeling

Bones develop during skeletal growth in predetermined sequences. Bone modeling is the process responsible for creating bone shape. Long bones of children increase in length and diameter through modeling. This modeling process is adaptive and involves both generalized and continuous growth. In addition, modeling involves the re-shaping of bone under the governance of the bone cells

(osteoblasts and osteoclasts) until adult bone morphology is attained. Bone modeling is the process of continuous change in bone shape, length, and width during an individual's growth until skeletal maturity is reached. Resorption and formation in bone modeling processes occur on distinct bone surfaces.

Remodeling

Bone remodeling is the process of local, coupled bone resorption and formation, maintaining skeletal mass and morphology in the mature adult. The term *remodeling*, or *bone turnover*, refers to the sequential processes of bone resorption and subsequent formation to maintain mineral homeostasis and skeletal integrity (Epstein 1988). The hallmark of bone remodeling is the coordinated local coupling of both resorption and formation processes. Bone remodeling involves the removal and internal restructuring of previously existing bone, and maintenance of tissue mass and architecture in the adult skeleton. Bone metabolism in health consists of a dynamic and continuous remodeling process normally maintained in a tightly coupled balance between resorption of old or damaged bone and the formation of new bone. The coupling of bone formation to bone resorption is based on histologic evidence indicating that, in the bone-remodeling cycle, osteoclastic resorption is followed, after the reversal phase, by osteoblastic activity that replaces the resorbed bone (Parfitt 1982). Bone remodeling is initiated by the destruction of the osteoid tissue that lines the bone matrix by the collagenase of the osteoblasts.

Osteoclasts normally take approximately 10 days to resorb bone. A lacunae is filled with osteoid by the osteoblasts in a period of approximately 80 days; the bone subsequently becomes mineralized to complete the 90- to 120-day remodeling cycle. Because these packets of remodeling are discrete geographically and chronologically, it appears likely that they are regulated by local factors produced in the bone marrow environment (Mundy 1987).

In the adult human skeleton, approximately 5–10% of the existing bone is replaced every year. As bone is a dynamic tissue, a constant flux exists with approximately 15–20% of the skeleton involved in the remodeling process at any one time. The turnover of cortical bone in most areas is probably

BUSINESS REPLY MAIL
FIRST CLASS MAIL   PERMIT NO. 78   WOBURN, MA

POSTAGE WILL BE PAID BY ADDRESSEE

DIRECT MAIL DEPARTMENT
BUTTERWORTH-HEINEMANN
225 WILDWOOD AVE
PO BOX 4500
WOBURN MA 01888-9930

NO POSTAGE
NECESSARY
IF MAILED
IN THE
UNITED STATES

At Butterworth-Heinemann, we are dedicated to providing you with quality service. So that we may keep you informed about titles relevant to your field of interest, please fill in the information below and return this postage-paid reply card. Thank you for your help, and we look forward to hearing from you!

What title have you purchased? ⌷

Where was the purchase made? ⌷

Name ⌷

Job Title ⌷

Institution ⌷

Address ⌷

Town/City ⌷

State/County ⌷

Zip/Postcode ⌷

Country ⌷

Telephone ⌷

email ⌷

☐ Please keep me informed about other books and information services on this and related subjects.

(FOR OFFICE USE ONLY)

BUTTERWORTH-HEINEMANN IS ON THE WEB – http://www.bh.com/

US1
US1

close to 5% per year, whereas the turnover of cancellous bone can reach up to 20% per year. Cancellous bone is more metabolically active than cortical bone because of its greater surface area on which bone cells may act.

Activation, Reversal, Formation

Based on the activation, reversal, formation (ARF) concept, a close anatomical and functional relationship exists between bone forming and resorbing cells at remodeling sites. Bone remodeling takes place on bone surfaces in discrete packets known as *basic multicellular* or *bone metabolism units* (BMUs) (Christenson 1997; Rodan 1998). Global bone metabolism manifests as the cumulative behavior of multiple BMUs so that defects in bone formation or resorption processes result in substantial changes in functional skeletal integrity. Bone remodeling may be influenced by mechanical forces applied to the skeleton, by local humoral factors, and by circulating hormones such as estrogens, androgens, calcitonin, parathyroid hormone, and 1,25-dihydroxyvitamin D_3 (see Chapter 4).

Markers of Bone Metabolism (Formation and Resorption)

The regulation of structure and cyclical metabolism of bone by hormones (Chapter 4) is reflected by markers of bone formation, resorption, and turnover. Bone formation and resorption are tightly controlled by systemic hormones and local factors produced by bone cells (e.g., the osteoblast). Bone is, therefore, a complex tissue constantly undergoing an integrated process of remodeling involving different factors and substances. Many cell-derived growth regulatory factors inherent to skeletal tissues exist, including prostaglandins, cytokines, and growth factors. For example, studies have demonstrated that insulin-like growth factor I is a critical differentiative factor for osteoblasts and is important as a coupling agent for bone cells (Crawford-Sharpe and Rosen 1999). These substances, produced by the osteoblast, have potent effects on skeletal metabolism. Bone biomarkers are useful to monitor bone diseases associated with increased bone resorption, such as malignant disease, primary hyperparathyroidism,

Table 2-2. Influence of Cytokines and Local Growth Factors on Bone

Cytokine, Eicosanoid, or Peptide Growth Factor	Effect on Bone
Epidermal growth factor (EGF) Interleukins (IL-1, IL-6) Leukotrienes (LT) Platelet-derived growth factor (PDGF) Tumor growth factor (TGF-α) Tumor necrosis factor (TNF-α)	Bone resorption (matrix reduction)
Fibroblast growth factor (FGF) Insulin-like growth factor (IGF-I, IGF-II) Prostaglandins (PGE) Transforming growth factor (TGF-β)	Bone formation
Fibroblast growth factor (FGF) Insulin-like growth factor (IGF-I, IGF-II) Transforming growth factor (TGF-β)	Collagen synthesis

Source: Adapted from BA Watkins. Regulatory effects of polyunsaturates on bone modeling and cartilage function. World Rev Nutr Diet 1998;83:38–51.

and Paget's disease. A number of excellent reviews provide an overview of the influence of cytokines, eicosanoids, and other growth factors on bone formation and resorption processes (Table 2-2) (Canalis et al. 1987; Jilka 1998; Mundy 1995; Pacifici 1996; Watkins 1998; Weryha and Leclère 1995).

The rate of formation or degradation of the bone matrix can be assessed by either measuring the enzymatic activity of the bone-forming or resorbing cells, such as alkaline (derived from osteoblasts) or acid (derived from osteoclasts) phosphatase activity, or by measuring bone matrix components that are released into the circulation during formation or resorption. Products or by-products of bone metabolism may indicate aberrations in bone formation and resorption processes. Markers of bone resorption of bone that are reflected in the degradation of type I collagen include N-telopeptides, C-telopeptides, fasting urinary calcium and hydroxyproline, pyridinoline and pyridinoline-containing peptides (collagen cross-links) in the plasma, urinary pyridinoline and deoxypyridinoline, tartrate-resistant acid phosphatase (TRAP), hydroxylysine glycosides, and urinary hydroxylysine glycosides (Christenson 1997; Delmas

1995). Bone formation markers represent osteoblast activity and include bone-specific alkaline phosphatase and the N-terminal and C-terminal extension peptides of procollagen I, all indicative of the formation of organic matrix in bone. Bone Gla protein (BGP or osteocalcin), produced by osteoblasts but also released during osteoclastic degradation, may indicate either formation of bone when resorption and formation are coupled, or turnover when they are uncoupled (Christenson 1997).

Bone biomarkers may indicate changes in bone metabolism more rapidly than bone mineral density evaluation or other imaging techniques (see Chapter 6). Although bone density measurement may be important clinically, efficacy of intervention may be less immediate than biochemical markers of bone metabolism whose measurement may provide more real-time assessment of bone resorption, formation, and turnover.

Summary

The skeleton is comprised of dynamic tissue that undergoes constant remodeling. Bone modeling is the process of continuous change in bone shape, length, and width until skeletal maturity is reached. *Remodeling*, or *bone turnover*, refers to the sequential processes of bone resorption and subsequent bone formation for maintenance of mineral homeostasis and skeletal integrity. Remodeling allows the skeleton to respond to the physical stimuli or stresses placed on it, and also to repair structural damage caused by fatigue, failure, or trauma. In normal bone remodeling, the processes of bone resorption and bone formation are usually closely coupled via local humoral factors. When the tightly connected sequence of bone remodeling is disturbed, such as with age or disease, the bone cell activity becomes uncoupled. Bone remodeling is regulated at a local level by mechanical forces applied to the skeleton, by paracrine factors, and by autocrine factors (e.g., cytokines); it is also regulated at an endocrine level by hormones.

Osteoblasts are bone cells responsible for bone formation; they synthesize and secrete the bone matrix. Osteoblasts originate in the pluripotential mesenchymal stromal cells of the bone marrow. Osteocytes are thought to have a communicative role in the mechanically adaptive control of bone architecture that requires feedback about its relationship with parameters of loading. Osteoclasts are multinucleate cells derived from the monocyte-macrophage lineage. Osteoclasts resorb mineralized bone by releasing acidic enzymes, a process involving cell-to-cell communication with the osteoblast.

References

Azria M. The value of biomarkers in detecting alterations in bone metabolism. Calcif Tissue Int 1989;45:7–11.

Bätge B, Diebold J, Stein H, et al. Compositional analysis of the collagenous bone matrix: a study of adult normal and osteopenic bone tissue. Eur J Clin Invest 1992;22:805–812.

Bidwell JP, Alvarez M, Feister H, et al. Nuclear matrix proteins and osteoblast gene expression. J Bone Mineral Res 1998;13:155–167.

Blair HC. How the osteoclast degrades bone. Bioessays 1998;20:837–846.

Boskey AL. Noncollagenous matrix proteins and their role in mineralization. Bone Miner 1989;6:111–123.

Burkhardt R, Kettner G, Böhm W, et al. Changes in trabecular bone, hematopoiesis and bone marrow vessels in aplastic anemia, primary osteoporosis and old age: a comparative histomorphometric study. Bone 1987;8:157–164.

Bushinsky DA. Internal Exchanges of Hydrogen Ions: Bone. In DW Seldin, G Giebisch (eds), The Regulation of Acid-Base Balance. New York: Raven Press, 1990;69–88.

Butler WT. The nature and significance of osteopontin. Connect Tissue Res 1989;23:123–136.

Canalis E, Lorenzo J, Burgess WH, Maciag T. Effects of endothelial cell growth factor on bone remodeling in vitro. J Clin Invest 1987;79:52–58.

Chen J, Shapiro HS, Sodek J. Developmental expression of bone sialoprotein mRNA in rat mineralized connective tissues. J Bone Miner Res 1992;7:987–997.

Chen J, Singh K, Mukherjee BB, Sodek J. Developmental expression of osteopontin (OPN) mRNA in rat tissues: evidence for a role for OPN in bone formation and resorption. Matrix Vol 1993;13:113–123.

Christenson RH. Biochemical markers of bone metabolism: an overview. Clin Biochem 1997;30:573–593.

Crawford-Sharpe G, Rosen CJ. Insulin like growth factor I and the skeleton: new perspectives. Endocrinologist 1999;9:81–86.

Delaissé JM, Vaes G. Mechanism of Mineral Solubilization and Matrix Degradation in Osteoclastic Bone Resorption. In BR Rifkin, CV Gay (eds), Biology and Physiology of the Osteoclast. Boca Raton, FL: CRC Press, 1992;289–314.

Delmas PD. Biochemical markers of bone turnover. Acta Orthop Scand 1995;66(Suppl 266):176–182.

Epstein S. Serum and urinary markers of bone remodeling:

assessment of bone turnover. Endocrine Rev 1988;9: 437–445.

Epstein S. Bone-derived proteins. Trends Endocrinol Metab 1989;Sept/Oct:9–14.

Fiore CE, Foti R, Fragetta C, et al. Clinical relevance of the measurement of non-collagen bone proteins in serum of senile osteoporotics. Arch Gerontol Geriatr 1991; (Suppl 2):475–480.

Geneser F. Textbook of Histology. Philadelphia: Lea & Febiger, 1986;219–257.

Glowacki J, Rey C, Glimcher MJ, et al. A role for osteocalcin in osteoclast differentiation. J Cell Biochem 1991; 45:292–302.

Green JR, Reeve J, Tellez M, et al. Skeletal blood flow in metabolic disorders of the skeleton. Bone 1987;8:293–297.

Hauschka PV, Mavrakos AE, Iafrati MD, et al. Growth factors in bone matrix, isolation of multiple types by affinity chromatography on heparin-sepharose. J Biol Chem 1986;261:12665–12674.

Hultenby K, Reinholt FP, Oldberg A, Heinegard D. Ultrastructural immunolocalization of osteopontin in metaphyseal and cortical bone. Matrix Vol 1991;11:206–213.

Ingram RT, Clarke BL, Fisher LW, Fitzpatrick LA. Distribution of noncollagenous proteins in the matirx of adult human bone: evidence of anatomic and functional heterogeneity. J Bone Miner Res 1993:8:1019–1028.

Jilka RL. Cytokines, bone remodeling, and estrogen deficiency: a 1998 update. Bone 1998;23:75–81.

Jilka RL, Weinstein RS, Bellido T, et al. Osteoblast programmed cell-death (apoptosis): modulation by growth-factors and cytokines. J Bone Miner Res 1998;13:793–802.

Lanyon LE. Osteocytes, strain detection, bone modeling and remodeling. Calcif Tissue Int 1993;53(Suppl 1):S102–S107.

Lazenby RA. Continuing periosteal apposition. I. Documentation, hypotheses, and interpretation. Am J Phys Anthro 1990;82:451–472.

Mundy GR. Bone resorption and turnover in health and disease. Bone 1987;8:S9–S16.

Mundy GR. Immune system and bone remodeling. Trends Endocrinol Metab 1990;1:307–311.

Mundy GR. Bone Remodeling and Its Disorders. London: Dunitz, 1995;1–38.

Ninomiya JT, Tracy RP, Calore JD, et al. Heterogeneity of human bone. J Bone Miner Res 1990;5:933–938.

Oreffo ROC, Bord S, Triffitt JT. Skeletal progenitor cells and aging human populations. Clin Sci 1998;94:549–555.

Pacifici R. Estrogen, cytokines and the pathogenesis of postmenopausal osteoporosis. J Bone Miner Res 1996;11: 1043–1051.

Parfitt AM. The coupling of bone formation to bone resorption: a critical analysis of the concept and of its relevance to the pathogenesis of osteoporosis. Metab Bone Dis Rel Res 1982;4:1–5.

Payne R. Mechanisms and management of bone pain. Cancer Suppl 1997;80:1608–1613.

Rodan GA. Control of bone formation and resorption: biological and clinical perspective. J Cell Biochem 1998; 30–31S:55–61.

Rodan GA, Noda M. Gene expression in osteoblastic cells. Curr Rev Eukaryotic Gene Expression 1991;1: 85–98.

Sharrock WJ. Bone and the hematopoietic and immune systems: a report of the proceedings of a scientific workshop. J Bone Miner Res 1998;13:537–543.

Singh I. The architecture of cancellous bone. J Anat 1978; 127:305–310.

Suda T, Nakamura I, Eijiro J, Takahashi N. Regulation of osteoclastic function. J Bone Miner Res 1997;12: 869–879.

Tanaka H, Hruska KA, Seino Y, et al. Disassociation of the macrophage-maturational effects of vitamin D from respiratory priming. J Biol Chem 1991;266: 10888–10892.

Teitelbaum SL, Tondravi MM, Ross FP. Osteoclasts, macrophages and the molecular mechanisms of bone resorption. J Leukocyte Biol 1997;61:381–388.

Termine JD. Cellular activity, matrix proteins and aging bone. Exper Gerontol 1990;25:217–221.

Volpi M, Katz EP. On the adaptive structures of the collagen fibrils of bone and cartilage. J Biomech 1991;24(Suppl 1):67–77.

Watkins BA. Regulatory effects of polyunsaturates on bone modeling and cartilage function. World Rev Nutr Diet 1998;83:38–51.

Weryha G, Leclère J. Paracrine regulation of bone remodeling. Horm Res 1995;43:69–75.

Yoo JU, Barthel TS, Nishimura K, et al. The chondrogenic potential of human bone-marrow–derived mesenchymal progenitor cells. J Bone Joint Surg 1998;80-A:1745–1757.

Young MF, Kerr JM, Ibaraki K, et al. Structure, expression and regulation of the major noncollagenous matrix proteins of bone. Clin Ortho 1992;281:275–294.

Chapter 3
Mineralization of Calcified Tissue

Marc D. Grynpas

The deposition of a mineral phase in various tissues occurs in most living organisms from the mineralization of the mollusk's shell to the mineralization of the human skeleton. This complex process is always under cellular control. The breakdown of these control mechanisms can lead to pathologic calcification of many tissues (e.g., skin, kidney, arteries, breast, brain). The chemical and physical mechanisms leading to the deposition of a solid mineral phase into an organic matrix are governed by the same laws as those of any solid precipitating from a solution. Problems arise from the fact that the extracellular matrix of calcified tissues is very different from aqueous solutions for two main reasons: (1) They provide a tridimensional framework on which the solid inorganic phase (the crystals) can be deposited, grow, and be ordered and (2) the solid network of macromolecules regulates the flow of water, anions, cations, solutes, and small molecules involved and therefore controls the kinetics of crystal formation and dissolution.

Requirements for Mineralization

The body fluids are the sources of the ions, which form the calcium phosphate crystals of calcified tissues. The concentration of calcium in body fluid is very constant at 2.5 mM. Only approximately one-half of the calcium is in a biologically active or free or ionic form; the remainder is either protein bound or complexed to small molecules such as citrate, bicarbonate, inorganic phosphate (P_i), and pyrophosphate. The level of inorganic phosphate in serum is more variable. In adult humans, the level is approximately 1 mM (2 mM in newborns). Most of this phosphate is free or ionic. Due to the pH, temperature, and ionic strength of the serum, the phosphate ions are present in the following ionized form: 80% HPO_4, 20% H_2PO_4, and less than 0.01% PO_4 (Neuman 1980). This implies that the degree of saturation of body fluids with respect to Ca and PO_4 can be expressed as a simple ion product: $(Ca^{++}) \times (P_i) = (1.3 \text{ mM} \times 1 \text{ mM}) = 1.3 \text{ mM}^2$.

To mineralize a tissue, it is necessary to (1) increase the level of concentration of Ca and PO_4 ions to help precipitate a Ca × PO_4 solid phase; (2) remove locally the circulating inhibitors of calcification, such as Mg, citrate, pyrophosphate, and many macromolecules; and (3) increase the concentration of promoters of mineralization, such as macromolecules, which, due to their conformation, act as nucleators of Ca × PO_4 crystals (Table 3-1).

Nature of the Mineral Phase of Hard Tissue

Many forms of calcium phosphate can exist in the conditions found in body fluids (Table 3-2). Of all these compounds, only hydroxyapatite (HA) is stable at neutral or basic pH. All the other compounds are stable in the neutral to acid range. In

Table 3-1. Requirements for Mineralization

1. Increase of Ca × PO$_4$ by cells
   Alkaline phosphatase
   Mitochondrial granules
   Matrix vesicle
2. Decrease of calcification inhibitors
   Pyrophosphates
   Magnesium
   Proteoglycans
   Other macromolecules
3. Increase of calcification promoters
   Phosphoproteins
   Phospholipids
   Proteoglycans
   Other macromolecules
   Collagen?

an aqueous environment at pH 7.4, all the compounds except HA are unstable and undergo a conversion to HA. Structurally, these compounds have many similarities and can therefore transform into each other or form sandwich structures in which crystal such as octacalcium phosphate (OCP) and HA may be mixed. Because the HA lattice is extremely complex (the unit cell comprises 42 atoms) and because the Ca/P molar ratio of newly formed bone is closer to 1 than to 1.66 (the molar ratio of HA), it has been postulated that the initial mineral phase deposited in calcified tissue is not HA but a precursor phase. Three different theories on the nature of the initial phase of bone mineral exist. The precursor phases theory states that there is an initial phase that is deposited in tissue with a lower Ca/P ratio than HA and, with time, converts to poorly crystalline HA (PCHA). Of these precursor phases, the OCP proposed by Brown (1966) is the foremost candidate for conversion. OCP has a low Ca/P ratio of 1.33 and a structure composed of phosphate rich layer alternating with water rich

layers (Brown and Chow 1976), which is similar to HA and forms plate-like crystals similar to those found in bone.

Another theory, the amorphous calcium phosphate (ACP) theory, states that bone mineral is initially deposited as an amorphous compound that slowly transforms itself into poorly crystalline HA over time. The theory, first proposed by Termine and Posner (1967), explains the changes in the chemistry and structures of bone crystals with maturation and aging. However, it was shown by Grynpas et al. (1984) that even in 17-day-old chick embryo it was not possible to detect ACP by x-ray radial distribution function. The most likely form of bone mineral crystals is a single apatite phase of variable chemical composition, which gradually becomes more crystalline as the crystals grow and finally approaches the Ca/P ratio of HA. The change in molar ratio and chemistry of the bone mineral can be explained by the changing size of the crystals alone. Whereas the surface layer of newly formed crystals is 50% of the crystal volume, the surface layer of the mature crystals (assuming a doubling in size) makes up only 25% of the volume, which can explain the changes in the chemistry of bone mineral (Glimcher et al. 1981).

The word *apatite*'s Greek root means to deceive. The appropriately named lattice of apatite allows for many substitutions, among the most important are Sr, Fe, Pb, Zn, Mg, Na for Ca; F and Cl for OH; and CO$_3$ for PO$_4$. The substitution of CO$_3$ for PO$_4$ is important because bone is involved in the body pH regulation by the release or absorption of bicarbonate ions (Green and Kleeman 1991). Because of these substitutions and of the chemical composition of bone, bone can be considered an infinite reservoir of not only Ca and PO$_4$, but also of many other chemical elements.

Table 3-2. Candidates for Biological Calcium Phosphates

Name	Formula	Ca/P (molar)	Zone of Stability
Hydroxyapatite (HA)	$Ca_{10}(PO_4)_6(OH)_2$	1.66	pH >7.0
Tricalcium phosphate (TCP)	$Ca_3(PO_4)_2$	1.5	7.0 > pH > 5.0
Amorphous calcium phosphate (ACP)	$Ca_9(PO_4)_6$ (variable)	1.3–1.5	—
Octocalcium phosphate (OCP)	$Ca_8H_2(PO_4)_6 5(H_2O)$	1.33	7.0 > pH > 5.0
Brushite (dicalcium phosphate dihydrate [DCPD])	$Ca HPO_4 2(H_2O)$	1.00	pH <5.0

Table 3-3. Bone Histogenesis: Some Definitions

Bone Formation Process	Description
Intramembranous bone formation	The periosteal column of long bones and the flat bones of the skull and face are formed by intramembranous bone formation, which is initiated with the condensation of an island of mesenchymal cells that differentiate into osteoblasts. These osteoblasts produce an extracellular matrix that mineralizes. No prior cartilage formation occurs.
Endochondral bone formation	Bone formation occurs on a cartilage model that is formed by chondroblasts. This cartilage model becomes vascularized and subsequently resorbed by multinucleated cells. Bone develops around the cartilage scaffold to form the midshaft regions of long bones (diaphyseal region). Epiphyseal plates (growth plates) are formed from hypertrophic chondrocytes at each end of the cartilage scaffold. This type of bone formation is considered to be the means by which fractures repair.

Location of Mineral Crystals

Mineralization occurs in two main forms (Table 3-3):

1. Endochondral calcification, in which bone forms via a temporary structure such as calcified growth plate cartilage. This process accounts for most of the longitudinal growth of long bone and stops when the epiphysis closes, at the end of adolescence.
2. Membranous bone formation, in which bone is formed by direct mineral deposition onto a pre-formed organic bone matrix without going through a temporary cartilage structure. This process accounts for most of the lateral growth of long bones and the formation of flat bones.

In the endochondral calcification system, specialized cells from cartilage (the growth plate chondrocytes) transform from a resting zone to a zone of proliferation, then to a zone of hypertrophy, and finally to a zone of calcification (Figure 3-1). In the growth plate, the environment appears to select the function and fate of these cartilage cells as the calcified cartilage is subsequently removed and replaced by bone (Bianco et al. 1998). The matrix in which the crystals are deposited consists of thin fibrils of mainly type II collagen, a meshwork of large proteoglycans, and other macromolecules. In this matrix, the crystals are distributed randomly, forming clumps or aggregates of small needles or plates. No specific relation between the crystals and the organic matrix exists.

In membranous bone formation, osteoblasts (bone-forming cells) synthesize an organic matrix, consisting mainly of large type I collagen fibrils, non-collagenous proteins, and small proteoglycans. As an essential distinction from the endochondral system, in membranous bone formation the mineral crystals have a specific relation to the collagen matrix. The long axis of the crystals (thin plates or needles) is parallel to the long axis of the collagen fibrils. Studies have shown that the first crystals go into the hole zone of the collagen fibrils. But as mineralization increases, not enough room exists in the collagen to accommodate the entire mineral mass; therefore, some mineral crystals accumulate extrafibrillarly (Simmons and Grynpas 1990).

Among the techniques providing sufficient resolution to analyze the biologically formed mineral crystals are electron microscopy, electron diffraction, x-ray diffraction, infrared spectroscopy, Raman spectroscopy, small-angle x-ray scattering, nuclear magnetic resonance spectroscopy, and atomic force microscopy. In the determination of crystal size, different diffraction techniques result in different measurements. X-ray, electron, and neutron diffraction, for example, may give an average crystal size (10–25 nm in length and 4–10 nm in width/cross section) that is smaller than that observed by direct electron microscopy. The reason for the difference in measurements may be that the crystals observed by electron microscopy are not single crystals but crystal aggregates. Also, conventional electron microscopy techniques can modify the crystals themselves by (1) translocating ions, (2) removing Ca and PO_4 ions, and (3) recrystalizing these ions in other places. This modification is due to the preparation of samples for electron microscopy, which involves aqueous solutions and dehydration. To

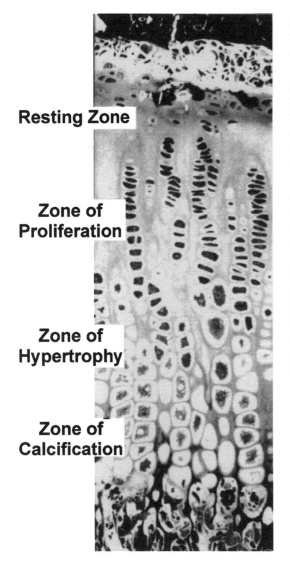

Resting Zone

Zone of Proliferation

Zone of Hypertrophy

Zone of Calcification

Figure 3-1. The growth plate.

maintain the crystals in their native state, new methods have been devised, such as non-aqueous fixation and embedding, or slam freezing and freeze substitution of samples. Finally, spectroscopic methods, such as infrared, Raman, or nuclear magnetic resonance spectroscopy, give us information about the changing atomic environment around the phosphates and carbonate groups of apatite (Dickson 1984).

Mechanisms of Calcification

The research on the mechanisms responsible for the deposition of inorganic crystals on an organic matrix in a living organism has a long history. A wealth of information exists regarding the matrix and the mineral deposits in invertebrate exoskeletons, in bones and teeth, and in pathologic calcifications (e.g., kidney and salivary stones, atherosclerotic plaques). The research focuses on the mineral and matrix characterization, gene expression and regulation for the protein constituents, and in vitro and in vivo models. Despite all these efforts, it is still not known why mineralization occurs in some tissue and not in others.

Two main schools of thought about mineralization exist: (1) cell-induced mineralization, commonly called the matrix vesicle theory, and (2) matrix-induced mineralization. According to the matrix vesicle theory, the cell translocates insoluble mitochondrial granules of calcium phosphate to the plasma membrane. The ions are included in a vesicle with a trilaminar membrane that is exocytosed into the extracellular milieu. The matrix vesicles contain acidic phospholipids, alkaline phosphatase, and non-collagenous proteins/proteolipids. The first crystals are formed on rupture of the membrane and give rise to the initial nidus of calcification. This process has been detailed mainly in calcifying cartilage (Anderson 1969), but it is claimed by its proponents to be true for bones and teeth as well. It has also been shown that in many systems (e.g., cell culture and in vivo) matrix vesicles are not present; therefore, there must be other mechanisms that bring about mineralization.

According to the matrix-induced theory of mineralization, cells create an environment that favors the deposition of crystals at a given place and time. To test these theories, many systems both in vitro and in vivo have been devised. The in vitro system usually consists of a supersaturated solution of calcium phosphates in which potential promoter or inhibitor proteins are added to determine the changes in $Ca \times PO_4$ concentration induced over time. These systems have been modified to replace aqueous solutions by agarose or collagen gels because the movements of ions, and therefore the kinetics of crystal formation, are very different in the presence of even a very diluted solution of macromolecules (Hunter 1992). In addition, many cell culture or organ culture systems have been devised to study the mechanisms of mineralization and the expression of genes from particular proteins that are believed to be involved in mineralization.

Mineralizing tissues have also been studied in vivo (e.g., embryonic chick, turkey tendon, and rat growth plate cartilage). However, different systems

Table 3-4. Proteins Involved in Mineralization

Protein	Effect	System
Osteopontin	Inhibitor	Bone
		Kidney stone
Phosphoryn	Promoter	Dentin
Bone sialoprotein	Promoter	Bone
Acidic phospholipid and proteolipids	Promoter	Calcifying cartilage
Aggrecan	Promoter Inhibitor	Calcifying cartilage
Osteocalcin	Inhibitor	Bone
Collagen I	Promoter Inhibitor	Tendon

may provide contradictory results. A particular protein in solution may be an inhibitor of mineralization but when it is immobilized in a solid matrix, it may be a promoter. Some proteins promote mineralization at low concentration and inhibit it at high concentration. Often, chemical modifications of some residues, such as dephosphorylation, deprive a given protein of its promoting or inhibiting activity. Table 3-4 lists proteins with their putative actions in the mineralization of tissues. It is important to realize that a protein that is present at sites of mineralization and increases in concentration with increased mineralization is not a proof that this protein is responsible for mineralization. This was demonstrated in vivo when a knock-out mice model (a mouse lacking the gene for a given protein) that lacked the proteins deemed essential for mineralization showed no phenotype and exhibited a normal mineralization of their bones (Boskey 1996).

Summary

In conclusion, the mineralization of living tissue is a ubiquitous and essential phenomenon in biology. Such an important biological phenomenon must have built-in redundancy and, therefore, it is possible that more than one mechanism leads to the mineralization of a particular tissue at a specific moment in the life of the organism. Due to the complexity of the system and the inadequacy of many model systems, we still do not know the exact mechanisms by which calcified tissues mineralize.

References

Anderson HC. Vesicle associated with calcification in the matrix of epiphyseal cartilage. J Cell Biol 1969;4:59.

Bianco P, Descalzi Cancedda F, Riminucci M, Cancedda R. Bone formation via cartilage models: the "borderline" chondrocyte. Matrix Biol 1998;17:185.

Boskey AL. Matrix proteins and mineralization: an overview. Conn Tissue Res 1996;35:357.

Brown WE. Crystal growth of bone mineral. Clin Orthop Rel Res 1966;44:205.

Brown WE, Chow LC. Chemical preparation of bone mineral. Ann Rev Mat Sci 1976;6:213.

Dickson GR. Methods of Calcified Tissue Preparation. Amsterdam, The Netherlands: Elsevier 1984;79.

Glimcher MJ, Bonar LC, Grynpas MD, et al. Recent studies of bone mineral: is the amorphous calcium phosphate theory valid? J Crystal Growth 1981;53:100.

Green J, Kleeman CR. Role of bone in regulation of systemic acid base balance. Kidney Int 1991;39:9.

Grynpas MD, Bonar LC, Glimcher MJ. Failure to detect an amorphous calcium phosphate solid phase in bone mineral—a radial distribution function study. Calcif Tissue Int 1984;36:291.

Hunter GK. Bone Metabolism and Mineralization. In BK Hall (ed), Bone (vol 4). Boca Raton, Florida: CRC Press, 1992;225.

Neuman WF. Fundamental and Clinical Bone Physiology. Philadelphia: Lippincott, 1980;83.

Simmons DJ, Grynpas MD. The Osteoblast and Osteocyte. In BK Hall (ed), Bone (vol 1). Boca Raton, Florida: CRC Press, 1990;193.

Termine JD, Posner AS. Amorphous/crystalline interrelationships in bone mineral. Calcif Tissue Int 1967;1:8.

Chapter 4

Physiology and Biochemistry
of Bone Tissue

Mineral Homeostasis: Calcium, Phosphorus, and Other Mineral Ion Balance

Bone is a reservoir for minerals that are essential to maintaining systemic inorganic ion homeostasis. A significant function of bone is to act as a buffer, maintaining plasma calcium and phosphate levels within a narrow physiologic range. Bone is a reservoir of calcium, magnesium, and sodium. Disturbed bone mineral metabolism may manifest in such disorders as Paget's disease, osteomalacia (rickets), and osteoporosis. These conditions receive attention in Chapter 12.

Endocrine Regulation of Bone

Both systemic hormones and cytokines generated in the bone cell microenvironment affect bone mineral metabolism and tissue remodeling processes via control of bone cell activity. Hormones and certain dietary lipids modulate the autocrine and paracrine cellular relationships via cytokines and growth regulatory factors produced locally by bone, and marrow cells within the bone itself. The definitions of autocrine and paracrine are as follows:

Paracrine: Intercellular communication involving the local diffusion of regulating substances from one cell to another nearby cell.
Autocrine: Intracellular communication whereby a single cell produces regulating substances

that, in turn, act on receptors on or within the same cell.

The principal hormones involved in regulating bone metabolism are PTH, vitamin D, and calcitonin, which influence extracellular fluid levels of calcium and phosphate, in part by their effects on the kidney and intestine (Table 4-1). In addition, the steroid hormones (e.g., glucocorticoids, growth hormone, estrogen, progesterone, and androgens) largely direct development and homeostasis of bone, in both normal and pathologic states.

Systemic Hormones

Parathyroid Hormone

The principal action of PTH is to mobilize bone mineral to increase the calcium concentration of extracellular fluid. PTH is produced by the parathyroid glands situated in the neck and is regulated by levels of serum calcium and $1,25(OH)_2D_3$. It stimulates bone turnover, renal phosphorus excretion, and renal calcium reabsorption. The net effect of PTH is to raise serum calcium and $1,25(OH)_2D_3$ levels and decrease serum phosphorus levels. PTH is classically considered to be a bone catabolic agent by virtue of its calcium regulating function. PTH may act on both the osteoclast and the osteoblast, however, having inherently different effects determined, in part, by whether its administration is continuous

Table 4-1. Blood Levels of Calcium (Ca) and Phosphate as a Result of the Effect of Calciotropic Hormones on Target Tissues

Hormone	Ca, P_i	Ca, P_i	Ca, P_i	Ca, P_i
PTH	↑, ↑	—	↑, ↓	↑, ↓
1,25(OH)$_2$D$_3$	↑, ↑	↑, ↑	—	↑, ↑
CT	↓, ↓	—	↓, ↓	↓, ↓
Target organ	Bone	Gut	Kidney	Net effect

CT = calcitonin; P_i = inorganic phosphate; PTH = parathyroid hormone; ↑ = increased level; ↓ = decreased level.

or intermittent (Chevalley and Rizzoli 1999). When delivered intermittently at low doses, PTH stimulates cortical and cancellous bone growth without effects on resorption in animal and clinical studies, demonstrating a selective anabolic response of bone cells to PTH. In contrast, when administered continuously, PTH behaves as a catabolic agent by causing an increase in osteoclastic bone resorption and suppressing bone formation (Morley et al. 1997; Mundy 1995).

Vitamin D

Vitamin D (1,25-dihydroxyvitamin D [1,25(OH)$_2$D$_3$]) is produced in the kidney and is regulated by serum levels of calcium, phosphorus, PTH, and the sex steroid hormones. It stimulates intestinal calcium and phosphorus absorption and, in concert with PTH, regulates bone turnover and renal excretion of calcium and phosphorus. The net effect of vitamin D is to raise serum levels of calcium and phosphorus and decrease PTH levels. Low levels of vitamin D attributed to dietary or sunshine deficiency or malabsorption of fat-soluble vitamins may result in osteomalacia (in adults) or rickets (in children) (see Chapter 12).

Calcitonin

Calcitonin (CT) is a 32–amino acid peptide hormone secreted mainly by the chief cells (C-cells) in the thyroid gland also found in the neck. Its main biological effect is to inhibit the osteoclastic resorption of bone, therefore its action directly opposes that of PTH. CT promotes fracture and wound healing and also behaves as an antihypertensive agent (Deftos 1993; Driessens et al. 1981). Secretion of

CT is maintained by the ambient serum calcium but can be affected by age and gender (Deftos 1993). Degradation of CT occurs in the kidney, thyroid gland, liver, and bone. CT can also be used clinically to reduce the elevated calcium levels found in some diseases such as Paget's disease, osteoporosis and, most notably, cancer. These conditions are discussed in Chapters 11 and 12.

Other Hormones Regulating Bone Metabolism

Other hormones that direct bone cell behavior include growth hormone, glucocorticoids, and sex steroid hormones (i.e., estrogen, progesterone, and androgens). These hormones are not under negative feedback control by concentrations of calcium in the extracellular fluid. Many substances that affect bone cell function are influenced by these hormones, including cytokines and growth regulatory factors, produced locally by bone and marrow cells within the bone itself.

Growth Hormone

The secretion of growth hormone (GH) is controlled by the hypothalamus. The importance of GH for normal skeletal growth during childhood and adolescence is well established (Parfitt 1991). GH is the most important hormone in the control of linear growth of long bones via its effects on epiphyseal growth. It is unclear how much of the effect of GH on bone remodeling is due to local or systemic production of insulin-like growth factors, and how much can be attributed to the direct effects of GH on bone (Tapanainen et al. 1991). However, GH has been shown to directly stimulate proliferation of human osteoblasts in vitro (Langdahl et al. 1998) and their synthesis of insulin-like growth factor I (Chapurlat and Delmas 1999). Adults with GH deficiency commonly have subnormal bone mineral density and an increased risk of fractures, which can be reversed by the administration of GH (Kann et al. 1998).

Corticosteroids

Corticosteroids are produced in the adrenal gland. The net effect of corticosteroids on bone is catabolic. Glucocorticoids act by inhibiting mature osteoblast function and preventing the transformation of preosteoblasts to osteoblasts (Watrous and Andrews 1989). Excess corticosteroids promote loss of bone (osteopenia).

Sex Steroid Hormones: Estrogen, Progesterone, and Androgens

The sex steroid hormones are major regulators of bone metabolism, and have an anabolic effect. In both sexes, osteoblasts respond via a receptor-mediated mechanism to estrogen (Benz et al. 1991; Colston et al. 1989; Colvard et al. 1989a; Colvard et al. 1989b; Ernst et al. 1989; Komm et al. 1988; Masuyama et al. 1992) progesterone, and androgens (Orwoll et al. 1991), demonstrating that the sex steroid hormones directly influence the regulation of bone remodeling activity. The sex steroid hormones may also act to regulate bone tissue indirectly via their influence on the calciotropic (calcium mobilizing) hormones such as parathyroid hormone, calcitonin, and vitamin D.

Estrogen.   Estrogen plays a major role in bone mineral homeostasis, modulating bone turnover by maintaining a balance, in both males and females, between bone formation and resorption. Sources of estrogen in the female include the ovary and the peripheral conversion of sex steroid precursors derived from the adrenals. The predominant estrogen in premenopausal females is estradiol, which is produced in the ovary. In the postmenopausal state when there is cessation of ovarian function, estrogens are derived almost exclusively from the peripheral conversion in adipose tissue of the androgen androstenedione to estrone (a less potent form of estrogen), a reaction mediated by the aromatase enzyme complex (Utian 1989). Extraglandular aromatization of circulating androgen is therefore the major source of estrogen in both males and postmenopausal females. The osteoblast itself possesses aromatase and other estrogen-converting substances (Purohit et al. 1992; Shozu and Simpson 1998), suggesting that bone is, in itself, an extraglandular source of local estrogen that plays an important role in bone mineral metabolism via autocrine and paracrine actions. Pubertal development in boys, involving growth and mineralization and epiphyseal closure of long bones, that was previously

attributed to the actions of androgens is, in fact, mediated in part by estrogens (Sharpe 1998; Simpson et al. 1999; Vanderschueren et al. 1998).

Estrogen is an antiresorptive agent that slows bone turnover by ultimately suppressing resorption. Both the osteoclast and osteoblast-like cells possess estrogen receptors (Benz et al. 1991; Komm et al. 1988). Some of the skeletal effects of estrogen on bone may also be mediated by increased production of bone morphogenic proteins (Rickard et al. 1998). In fact, the mechanism by which estrogen regulates bone remodeling illustrates the extensive role it plays in modulating the production of cytokines and growth factors from bone marrow and bone cells. These factors induce antiosteoclastic behavior via the modulation of osteoblastic production of different substances, including interleukin 1 (IL-1), IL-6, and transforming growth factor-beta (TGF-β), which in turn regulate osteoclastogenesis and bone resorption activity (Ribot and Tremollieres 1995). More specifically, the role of estrogen may be in down-regulating the production of several cytokines (IL-1, IL-6, tumor necrosis factor [TNF], macrophage colony stimulating factor [M-CSF], and granulocyte M-CSF [GM-CSF]), which are capable of independently or co-operatively regulating bone resorption and osteoclastogenesis (Pacifici 1996).

Estrogen deficiency, experienced at menopause in females, is known to play a significant role in the pathogenesis of postmenopausal osteoporosis. Bone is affected by waning levels of estrogen at menopause due to a decline in ovarian function. The number of follicles in the ovaries decreases and less estrogen and progesterone is synthesized.

Progesterone.   Progesterone is normally produced as a result of its combined secretion from the adrenal gland and ovaries. Peripheral conversion of steroids to progesterone occurs only during pregnancy. Progesterone receptors have been detected in osteoblast-like cells and progesterone also has considerable affinity for the androgen receptor. This suggests progesterone bioactivity in osteoblastic cells could be mediated via interactions of progestins with either androgen or progesterone receptors (Orwoll et al. 1991). The estrogen receptor also cooperates functionally with the progesterone receptor (Bradshaw et al. 1991). Both estrogen and progesterone have been shown to induce proliferation and differentiation of osteoblast-like cells in vitro (Scheven et al. 1992).

Androgens: Androstenedione, Dehydroepiandrosterone, and Testosterone.   Bone is a target organ of the androgens. Androgens have important effects on the human skeleton; they affect both bone maturation and homeostasis of mature bone in both genders (Hansen and Tho 1999). Dehydroepiandrosterone (DHEA) like androstenedione, is a weak androgen and possesses only 3% of the potency of testosterone (Spector et al. 1991). DHEAS is the sulfated ester of DHEA and is derived exclusively from the adrenal glands. More than 99% of the circulating DHEA in humans is found in the sulfated form. It is the most abundant circulating steroid hormone. Testosterone and its anabolic steroid analogues inhibit bone loss, with androgen deficiency resulting in severe osteopenia in both sexes (Wong et al. 1993). Testosterone may be involved in the stimulation of the biological response to vitamin D in the classic target organs such as the intestine and bone, identifying another factor in the pathogenesis of osteoporosis, particularly in hypogonadal men (Otremski et al. 1997).

Androgens are common precursors of estrogen in both sexes. Peripheral aromatization of testosterone and androstenedione is the principal source for circulating estrogens in men and postmenopausal or surgically menopausal women (Schweikert et al. 1995). In fact, in men, almost all of the circulating estrogens are derived from peripheral conversion of androgens. Androgens have the unique characteristic that they may be converted within the target cell into either the nonaromatizable 5-alpha dihydrotestosterone or into estrogens. The androgen effects on bone may therefore be expressed via activation of the androgen or the estrogen receptor. It is believed that the skeletal actions of the androgens are mediated either directly, via the androgen receptor in the osteoblast, or indirectly, as a prohormone via the estrogen receptor after aromatization to estrogens (Colvard et al. 1989a; Colvard et al. 1989b; Kasperk et al. 1989; Kasperk et al. 1990; Orwoll et al. 1991; Masuyama et al. 1992; Vanderschueren and Bouillon 1995; Vanderschueren et al. 1998). In the growth plates of developing bone in both genders, androgen receptors have been observed to be predominantly expressed in hypertrophic chondrocytes as well as in osteoblasts at sites of bone formation, as observed in osteophytes taken from adult bone of both gen-

ders (Abu et al. 1997). Therefore, androgen receptors are present and widely distributed in normal developing human bone (representing skeletal maturation) and osteophytic bone (representing new bone development), providing evidence for direct action of the androgens on bone formation in both genders. Human osteoblast-like cells also appear to have the capacity to convert the weak androgen androstenedione into the more potent biological androgens, testosterone, and dihydrotestosterone (Bruch et al. 1992). A direct effect of androgens on osteoclasts has not yet been demonstrated (Vanderschueren and Bouillon 1995). Androgens may, however, affect bone resorption indirectly by inhibiting the recruitment of osteoclast precursors from bone marrow, by causing decreased amounts of IL-6 and prostaglandin E_2 (PGE_2) to be secreted (Marks and Miller 1993), by developing an altered sensitivity of marrow cells or osteoblasts for bone resorption-stimulation factors such as PTH, or by a combination of the three (Vanderschueren and Bouillon 1995).

Androgens also influence skeletal homeostasis in adult women, although the androgens' mode of action may again be related to their conversion into estrogens (Gasperino 1995). In women, androgen and estrogen metabolism and production occur in several tissues:

1. Ovaries in premenopausal women
2. Adrenal cortex
3. Adipose tissue
4. Bone cells

In the premenopausal woman, the adrenal gland is the major source of circulating androgens, such as androstenedione, whereas the major androgen products of the ovary are DHEA and androstenedione. Androgenic hormones appear to be among the most important determinants of peak cancellous bone density in young women (Buchanan et al. 1988). In postmenopausal women, serum androgen concentrations have significant protective effects on bone mass. Pathologic androgen excess in women may lead to a condition known as *hirsutism*. Whereas androgens influence bone and mineral metabolism in both genders, higher serum androgen levels in men exert potent osteoanabolic effects. Higher androgen levels in concert with higher androgen receptor expression at certain skeletal sites are thought to contribute to the sexual dimorphism of the skeleton (Kasperk et al. 1997).

Nutrition and Bone

The maximum amount of bone mass attained during bone growth, and the achievement of *peak bone mass* (discussed in detail in Chapter 5) is determined from early childhood by both heritable and environmental factors. Dietary calcium, saturated fat, fiber, and vitamin C have been associated with cortical and cancellous bone mineral density in healthy children and adolescents (Gunnes and Lehmann 1995). The interaction of gene polymorphisms (e.g., vitamin D receptor) and environmental factors (e.g., diet) likely provide an insight to the complex development of bone mineral mass (Ferrari et al. 1998).

Calcium

Calcium is essential to fuel many metabolic processes and its involvement with phosphate salts provides the basis for the mechanical rigidity of bones and teeth. In fact, 99% of the body's calcium reserves are found in bone and teeth. Calcium is needed for normal growth and consolidation of the skeleton. Peak bone mass (Chapter 5) is an important determinant of bone mass later in life and inherently a determinant of the risk of fracture, making sufficient calcium intake during growth important (Barr and McKay 1998). Calcium found in the skeleton plays an essential role in meeting the metabolic needs of the body in states of calcium deficiency. Such conditions manifest under certain metabolic fluxes or disease states as calcium is readily lost via the bowel, kidneys, and skin. In adults, calcium deficiency may cause mobilization of calcium from bone and is conducive to the osteopenic state. The effect of decreased levels of calcium and the sex steroid hormones is believed to be additive (Nordin 1997). Of some debate is the definitive role of calcium in attaining peak bone density and its role in determining the subsequent rate of bone loss. It has been suggested that calcium intake has a greater effect on bone mass before puberty than during or after the adolescent growth spurt (Johnston et al. 1992). The role of calcium in the etiology of certain metabolic bone diseases, such as osteoporosis, and subsequent fractures is controversial (Nordin et al. 1999). One study did find an inverse association of dietary calcium with subsequent risk of hip fracture, however, recommending an increased dietary calcium intake in older men and women to prevent injury (Holbrook et al. 1988).

Calcium balance is determined by calcium ingestion and absorption, coupled with excretion in feces and urine. Although other nutrients may alter calcium absorption and excretion, the factor determining calcium availability is calcium ingestion. The Recommended Dietary Allowance (RDA) for calcium is greatest, namely 1,200 mg per day, during adolescence (11–18 years of age) and early adulthood (19–24 years of age). People of all ages have the same calcium requirement except when women are pregnant, lactating or are postmenopausal. The RDA for children (1–10 years) and adults 25 years and older is 800 mg per day (National Research Council 1989).

Calcium and Age-Related Conditions of Bone

Whether menopausal changes in calcium metabolism are the cause or the result of postmenopausal bone loss is debated (Nordin 1997). The rise in obligatory calcium excretion at menopause causes an increase in the theoretical calcium requirement in postmenopausal women to approximately 1,000 mg or 1,200 mg if calcium absorption declines at the same time. Levels of the markers of bone turnover were reduced in one population of postmenopausal women taking calcium supplementation, with the greatest effect seen in women who had a previously low intake of dietary calcium (Fardellone et al. 1998).

Fluoride

Dietary fluoride obtained from food and water is absorbed efficiently, without regulation, at both the stomach and small intestine. In young healthy individuals, approximately one-half of absorbed fluoride is rapidly taken up by developing bone and teeth and the remainder is excreted in the urine in an increasing manner as bone growth slows (Cerklewski 1997). The vast majority of total body fluoride is found in the skeleton. Fluoride has an important role in the mineralization process of both skeletal bone and teeth; it is recognized as a beneficial trace element for dental health in humans. Fluorosis occurs when toxic levels of fluoride exist, indicating that as a typical trace element, fluoride's action is biphasic in nature. Fluoride may have a mitogenic role in osteoblast cell proliferation; however, its role in the therapeutic treatment of osteoporosis has not been fully determined (Cerklewski 1997).

Dietary Fat

The impact of dietary lipids on bone formation and chondrocyte function has been of interest (Watkins 1998). Although the literature is limited, an association of saturated fat intake with improved bone modeling and bone mineral density (BMD) has been demonstrated in children. In a study of white children (8–11 years of age) and adolescents (11–17 years of age), BMD in the forearm was predicted by dietary saturated fat intake (Gunnes and Lehmann 1995). In the adult avian model, it was found that saturated fat significantly increased bone turnover rates as reflected by increased periosteal bone formation, total new bone formation, and increased intracortical porosity in cortical bone (Watkins 1998). It appears that the dietary ^{20}C and ^{22}C (n-3) fatty acids aid in modulating PGE_2 levels produced locally in bone to optimize bone formation and perhaps prevent excessive bone resorption (Watkins 1998). Essential fatty acid–deficient animals developed severe osteoporosis coupled with increased renal and arterial calcification (Kruger and Horrobin 1997). Essential fatty acids have been shown to increase calcium absorption at the gut due to an enhanced effect of vitamin D at this site. In addition, reduced urinary excretion of calcium, increased calcium deposition in bone and improvement in bone strength, and enhanced synthesis of bone collagen are associated with essential fatty acids (Kruger and Horrobin 1997).

Vitamin A

High dietary intake (>1.5 mg/day) of retinol (vitamin A) has been associated with decreased bone mineral density and spontaneous fractures of the hip (Melhus et al. 1998).

Vitamin D

Rickets is a condition induced by vitamin D deficiency that affects developing bone. Rickets and osteomalacia (the adult equivalent) are diseases of vitamin D deficiency characterized histologically by a failure of the organic matrix of bone to mineralize.

The discovery of vitamin D and its production in skin and foods by UV irradiation in the early part of the twentieth century led to the elimination of rickets as a major medical problem (DeLuca 1988). Osteomalacia is discussed further in Chapter 12.

Vitamin E

Dietary vitamin E may also play a protective role against bone loss (Cohen and Meyer 1993) and may be of benefit for optimal bone health in the elderly (Maenpaa et al. 1989) and general bone formation during skeletal growth (Xu et al. 1995).

Summary

Bone acts as a reservoir of minerals that are essential to maintaining systemic inorganic ion homeostasis. A significant function of bone is to act as a buffer, maintaining plasma calcium and phosphorus levels within a narrow physiologic range. Homeostatic control of the hormonal milieu is required to sustain bone metabolism so that the skeleton is able to maintain sufficient bone for calcium homeostasis, respond appropriately to the biomechanical demands imposed on it, as well as accomplish local repair. Both systemic hormones and cytokines generated in the bone cell microenvironment affect bone mineral metabolism and tissue remodeling processes via control of bone cell activity. The principal hormones involved in bone metabolism are parathyroid hormone (PTH), vitamin D, and calcitonin, which not only impact on extracellular fluid levels of calcium and phosphate, but also on the kidney and intestine. In addition, there are the steroid hormones (glucocorticoids, growth hormone, estrogen, progesterone, and the androgens) that can influence development and homeostasis of bone, in both normal and pathologic states. These steroid hormones are not under negative feedback control by concentrations of calcium in the extracellular fluid.

The principal action of PTH is to mobilize bone mineral to increase the calcium concentration of extracellular fluid. PTH is produced by the parathyroid glands situated in the neck and is regulated by levels of serum calcium and $1,25(OH)_2D_3$. Vitamin D $(1,25[OH]_2D_3)$ is ultimately produced in the kidney and is regulated by serum levels of calcium, phosphorus, PTH, and the sex steroid hormones. It stimulates intestinal calcium and phosphorus absorption and, in concert with PTH, regulates bone turnover and renal excretion of calcium and phosphorus. The main biological effect of calcitonin is to inhibit the osteoclastic resorption of bone and, therefore, its action directly opposes that of PTH. Growth hormone is the most important hormone in the control of linear growth of long bones via its effects on epiphyseal growth. Corticosteroids are produced in the adrenal gland and their net effect on bone is catabolic. Excess corticosteroids promote loss of bone (osteopenia).

Estrogen plays a major role in bone mineral homeostasis, modulating bone turnover by maintaining a balance between bone formation and resorption in both males and females. Sources of estrogen in the female include the ovary and the peripheral conversion of sex steroid precursors derived from the adrenals. Androgens may affect bone metabolism in both sexes either directly by stimulation of the androgen receptor or by their conversion into estrogens and stimulation of the estrogen receptor. Direct and/or indirect action (via aromatase activity) of estrogen has important effects on skeletal integrity in males. Androgens have important effects in both sexes, and they affect both bone maturation and homeostasis of mature bone.

References

Abu EO, Horner A, Kusec V, Triffitt JT. The localization of androgen receptors in human bone. J Clin Endocrinol Metab 1997;82:3493–3497.

Barr SI, McKay HA. Nutrition, exercise and bone status in youth. Int J Sport Nutr 1998;8:1224–1242.

Benz DJ, Haussler MR, Komm BS. Estrogen binding and estrogenic responses in normal human osteoblast-like cells. J Bone Miner Res 1991;6:531–541.

Bradshaw MS, Tsai SY, Leng X, et al. Studies on the mechanism of functional cooperativity between progesterone and estrogen receptors. J Biol Chem 1991;266:16684–16690.

Bruch HR, Wolf L, Budde R, et al. Androstenedione metabolism in cultured human osteoblast-like cells. J Clin Endocrinol Metab 1992;75:101–105.

Buchanan JR, Hospodar P, Myers C, et al. Effect of excess endogenous androgen on bone density in young women. J Clin Endocrinol Metab 1988;67:937–943.

Cerklewski FL. Fluoride bioavailability: nutritional and clinical aspects. Nutr Res 1997;17:907–929.

Chapurlat RD, Delmas PD. Growth hormone and bone tissue in adults. Presse Medicale 1999;28:559–562.

Chevalley T, Rizzoli R. Impact of parathyroid hormone on bone. Presse Medicale 1999;28:547–553.

Cohen ME, Meyer DM. Effect of dietary vitamin E supplementation and rotational stress on alveolar bone loss in rice rats. Arch Oral Biol 1993;38:601–606.

Colston KW, King RJB, Hayward J, et al. Estrogen receptors and human bone cells: immunocytochemical studies. J Bone Miner Res 1989;4:625–631.

Colvard D, Eriksen EF, Keeting PE, et al. Identification of androgen receptors in normal human osteoblast-like cells. Proc Natl Acad Sci U S A 1989a;86:854–857.

Colvard D, Spelsberg T, Eriksen E, et al. Evidence of steroid receptors in human osteoblast-like cells. Connect Tissue Res 1989b;20:33–40.

Deftos L. Calcitonin. In M Favus (ed), Primer on the Metabolic Bone Diseases and Disorders of Mineral Metabolism (2nd ed). New York: Raven Press, 1993.

DeLuca HF. The vitamin D story: a collaborative effort of basic science and clinical medicine. FASEBJ 1988;2:224–236.

Driessens MF, Vanhoutte PM, Mortier G. Effect of calcitonin, hydrocortisone and parathyroid hormone on canine bone blood vessels. Am J Physiol 1981;241:H91–H94.

Ernst M, Heath JK, Schmid C, et al. Evidence for a direct effect of estrogen on bone cells in vitro. J Steroid Biochem 1989;34:279–284.

Fardellone P, Brazier M, Kamel S, et al. Biochemical effects of calcium supplementation in postmenopausal women: influence of dietary calcium intake. Am J Clin Nutr 1998;67:1273–1278.

Ferrari S, Rizzoli R, Bonjour JP. Heritable and nutritional influences on bone-mineral mass. Aging Clin Exp Res 1998;10:205–213.

Gasperino J. Androgenic regulation of bone mass in women. Clin Ortho Related Res 1995;311:278–286.

Gunnes M, Lehmann EH. Dietary calcium, saturated fat, fiber and vitamin C as predictors of forearm cortical and trabecular bone mineral density in healthy children and adolescents. Acta Paediatr 1995;84:388–392.

Hansen KA, Tho SPT. Androgens and bone health. Semin Reprod Endocrinol 1998;16:129–134.

Holbrook TL, Barrett-Connor E, Wingard DL. Dietary calcium and risk of hip fracture: 14-year prospective population study. Lancet 1988;2:1046–1049.

Johnston CC, Miller JZ, Slemenda CW, et al. Calcium supplementation and increases in bone mineral density in children. N Engl J Med 1992;327:82–87.

Kann P, Peipkorn B, Schehler B, et al. Effect of long-term treatment with GH on bone metabolism, bone mineral density and bone elasticity in GH-deficient adults. Clin Endocrinol 1998;48:561–568.

Kasperk CH, Wergedal JE, Farley JR, et al. Androgens directly stimulate proliferation of bone cells in vitro. Endocrinology 1989;124:1576–1578.

Kasperk C, Fitzsimmons R, Strong D, et al. Studies of the mechanism by which androgens enhance mitogenesis and differentiation in bone cells. J Clin Endocrinol Metab 1990;71:1322–1329.

Kasperk C, Helmboldt A, Borcsok I, et al. Skeletal site-dependent expression of the androgen receptor in human osteoblastic cell-populations. Calcif Tissue Int 1997;61:464–473.

Komm BS, Terpening CM, Benz DJ, et al. Estrogen binding,

receptor mRNA, and biologic response in osteoblast-like osteosarcoma cells. Science 1988;241:81–83.

Kruger MC, Horrobin DF. Calcium metabolism, osteoporosis and essential fatty acids: a review. Progress Lipid Res 1997;36:131–151.

Langdahl BL, Kassem M, Moller MK, Eriksen EF. The effects of IGF-I and IGF-II on proliferation and differentiation of human osteoblasts and interactions with growth hormone. Eur J Clin Invest 1998;28: 176–183.

Maenpaa PH, Pirhonen A, Pirskanen A, et al. Biochemical indicators related to antioxidant status and bone metabolic activity in Finnish elderly men. Int J Vitam Nutr Res 1989;59:14–19.

Marks SC, Miller SC. Prostaglandins and the skeleton: the legacy and challenges of two decades of research. Endocrine J 1993;1:337–344.

Masuyama A, Ouchi Y, Sato F, et al. Characteristics of steroid hormone receptors in cultured MC3T3-E1 osteoblastic cells and effect of steroid hormones on cell proliferation. Calcif Tissue Int 1992;5:376–381.

Melhus H, Michaelsson K, Kindmark A, et al. Excessive dietary-intake of vitamin A is associated with reduced bone mineral density and increased risk for hip fracture. Ann Int Med 1998;129:770.

Morley P, Whitfield JF, Willick GE. Anabolic effects of parathyroid hormone on bone. Trends Endocrinol Metab 1997;8:225–231.

Mundy GR. Bone Remodeling and Its Disorders. London: M. Dunitz, 1995;39–65.

National Research Council. Recommended Dietary Allowances (10th ed). Washington, DC: National Academy Press, 1989;10–23,174–205.

Nordin BEC. Calcium and osteoporosis. Nutrition 1997;13: 664–686.

Nordin BEC, Need AG, Morris HA, Horowitz M. Biochemical variables in pre- and postmenopausal women: reconciling the calcium and estrogen hypotheses. Osteoporosis Int 1999;9:351–357.

Orwoll ES, Stribrska L, Ramsey EE, Keenan EJ. Androgen receptors in osteoblast-like cell lines. Calcif Tissue Int 1991;49:183–187.

Otremski I, Levran M, Salama R, Edelstein S. The metabolism of vitamin D3 in response to testosterone. Calcif Tissue Int 1997;60:485–487.

Pacifici R. Estrogen, cytokines and the pathogenesis of postmenopausal osteoporosis. J Bone Miner Res 1996;11: 1043–1051.

Parfitt AM. Growth hormone and adult bone remodelling. Clin Endocrinol 1991;35:467–470.

Purohit A, Flanagan AM, Reed MJ. Estrogen synthesis by osteoblast cell lines. Endocrinology 1992;131:2027–2029.

Ribot C, Tremollieres F. Stéroïdes sexuels et tissu osseux. Annales d'Endocrinologie (Paris) 1995;56:49–55.

Rickard DJ, Hofbauer LC, Bonde SK, et al. Bone morphogenetic protein-6 production in human osteoblastic cell lines: selective regulation by estrogen. J Clin Invest 1998;101:413–422.

Scheven BAA, Damen CA, Hamilton NJ, et al. Stimulatory effects of estrogen and progesterone on proliferation and differentiation of normal human osteoblast-like cells in vitro. Biochem Biophys Res Commun 1992;186:54–60.

Schweikert HU, Wolf L, Romalo G. Oestrogen formation from androstenedione in human bone. Clin Endocrinol 1995;43:37–42.

Sharpe RM. The roles of estrogen in the male. Trends Endocrinol Metab 1998;9:371–377.

Shozu M, Simpson ER. Aromatase expression of human osteoblast-like cells. Molecular Cell Endocrinol 1998; 139:117–129.

Simpson E, Rubin G, Clyne C, et al. Local estrogen biosynthesis in males and females. Endocr Related Cancer 1999;6:131–137.

Spector TD, Thompson PW, Perry LA, et al. The relationship between sex steroids and bone mineral content in women soon after the menopause. Clin Endocrinol 1991;34:37–41.

Tapanainen J, Tonnberg L, Martikainen H, et al. Short and long term effects of growth hormone on circulating levels of insulin-like growth factor-1 (IGF-I), and insulin: a placebo-controlled study. J Clin Endocrinol Metab 1991;73:71–74.

Utian WH. Biosynthesis and physiologic effects of estrogen and pathophysiologic effects of estrogen deficiency: a review. Am J Obstet Gynecol 1989;161:1828–1831.

Vanderschueren D, Boonen S, Bouillon R. Action of androgens versus estrogens in male skeletal homeostasis. Bone 1998;23(5):391–394.

Vanderschueren D, Bouillon R. Androgens and bone. Calcif Tissue Int 1995;56:341–346.

Watkins BA. Regulatory Effects on Polyunsaturates on Bone Modeling and Cartilage Function. In AP Simopoulos (ed), The Return of Fatty Acids in the Food Supply. Land-Based Animal Food Products and Their Health Effects. World Rev Nutr Diet. Basel, Germany: Karger, 1998;83:38–51.

Watrous DA, Andrews BS. The metabolism and immunology of bone. Semin Arthritis Rheum 1989;19:45–65.

Wong FHW, Pun KK, Wang C. Loss of bone mass in patients with Klinefelter's syndrome despite sufficient testosterone replacement. Osteoporosis Int 1993;3:3–7.

Xu H, Watkins BA, Seifert MF. Vitamin E stimulates trabecular bone formation and alters epiphyseal cartilage morphology. Calcif Tissue Int 1995;57:293–300.

Chapter 5
Changes in Bone across the Lifespan

Bone Histogenesis in Growth and Development

Bone is a specialized type of dense connective tissue that derives its origin from pluripotential cells of primitive mesoderm. An extensive review of the embryologic development of bone is beyond the scope of this book; however, two basic types of bone formation processes (intramembranous and endochondral ossification) are briefly described. Generally stated, specific bone development processes differ; however, the actual formation of bone in both intramembranous and endochondral ossification proceeds in the same manner (Figure 5-1).

Intramembranous Bone Formation

Intramembranous bone formation is typical of the flat bones of the skull, part of the mandible, and the clavicle, whereby a membranous compact plate of primitive fetal mesenchyme ossifies directly during development in utero. In intramembranous ossification, bone is formed directly from the innermost layer of the periosteum, and no intermediate cartilaginous phase occurs. Growth in the width of bone occurs by direct apposition by intramembranous bone formation processes.

Endochondral Bone Formation

Endochondral bone formation, the formation of calcified bone on a cartilage scaffold, occurs during skeletal development, postnatal growth, and fracture repair (Stevens and Williams 1999). Bones of the base of the skull, the vertebral column, the pelvis, and the extremities are formed as a result of ossification of a preformed hyaline cartilage model. A cartilage model begins as a condensation of mesenchyme during the embryonic period and results from the proliferation of chondrocytes. The cartilage cells mature and eventually calcify. In adults, endochondral ossification is the process by which a cartilage model is replaced by calcified bone, as in the healing of a long bone fracture.

Bone Mass in Growth, Development (Maturation), and Aging

Bone mass changes throughout life in three major phases: growth, consolidation, and involution (Riggs and Melton 1986). The growth phase, whereby the skeleton grows in length, occurs during childhood and adolescence. During this phase, the bones simultaneously expand in diameter and acquire their shape through modeling processes. During skeletal growth, up to 90% of the ultimate bone mass is deposited. Termination of skeletal growth occurs at the closure of the epiphyses. A phase of skeletal consolidation lasts for up to 15 years, when bone mass increases further, until the mid-30s, when it is considered that peak bone mass is attained. Involutional bone loss begins between the ages of 35 and 40 years, with the rate and onset of bone loss thought to be genetically predeter-

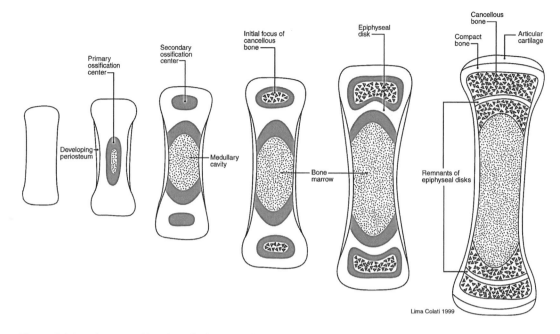

Figure 5-1. Development of long bone is the result of both endochondral and intramembranous ossification processes.

mined. Cortical and cancellous bone is lost with advancing age in both genders, although the rate of bone loss varies according to bone type (cancellous versus cortical) and anatomic site. The annual rate of cancellous bone loss ranges from approximately 0.6% to 2.4% in women, with a rapid loss in the first 10 menopausal years (Shipman et al. 1999), and 0.2% to 1.2% in men. The initial rate of cortical bone loss is 0.3–0.5% annually in both women and men, although this increases to 2–3% in women at menopause. A return to a slower rate of bone loss occurs approximately 10 years after menopause (Figure 5-2). Women may have an overall loss of 35–50% of cancellous bone mass and 25–30% of cortical bone mass, whereas men may lose 14–45% of cancellous bone mass and 5–15% of their cortical bone mass across the lifespan (Jackson and Kleerokoper 1990; Riggs and Melton 1986). Low bone mass is of great clinical concern, because it is associated with an increased risk of fracture.

Peak Bone Mass

Bone mass is acquired to the greatest extent between the ages of 14 and 20 years (Slemenda et al. 1990). In one cross-sectional study of the vertebrae from adolescent girls during the skeletal growth phase, bone mass increased most dramatically between ages 10 and 14 years, or until the first year after menarche, reaching 86% of adult bone mass values by age 14 (Sabatier et al. 1996). The potential determinants of peak bone mass include race, gender, hereditary factors, exercise, diet, smoking, alcohol consumption, and endocrine factors. In fact, age, level of physical activity, and family history are independent predictors of peak bone mineral density (BMD) (Rubin et al. 1999). Black populations have a higher bone mass than whites or Asians (Cohn et al. 1977). Men have more dense bone than women across the lifespan (Mazess 1982). In fact, at maturity women have approximately 20% lower peak bone mass compared to men. Some evidence exists that points to a strong genomic regulation over bone mass acquisition (Nguyen et al. 1998). Daughters of osteoporotic women have lower than expected bone mass and a greater concordance of bone mass exists between monozygotic than dizygotic twins (Seeman et al. 1989). It has been estimated that approximately 20% of adult peak bone mass is further influenced by environmental factors (Pocock et al. 1987). Bone mass is greater in young adults who exercise regularly than in more sedentary individuals, emphasizing the role of mechanical factors in the determination of

Figure 5-2. Dual energy x-ray absorptiometry profile. Note the regional decline in bone mass in women after 35–40 years. **A.** Femoral neck region. **B.** Lumbar spine region. (Courtesy of Sonia Bibershtein, B.Sc. [P.T.], Women's College Hospital, Toronto.)

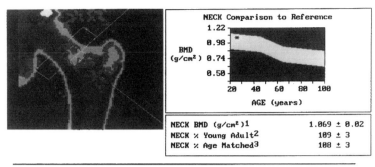

NECK BMD (g/cm²)[1]   1.069 ± 0.02
NECK % Young Adult[2]   109 ± 3
NECK % Age Matched[3]   108 ± 3

Age (years)........	26	Large Standard......	267.56	Scan Mode.......	Fast
Sex................	Female	Medium Standard.....	199.30	Scan Type...........	DPX-Alpha
Weight (lb)........	145.0	Small Standard......	142.21	Collimation (mm).....	1.68
Height (in)........	66	Low keV Air (cps)...	835851	Sample Size (mm).....	1.2x 1.2
Ethnic.............	White	High keV Air (cps)..	474649	Region height (mm)...	60.0
System............	8213	Rvalue (%Fat).......	1.343(24.6)	Region width (mm)....	15.0
Side..............	Left	Current (uA)........	3000	Region angle (deg)...	49

NECK   : BMC[5] (grams) = 4.78   AREA[5] (cm²) = 4.47
WARDS : BMC[5] (grams) = 2.13   AREA[3] (cm²) = 2.22
TROCH : BMC[3] (grams) = 10.82   AREA[5] (cm²) = 11.15

REGION	BMD[1] g/cm²	Young Adult[2] %	Z	Age Matched[3] %	Z
NECK	1.069	109	0.75	108	0.66
WARDS	0.957	105	0.36	103	0.22
TROCH	0.970	123	1.64	122	1.62

A

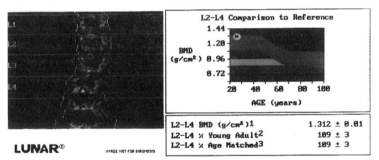

LUNAR®   (IMAGE NOT FOR DIAGNOSIS)

L2-L4 BMD (g/cm²)[1]   1.312 ± 0.01
L2-L4 % Young Adult[2]   109 ± 3
L2-L4 % Age Matched[3]   109 ± 3

Age (years)........	26	Large Standard......	267.56	Scan Mode.......	Fast
Sex................	Female	Medium Standard.....	199.30	Scan Type...........	DPX-Alpha
Weight (lb)........	145.0	Small Standard......	142.21	Collimation (mm).....	1.68
Height (in)........	66	Low keV Air (cps)...	835851	Sample Size (mm).....	1.2x 1.2
Ethnic.............	White	High keV Air (cps)..	474649	Current (uA)........	3000
System............	8213	Rvalue (%Fat).......	1.374(8.9)		

REGION	BMD[1] g/cm²	Young Adult[2] %	Z	Age Matched[3] %	Z
L1	1.254	111	1.04	111	1.01
L2	1.273	106	0.61	106	0.58
L3	1.356	113	1.30	113	1.27
L4	1.304	109	0.86	108	0.83
L1-L2	1.264	110	0.95	110	0.92
L1-L3	1.299	111	1.07	111	1.04
L1-L4	1.300	110	1.00	110	0.97
L2-L3	1.318	110	0.98	109	0.95
L2-L4	1.312	109	0.94	109	0.91
L3-L4	1.329	111	1.07	110	1.04

1 - See appendix E on precision and accuracy. Statistically 68% of repeat scans will fall within 1 SD.
2 - USA AP Spine Reference Population, Ages 20-45.
3 - Matched for Age, Weight(males 50-100kg; females 35-80kg), Ethnic.

B

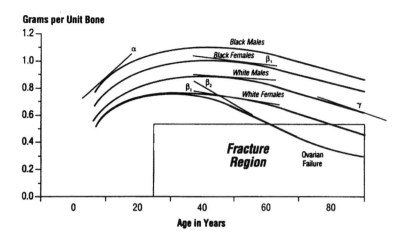

Figure 5-3. Schematic representation of effects of age, gender, and race on bone mass. (Reprinted with permission from CJ Rosen. Growth hormone, insulin-like growth factors, and the senescent skeleton: Ponce de Leon's fountain revisited? Cell Biochem 1994;56:350.)

bone mass (Nilson and Westlin 1971). Current levels of self-reported exercise were associated with BMD at the neck of the femur, greater trochanter, and Ward's triangle, supporting the view that exercise is beneficial to BMD levels (Torgerson et al. 1995). Lifestyle factors, including smoking and alcohol consumption during adolescence and early adult life, also have an adverse effect on peak bone mass (Mazess and Barden 1991). Furthermore, in one large population study, a significant and detrimental association was demonstrated between the history of women's mothers' smoking and BMD of their offspring (Torgerson et al. 1995). Hormonal factors appear to affect peak bone mass; early menarche, pregnancy, and the use of the oral contraceptive pill are all associated with a higher bone mass (Goldsmith and Johnston 1975; Stevenson et al. 1989).

Although bone loss with age is a universal phenomenon, not all individuals experience fractures at an advanced age. BMD is currently used as the strongest predictor of future fracture, the overall risk of which is determined by the peak bone mass, the age at which bone loss begins, and the rate at which bone loss progresses. An age-related alteration in bone remodeling processes as well as prior peak bone mass attained during the growth and maturation period are determining factors of bone mass in an elderly individual. Low bone mass with age is considered a natural part of aging. When loss of bone mass is associated with skeletal fragility, leading to an increased risk of fracture, the condition is referred to as *age-related* (type II or senile) *osteoporosis* (Johnston and Slemenda 1994). Age-related bone loss is a generalized phenomenon that affects the entire skeleton; however, the rate of bone loss dif-

fers from one site of the skeleton to another and between the different bony envelopes. In age-related osteoporosis, bone loss is global, affecting both cortical and cancellous bone and making the femoral neck particularly susceptible to fracture. Types I and II osteoporosis are further discussed in Chapter 12.

As the population ages, the prevalence of age and age-related disorders of bone rises. However, the mechanisms leading to age-related bone loss remain poorly understood. The functional decline in most biological systems, of which bone is one, appears to be regulated by genetic factors. The role of genetic factors in the development of skeletal fragility, in which one or more sets of genes control acquisition of peak bone mass, has been appreciated as well (Rosen 1994). Age-related bone loss is likely the result of the interactivity of genetic determinants as they relate with environmental and hormonal factors, lending support to the hypothesis that the genome regulates aging via homeostatic and integrative mechanisms. The rate of menopausal bone loss varies among women of different races and ethnic backgrounds, demonstrating the interactive influences of genetic and hormonal factors during this critical time (Figure 5-3). In men, aging is associated with a gradual decline in serum testosterone, the deficiency of which is considered one of the strongest independent risk factors for the development of age-related osteoporosis (Jackson et al. 1992).

Age-Related Changes in the Mineral of Bone

Reduced bone mass in both aging men and women is typically unrelated to mineralization defects per se.

During aging and other periods of known low remodeling activity, mineralization is shifted toward higher mineral densities (hypermineralization), which has the overall effect of influencing the material properties of bone, its role in terms of mechanical support and as an ion reservoir, and its ability to affect acid-base balance in the body (Grynpas 1993).

Changes in Bone Cell Behavior with Age

Age-related changes are reflected in an altered bone remodeling sequence that may be owing to a decline in osteoblast function that, in turn, leads to reduced bone formation. In young adults, at the termination of the skeletal growth phase, bone remodeling processes are balanced with closely coupled bone resorption and formation activity. With aging, a remodeling imbalance occurs and, ultimately, more bone is removed than is replaced. The change in the signals that trigger, control, and terminate the bone cell processes with aging is unclear (Table 5-1). The defect in bone formation that occurs in normal aging amounts to too small a work output by each new team of osteoblasts, resulting in incomplete refilling of resorption cavities. Whether too few osteoblasts are assembled, which would result from a defect in a coupling signal or from a deficiency of osteoblast precursors, or whether each osteoblast makes a subnormal amount of bone is unknown (Parfitt 1984). Human bone cells from older donors may produce less proteoglycan, fibronectin, and thrombospondin than those from younger controls (Fedarko 1992). An aberrant extracellular matrix created because of the change in nature and activity of human bone cells contributes to the altered macromolecular organization and, hence, the integrity of the skeleton.

A reduction in bone mass with aging may also be owing to reduction of the proliferative capacity of progenitor cells or their responsiveness to biological factors leading to alteration in subsequent differentiation (Oreffo et al. 1998). Three possible mechanisms have been hypothesized to explain the effects of aging on the osteoblast (Rosen 1994):

1. An aberrant recruitment of osteoprogenitor cells from pluripotential bone marrow stem cells occurs.
2. Reduced proliferation of osteoblast-like cells occurs, due either to lower growth factor production in marrow cells or resistance to paracrine,

Table 5-1. Age-Related Changes in Osteoblasts and Osteocytes

Osteoblasts	Osteocytes
↓ Cell proliferation	Atrophy
↓ Size	↓ Metachromasia in matrix collagen fibrils
Hyperchromic nucleus	↓ Matrix water content
	↑ Size of hydroxyapatite crystal

↓ = decreased; ↑ = increased.
Source: Adapted from EA Tonna. Skeletal aging and its effects on the osteogenic potential. Clin Orthop 1965;40:57–81.

autocrine, and endocrine growth factors. The production of skeletal growth factors may be normal with aging, but senescent osteoblasts may be resistant to their biological action, resulting in down-regulated growth factor receptors, impaired second messages, or the production of inhibitory growth factor–binding proteins.
3. Osteoblastic differentiation is impaired.

Changes in Bone with Aging: Confounding Factors

Confounding factors that may influence bone loss with age include calciotropic and sex steroid hormone changes (e.g., menopause in women, smoking, nutritional factors, an associated decline in physical activity levels).

Calciotropic Hormones and Changes in Mineral Regulation

Aging is accompanied by a myriad of effects on calcium homeostasis and metabolism. Aging alters the metabolism of vitamin D and calcium in several ways. Calcium availability may be reduced in the elderly because of decreased dietary intake of calcium and vitamin D, reduced solar exposure, and a decrease in the production of provitamin D by the skin (Bell 1995).

An age-related decline in dermal production of 7-dehydrocholesterol, the precursor of provitamin D_3, occurs so that synthesis of vitamin D_3 in the skin may be impaired (MacLaughlin and Holick 1985). Intake of vitamin D may be reduced and exposure to sunlight may be diminished in institutionalized or housebound individuals (Bouillon et al. 1987; Reid et al. 1986). A reduction in renal production of 1,25-dihydroxyvitamin D_3 (Tsai et al. 1984), intestinal absorption of calcium (Alevizaki et al. 1965; Francis et al. 1984), and ingestion of calcium (Gallagher et al. 1979) may also occur. In age-matched older individuals (>43–64 years of age), men demonstrated less variability in the physiologic control of Ca^{2+} than women during the women's peri- to postmenopausal years, suggesting that Ca^{2+} homeostasis is disrupted in the same age groups most vulnerable to bone loss (Watson et al. 1997).

A decreased sensitivity of the intestine to 1,25-dihydroxyvitamin D_3 and a decline in calcium absorption is typical in some older patients (Wémeau 1995). The combination of poor gastrointestinal absorption with suboptimal ingestion of calcium increases the likelihood of a negative calcium balance in these individuals. In response to the negative calcium balance, parathyroid hormone (PTH) secretion increases with the overall effect of increased bone resorption. An age-related increase in serum PTH has been considered a pathogenetic mechanism of age-related osteoporosis (Epstein et al. 1986; Riggs and Melton 1986). In addition, the decrease in calcitonin secretion in the elderly relates to a loss of sex steroids and calcitriol (Wémeau 1995).

Sex Steroid Hormones

In women, the production of sex steroid hormones of ovarian and adrenal origin (e.g., estrogens, androgens) declines with age (Crilly et al. 1981). One of the hallmarks in the chronobiology of reproductive aging in women is menopause, the cessation of ovulatory function. Serum estradiol levels are at their lowest values between the ages of 51 and 60 years, as the ovaries cease to function. Rapid falls in androgen (testosterone and androstenedione) levels also have been described in women, but they are less marked than the drop in estradiol (Rozenberg et al. 1988; Rozenberg et al. 1990). The less significant decline of androgens is attributed to the significant adrenal contribution to androgen production and the relatively smaller reduction in ovarian androgens after the menopause (Judd et al. 1982). Serum levels of dehydroepiandrosterone-sulfate (DHEAS), one of the adrenal androgens, fall to their minimal values between 60 and 70 years of age, constituting an "adrenopause" (Cumming et al. 1982).

Chronologic aging results in reduced gonadotropin secretion in women, although the precise mechanisms that account for the decline in neuroendocrine function remain unclear. Evidence shows gonadotropin secretion (based on diminished pituitary or hypothalamic function) is reduced during advanced age in postmenopausal women (Rossmanith et al. 1990; Rossmanith et al. 1991). Although growth hormone and insulin-like growth factor-I (IGF-I) change with age, it is uncertain whether these changes are extensively responsible for age-related bone loss.

Nutritional Changes

Appropriate daily calcium intake is estimated to be 800–1,200 mg per day for children 1–10 years of age, 1,200–1,500 mg per day for adolescents and persons up to 24 years old, 1,000 mg per day for premenopausal women, and as much as 1,500 mg per day for postmenopausal women not receiving estrogen treatment (Heaney et al. 1978; Kanders et al. 1988; National Research Council 1989; Nordin et al. 1979; Sandler et al. 1985). The role of dietary calcium, however, remains controversial when considering it as a factor in the pathogenesis of bone loss with age. Although evidence of a relationship between dietary calcium intake and bone mass exists, the relationship more likely relates to an effect on peak bone mass rather than on bone loss because other studies show no relationship between calcium intake, bone mass, and bone loss in postmenopausal women (Holbrook et al. 1988). Whereas various nutritional factors affect bone metabolism (see Chapter 4), calcium and vitamin D have received the greatest attention in terms of their potential use as therapeutic agents in potentiating and preserving bone mass (Chapuy et al. 1992; Reginster 1995). Although one study showed that the risk of femoral fracture was reduced in subjects with a higher dietary intake of calcium (Holbrook et al. 1988), other studies concluded that an increase in dietary calcium was seen as unlikely to produce a major effect on the rate of bone loss (Riggs et al. 1987) or risk of femoral fracture (Wooten et al. 1979). Because of the reduction in calcium absorption with advancing age, increasing the dietary calcium requirements further, it remains prudent to advise postmenopausal women to adhere to a diet rich in calcium. Although metabolic and physiologic responses to caffeine may not differ between older and younger individuals, it may have a greater impact on calcium metabolism and bone in older people; caffeine consumption may increase urinary calcium levels derived from an already compromised skeleton (Massey 1998).

Physical Activity

Physical activity is important to the skeleton at any age because the associated weightbearing and muscular activity stimulates bone formation and increases or at least stabilizes bone mass; immobilization leads to rapid bone loss (Krolner et al. 1983). The importance of physical activity in maintaining bone mass is further emphasized by several case control studies showing that patients in whom femoral fractures are sustained are habitually less active than control subjects (Holbrook et al. 1988). Cross-sectional studies in women up to age 85 years show that physically active women have a lower age-related rate of bone loss than less active women (Jacobson et al. 1984; Stillman et al. 1986). In view of the recognized benefits of weightbearing and exercise on bone and the deleterious effects of immobilization on the skeleton, it is clear that regular exercise and physical activity is encouraged and should be adopted as a lifelong practice. Advocacy for physical activity and good nutrition relies on the premise that the incidence of age-related changes in bone is modifiable if dietary and lifestyle patterns conducive to achieving the highest possible peak bone mass are adopted, during both the skeletal growth and other critical periods during which bone is vulnerable to change.

Physical Stimuli and Older Bone: Experimental Evidence

Although the effects of exercise or purposeful activity on bone are extensively addressed in Chapter 8, the mechanisms by which the older skeleton responds to physical activity merits attention within the context of this chapter.

The results of one animal study suggest that physical stimuli that are clearly osteogenic in the young adult skeleton are hardly acknowledged in older bone tissue (Rubin et al. 1992). Although substantial new bone formation was generated with exercise on periosteal and endosteal surfaces of young adult cortical bone in an avian model, no evidence of any renewed surface modeling was displayed (Rubin et al. 1992). Strains in the young adult avian skeleton perceived as osteogenic

were not sufficient to activate bone formation in the aging skeleton, resulting in no net change in properties of the skeletal area of the older bone tissue. The age-related modeling and remodeling differences observed in these experiments might not be the result of a disease process per se, but instead a reflection of compromised signal transduction pathways that attenuate the older skeleton's ability to respond to the osteogenic stimuli. The aging process could modulate the transformation of a physical signal to a tissue response. Gradients created by fluid pressure differentials as a result of functionally induced tissue deformation, and their bioelectric by-products, are essential signals to the regulation of skeletal mass, but may differ in the older skeleton (Pollack et al. 1977). With age, the surface-to-volume ratio of mineralized matrix diminishes (Bonar et al. 1983; Boskey and Posner 1984) in combination with the known age-induced increase in fluid viscosity (Bennett and Kaye 1981). The above cell-independent normal developments of aging may, in part, be responsible for the attenuated bone tissue response to these mechanical stimuli (Rubin 1992). The magnitude of the electrokinetic currents generated by deformation in loading might only be a fraction of that generated by younger adult bone; it has been hypothesized that modulated streaming potentials represent one way by which the normal processes of aging could compromise signal transduction pathways and, in turn, reduce bone tissue response to mechanical stimuli (Rubin 1992). Age-related modulation of the bone's capacity to respond to mechanical stimulation could also be the result of changes in the phenotype of the population of bone cells available (Tyan 1985). The osteogenic criteria that define Wolff's law (see Chapter 7) in a young responsive skeleton, therefore, may not be capable of counteracting the direct and indirect factors in the aging skeleton.

Changes in Quality and Quantity of Bone with Age

With advancing years, a decrease in the BMD occurs, as measured in a variety of ways, including dual energy x-ray absorptiometry (DEXA) and calcium bone index (CaBI). Decreases occur in the radiographic density of bone measured in vivo, the weight of the skeleton, and the physical density ratio (weight to volume) of individual bones and the mineral content (as measured by the percentage ash weight). Thus, bone loss with age is a problem

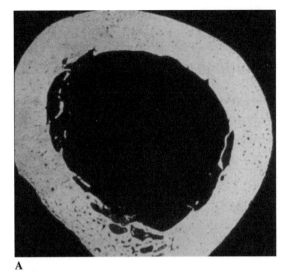

A

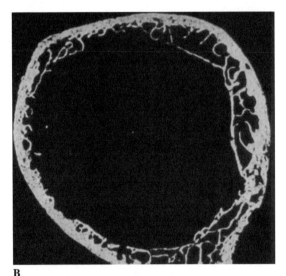

B

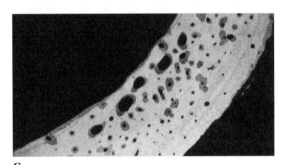

C

Figure 5-4. Changes in cortical bone with age. **A.** Young. **B.** Old. Note the increased trabecularization and decreased cortical width. **C.** Increased intracortical (size and number) porosity with age. (Courtesy of Dr. Marc Grynpas, Ph.D., Samuel Lunenfeld Research Institute, Mount Sinai Hospital, Toronto.)

of major concern. In addition, the overall change with age of BMD varies at different skeletal sites, with the loss of BMD in the vertebral body and in Ward's triangle of the femur (35%) reported to be approximately twice that in the posteroanterior spine and the femoral neck regions (18–21%) (Mazess et al. 1995).

Whereas the progressive loss of BMD is observed as part of the normal aging process, notable changes also occur in the quality and quantity of the internal architecture and connectivity of bone. Brittleness is greater and energy storage capacity of bone is reduced due to both the qualitative and quantitative changes in bone tissue with age. Specific changes occur in cortical and cancellous bone tissue.

Cortical

Prolonged reversal and refilling times increase porosity and reduce bone density in aging individuals (Martin and Burr 1989). Age-related osteoporosis (type II) is characterized by an overall decline in wall thickness of the resorption cavity (Pacifici and Avioli 1993). The bone remodeling cycle is imbalanced, with a reduction in bone formation due to a defect in osteoblastic function. Increased porosity may be caused by (1) increased numbers of haversian canals, (2) larger haversian canals, and (3) more resorption spaces and incompletely refilled osteons (Martin and Burr 1989), all of which create an overall volumetric deficit and decline in the structural integrity of cortical bone with age. The overall decrease in the total amount of bone tissue ultimately reduces the mechanical integrity of the bone. Significant differences in cortical porosity are evident between genders, caused mainly by higher values attained in the early postmenopausal years in women (Brockstedt et al. 1993).

The diaphysis of long bones increases in diameter throughout life, due to continuous periosteal growth (Garn et al. 1967; Nordin 1966). In many bones, net periosteal apposition continues slowly throughout life (Smith and Walker 1964). Periosteal expansion is linear from the third decade on, and it begins before significant net endosteal loss occurs (Figure 5-4). During the same period, the marrow cavity enlarges because of ongoing significant endosteal resorption, leading to a net decrease in cortical thickness in the

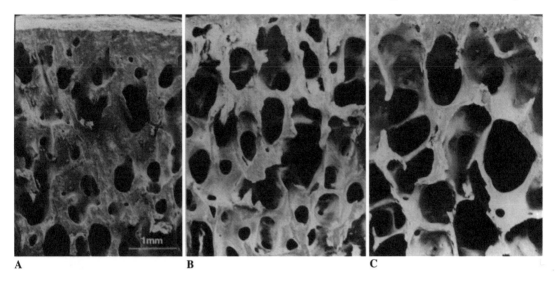

Figure 5-5. Age-related changes in cancellous bone obtained from women of three different age groups: 24 years (**A**), 63 years (**B**), and 89 years (**C**). (Courtesy of Dr. Marc Grynpas, Ph.D., Samuel Lunenfeld Research Institute, Mount Sinai Hospital, Toronto.)

axial and appendicular skeleton (Jee et al. 1991). Continuing periosteal apposition of lamellar bone leads to greater skeletal dimensions in older individuals and likely represents an effort at mechanical compensation for changes in the endosteal region (Lazenby 1990).

Cancellous

Width, number, and connectivity of the trabeculae in cancellous bone are reduced with age (Figure 5-5). As a result, a disruption in trabecular architecture and a net loss in cancellous bone volume occurs. The decrease in cancellous bone with advancing age is owing to both an increase in the distance between trabeculae and a decrease in the width of individual trabecular profiles (Weinstein and Hutson 1987). In men, a linear reduction in cancellous bone occurs; a similar trend occurs in women until menopause begins.

Vertebral cancellous bone loss in women may commence during or before the third decade, in contrast to radial cortical bone density, which does not decline during premenopausal years (Buchanan et al. 1988). At menopause, a marked acceleration in the rate of cancellous bone loss is observed. Old age is associated with a decline in bone mass in the cancellous bone of the vertebral bodies in both genders, although the rate and amount of the decline is greater in women. Vertebral cancellous bone density declines 45–50% in healthy people between ages 20 and 80 years (Mosekilde et al. 1987). Although the number and thickness of both the horizontal and vertical trabeculae decreases with age, the principal and most significant loss takes place at the horizontal trabeculae (Twomey et al. 1983). The trabeculae behave as cross-braces; their loss affects the vertebral bodies ability to bear and transmit body weight. The horizontal trabeculae thin and perforate within the network (Figure 5-6), leaving the vertical trabeculae unsupported and, therefore, subject to bending forces instead of the normal compressive forces (Kleerekoper et al. 1985; Mosekilde 1993). The loss of the vertical trabeculae is most marked below the nucleus pulposus of the intervertebral disk (IVD), the region of the disk most involved in transmitting compressive loads from one vertebra to the next (Twomey and Taylor 1987). The area of the bone immediately adjacent to the nucleus shows the largest number of microfractures in old age (Vernon-Roberts and Pirie 1973). This causes the vertebrae to become shorter, wider, and more concave at their endplate region in the lumbar spine (Twomey and Taylor 1988); wedge or anterior compression fractures are common (Twomey and Taylor 1994). With advancing age, progressive spinal deformities, such as spinal kyphosis, may present as a

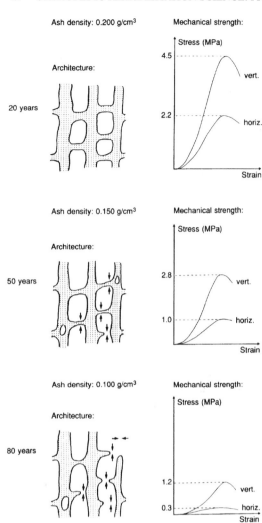

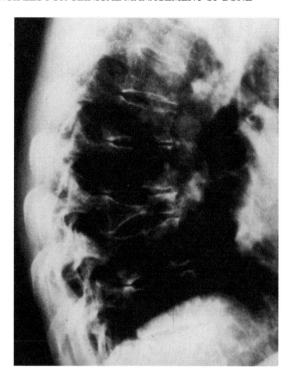

Figure 5-7. With advancing age in both genders, progressive spinal deformities (spinal kyphosis) may present as a result of a single or series of vertebral body fractures.

Figure 5-6. Typical relationship between ash density, architecture, and mechanical strength (vertical and horizontal) for vertebral trabecular bone obtained from three different age groups: 20 years, 50 years, and 80 years. (MPa, megapascal.) (Reprinted with permission from L. Mosekilde. Normal age-related changes in bone mass, structure, and strength—consequences of the remodeling process. Dan Med Bull 1993;40:76.)

result of a single or series of vertebral body fractures (Figure 5-7).

The selective loss of horizontal trabeculae, in addition to the hormonal deficiencies known to exist in old age, suggests that mechanical factors are important in age-related bone loss. The biomechanical competence of vertebral trabecular bone depends not only on bone mass, but also on the continuity of the trabecular lattice, which changes with increasing age (Mosekilde et al.

1987). The age-related decline in bone biomechanical competence is more pronounced than the decline in bone mass. This discrepancy is caused by the structural changes in the three-dimensional trabecular network, indicating that quantitative and qualitative changes in bone tissue are of great importance.

Age-Related Changes in Bone Biomechanics

Cortical Bone

Aging adversely affects the elastic and ultimate properties of human cortical bone (Zioupas and Currey 1998). Stiffness and strength diminishes in aging bone. Thus, aging bone may be less tough (the amount of energy required to fracture a specimen is decreased) because it is capable of a lesser degree of postyield and prefailure damage (Courtney et al. 1996); however, a combination of the hypotheses that the increased intrinsic fragility of aging bone is caused by its ability to absorb less postyield damage and a reduced ability to hinder the onset of a macrocrack is favored by others (Zioupos and Currey 1998).

Cancellous Bone

The inability of spinal vertebral bodies to cope with sustained loading is incurred as a result of age-related biochemical and morphologic changes, the altered shape of lumbar disks, and a deterioration in spinal posture and flexibility.

Young adult vertebral bodies can resist typical vertical compressive forces of body weight because of the arrangement of the trabeculae. The architecture of load-bearing vertebral trabecular bone of a young adult is characterized by thick vertical plates and columns reinforced by relatively thinner horizontal trabeculae. With age, the vertical plates are successively perforated during remodeling processes and converted into columns; the horizontal trabeculae are disconnected and often disappear (Parfitt 1984). Normal loss of cancellous bone with age occurs predominantly by a process that removes entire structural elements of bone, leaving those that remain more widely separated but only slightly reduced in thickness; this transforms the mainly continuous trabecular network characteristic of a young person into the mainly discontinuous network characteristic of the elderly (Parfitt et al. 1983). In cancellous bone, the compressive strength of normal vertebral trabecular bone (expressed as maximum load per unit cross-sectional area) is reduced by 70–85% across the lifespan (Mosekilde et al. 1985).

Gender Differences in Skeletal Remodeling

In men, bone loss accelerates at most skeletal sites after age 50 years. It is associated with a decline in markers of bone turnover, with a relative decrease in bone formation compared to bone resorption, and with falling levels of free androgens (Jackson et al. 1992; Wishart et al. 1995). Ten to fifteen percent of all vertebral fractures and 20–25% of all hip fractures occur in men (Cummings et al. 1985; Seeman et al. 1983). In women, menopause accounts for one-third of the bone loss, whereas the remaining two-thirds may be attributed to other age-related factors across the lifespan (Luisetto et al. 1993).

Age-Related Pathology of Bone

The incidence of disorders such as osteomalacia, osteoporosis, and Paget's disease increase with age. These disorders are three major bone-deforming diseases that manifest in the elderly population and, in turn, adversely affect the quality and quantity of bone. Bone disease has high prevalence in adults, making an understanding of bone metabolism and aberrations even more important for assessing fracture risk and monitoring therapy. Bone-deforming conditions are discussed in greater detail in Chapter 12.

Clinical Outcome: Implications for Physical Rehabilitation

Given that conditions such as osteoarthritis, osteoporosis, and hip and spine fracture are considered strong predictors of impaired function (Ensrud et al. 1994), it is critical for the physical rehabilitation professional to have extensive knowledge of the underlying pathophysiologic conditions of bone that are associated with age. In the first decade of the twenty-first century, North American society will observe the consequences of the growth of an older population. Musculoskeletal disorders in this elderly population are widespread and have ramifications on public health service both from a preventive and rehabilitation perspective. The prevention of age-related diseases of bone by maximizing bone mass is critical. Because of the current inability of pharmacologic agents to restore bone mass once it is lost, the focus must be on maximizing peak bone mass during the years of skeletal growth and maintaining it in years that follow. Although peak bone mass is, in part, genetically determined, bone health can be modified by lifestyle choices such as nutrition, adequate calcium intake, and adoption of weightbearing exercise.

The incidence of fractures increases with advancing age and is higher in women than in men. This difference is thought to be owing to women's lower initial peak bone mass and more rapid bone loss at menopause. Patients with age-related femoral fracture were less physically active than control subjects in a number of studies (Chalmers and Ho 1970; Cooper et al. 1988; Holbrook et al. 1988). Femoral fractures are the most important fracture in the elderly; they are known to cause greater mortality, higher morbidity, and health care expenditure than all other fractures combined (Holbrook et al. 1988).

Forearm fractures are the most common fracture in people younger than 75 years, with their incidence rising steeply in women during menopause.

As humans experience increased incidence of fractures with age, consideration must be given to extraosseous factors, such as reduced proprioceptive efficiency, impaired reflexes, reduced cushioning by fat, as well as osseous factors such as quantitative changes in the shape and size of the bones (diameter and cortical thickness) and a deterioration of the quality of the bone material. Further attention to both the bone quality and bone quantity (bone mass) has important ramifications in the quest for prediction of fracture in an individual. According to present trends, 16–20% of Canadians will exceed the age of 65 years by 2031 (Shephard 1989). Therefore, substantial opportunity exists for preventive practice by rehabilitation specialists with an interest in the geriatric field. This effort has the far-reaching effect of optimizing bone health that may, in turn, reduce societal demands for the institutional care of age-related fractures.

many contributing factors that become of great relevance to an aging population. Of these, inactivity and bed rest; decreased nutritional intake; drug-induced, genetic, and other confounding chronic illnesses; and reduction in endocrine activity are huge contributing and interrelated factors associated with age. Therefore, maintenance of bone mass, and the factors controlling its decline, are multifactorial.

The mechanical properties of an individual bone are determined by the amount and distribution of bone mineral, the bone matrix quality (skeletal architecture), and the interactive qualities between the two. In cancellous bone, aging is associated with a reduction in bone mass and a disruption of internal architecture with a particular loss of horizontal trabeculae. In cortical bone, there is an age-related increase in intracortical porosity, increased periosteal diameter, and increased marrow diameter and a net decrease in cortical thickness. An increased prevalence of disorders such as osteomalacia, osteoporosis, and Paget's disease also adversely affect the quality of bone.

Summary

An age-related decline in bone mass is universal. Bone loss is considered to begin between the ages of 35 and 40 in both sexes, a time at which bone maintenance and factors controlling its decline are considered multifactorial. Aging, as distinct from disease, results in specific and typical changes across all bone compartments, causing altered tissue characteristics in all humans that ultimately alter the mechanical competence of the skeleton. It is, however, difficult to clearly distinguish intrinsic changes in bone due to aging alone compared to aging changes due to extrinsic and preventable factors. The onset of bone loss is thought to be predetermined and may be related to a decline in osteoblast function leading to impaired new bone formation. Other possible factors include menopause, physical inactivity, nutritional factors, and a declining calcium absorption performance.

Bone loss with age is universal and may be attributed to a wide number of systemic factors that indirectly or directly regulate skeletal homeostasis. Many of these systems also are affected by their own inherent age-related changes (e.g., renal and intestinal systems). To promote negative bone balance, there are

References

Alevizaki CC, Ikkos DG, Singhelakis P. Progressive decrease of true intestinal calcium absorption with age in normal man. J Nucl Med 1965;14:760–762.

Bell NH. Vitamin D metabolism, aging and bone loss [editorial]. J Clin Endocrinol Metab 1995;80:1051.

Bennett G, Kaye M. Homeostatic removal of senescent murine erythrocytes by splenic macrophages. Exp Hematol 1981;9:297–307.

Bonar LC, Roufosse AH, Sabine WK, et al. X-ray diffraction studies of the crystallinity of bone mineral in newly synthesized and density fractionated bone. Calcif Tissue Int 1983;35:202–209.

Boskey AL, Posner AS. Bone structure, composition and mineralization. Orthop Clin N Am 1984;15:597–643.

Bouillon RA, Auwerx JH, Lissens WD, Pelemans WK. Vitamin D status in the elderly: season substrate deficiency causes 1,25-dihydroxycholecalciferol deficiency. Am J Clin Nutr 1987;45:755–763.

Brockstedt H, Kassem M, Eriksen EF, et al. Age and sex-related changes in iliac cortical bone mass and remodeling. Bone 1993;14:681–691.

Buchanan JR, Myers C, Lloyd T, Greer RB. Early vertebral trabecular bone loss in normal premenopausal women. J Bone Miner Res 1988;3:583–587.

Chalmers J, Ho KC. Geographical variations in senile osteoporosis: the association of physical activity. J Bone Joint Surg 1970;52:667.

Chapuy M, Arlot M, Duboeuf F, et al. Vitamin D_3 and calcium to prevent hip fractures in elderly women. N Engl J Med 1992;327:1637–1642.

Cohn S, Abesamis C, Yasumura S, et al. Comparative skeletal mass and radial bone mineral content in black and white women. Metabolism 1977;26:239–252.

Cooper C, Barker D, Wickham C. Physical activity, muscle strength, and calcium intake in fracture of the proximal femur in Britain. BMJ 1988;297:1443–1446.

Courtney AC, Hayes WC, Gibson LJ. Age-related differences in post-yield damage in human cortical bone. Experiment and model. J Biomech 1996;29:1463–1471.

Crilly RG, Francis PM, Nordin BEC. Steroid hormones, ageing and bone. Clin Endocrinol Metab 1981;10:115–139.

Cumming DC, Rebar RW, Hopper BR, Yen SSC. Evidence for an influence of the ovary on circulating dehydroepiandrosterone sulfate levels. J Clin Endocrinol Metab 1982;54:1069–1071.

Cummings SR, Kelsey JL, Nevitt MC, O'Dowd KJ. Epidemiology of osteoporosis and osteoporotic fractures. Epidemiol Rev 1985;7:178–208.

Ensrud KE, Nevitt MC, Yunis C, et al. Correlates of impaired function in older women. J Am Geriatr Soc 1994;42:481–489.

Epstein S, Bryce G, Hinman JW, et al. The influence of age on bone mineral regulating hormones. Bone 1986;7:421–425.

Fedarko NS. Age-related changes in hyaluronin, procollagen, collagen and osteonectin synthesis by human bone cells. J Cell Physiol 1992;151:215–227.

Francis R, Peacock M, Barkworth S. Renal impairment and its effects on calcium metabolism in elderly women. Age Ageing 1984;13:14–20.

Gallagher JC, Riggs BL, Eisman J, et al. Intestinal calcium absorption and serum vitamin D metabolites in normal subjects and osteoporotic patients: effect of age and dietary calcium. J Clin Invest 1979;64:729–736.

Garn SM, Rohmann CG, Wagner B, Oscole W. Continuing bone growth throughout life: a general phenomenon. Am J Phys Anthropol 1967;26:313–317.

Goldsmith N, Johnston J. Bone mineral: effects of oral contraceptives, pregnancy and lactation. J Bone Joint Surg 1975;57A:657–668.

Grynpas M. Age and disease-related changes in the mineral of bone. Calcif Tissue Int 1993;53(Suppl 1):S57–S64.

Heaney R, Recker R, Saville P. Menopausal changes in calcium balance performance. J Lab Clin Med 1978;92:953–993.

Holbrook T, Barrett-Connor E, Wingard D. Dietary calcium and risks of hip fracture: 14 year prospective population study. Lancet 1988;2:1046–1049.

Jackson JA, Kleerekoper M. Osteoporosis in men: diagnosis, pathophysiology and prevention. Medicine (Baltimore) 1990;69:139–152.

Jackson JA, Riggs MW, Spiekerman AM. Testosterone deficiency as a risk factor for hip fractures in men: a case control study. Am J Med Sci 1992;304:4–8.

Jacobson PC, Beaver W, Grubb SA, et al. Bone density in women: college athletes and older athletic women. J Orthop Res 1984;2:328.

Jee WSS, Li X, Schaffler MT. Adaptation of diaphyseal structure with aging and increased mechanical usage in the adult rat: a histomorphometrical and biomechanical study. Anat Rec 1991;230:332–338.

Johnston CC Jr, Slemenda CW. Osteoporosis in the Elderly. In DF Apple, CH Wilson (eds), Prevention of Falls and Hip Fractures in the Elderly. Rosemont, IL: American Academy of Orthopaedic Surgeons, 1994;33–37.

Judd HL, Judd GE, Lucas WE, Yen SSC. Endocrine function of postmenopausal ovary: concentrations of androgens and oestrogens in ovarian and peripheral vein blood. J Clin Endocrinol Metab 1982;39:1020–1024.

Kanders B, Dempster D, Lindsay R. Interaction of calcium nutrition and physical activity on bone mass in young women. J Bone Miner Res 1988;3:145–149.

Kleerekoper M, Villanueva AR, Stanciu J, et al. The role of three-dimensional trabecular microstructure in the pathogenesis of vertebral compression fractures. Calcif Tissue Int 1985;37:594–597.

Krolner B, Toft B, Nielsen S, Tondevold E. Physical exercise as prophylaxis against involutional bone loss: a controlled trial. Clin Sci 1983;64:541–546.

Lazenby RA. Continuing periosteal apposition I: documentation, hypothesis, and interpretation. Am J Phys Anthro 1990;82:451–472.

Luisetto G, Zangari M, Tizian L, et al. Influence of aging and menopause in determining vertebral and distal forearm bone loss in adult healthy women. Bone Miner 1993;22:9–25.

MacLaughlin J, Holick MF. Aging decreases the capacity of human skin to produce vitamin D_3. J Clin Invest 1985;76:1536–1538.

Martin RB, Burr DB. Aging Effects. In RB Martin, DB Burr (eds), Structure, Function and Adaptation of Compact Bone. New York: Raven Press, 1989;214–231.

Massey LK. Caffeine and the elderly. Drugs Aging 1998;13:43–50.

Mazess RB. On aging bone loss. Clin Orthop 1982;165:239–252.

Mazess RB, Barden HS. Bone density in premenopausal women: effects of age, dietary intake, physical activity, smoking and birth control pills. Am J Clin Nutr 1991;53:132–142.

Mazess RB, Barden HS, Eberle RW, Denton MD. Age-changes of spine density in posterior-anterior and lateral projections in normal women. Calcif Tissue Int 1995;56:201–205.

Mosekilde LI. Normal age-related changes in bone mass, structure and strength: consequences of the remodelling process. Dan Med Bull 1993;40:65–83.

Mosekilde LI, Mosekilde LE, Danielsen CC. Biomechanical competence of vertebral trabecular bone in relation to ash density and age in normal individuals. Bone 1987;8:79–85.

Mosekilde LI, Viidik A, Mosekilde LE. Correlation between

the compressive strength of iliac and vertebral trabecular bone in normal individuals. Bone 1985;6:291–295.

National Research Council. Recommended Dietary Allowances (10th ed). Washington, DC: National Academy Press, 1989;174–184.

Nguyen TV, Howard GM, Kelly PJ, Eisman JA. Bone mass, lean mass, and fat mass: same genes or same environments. Am J Epidemiol 1998;147:3–16.

Nilson BE, Westlin N. Bone density in athletes. Clin Orthop 1971;77:179–182.

Nordin B. International patterns of osteoporosis. Clin Orthop 1966;45:17–30.

Nordin B, Horsman A, Marshall D, et al. Calcium requirement and calcium therapy. Clin Orthop 1979;140:216–239.

Oreffo ROC, Bord S, Triffitt JT. Skeletal progenitor cells and aging human populations. Clin Sci 1998;94:549–555.

Pacifici R, Avioli L. Effects of Aging on Bone Structure and Metabolism. In CV Avioli (ed), The Osteoporotic Syndrome. New York: Wiley Liss, 1993;1–16.

Parfitt AM. Age-related structural changes in trabecular and cortical bone: cellular mechanisms and biomechanical consequences. Calcif Tissue Int 1984;36:123–128.

Parfitt AM, Mathews CHE, Villanueva AR, et al. Relationships between surface, volume and thickness of iliac trabecular bone in aging and in osteoporosis. J Clin Invest 1983;72:1396–1407.

Pocock NA, Eisman JA, Hopper JL, et al. Genetic determinants of bone mass in adults. J Clin Invest 1987;80:706–710.

Pollack SR, Korostoff E, Fineberg M, et al. Stress-generated potentials in bone: effects of collagen modification. J Biomed Mater Res 1977;11:677–700.

Reginster JYL. Treatment of bone in elderly subjects: calcium, vitamin D, fluoride, bisphosphonates, calcitonin. Horm Res 1995;43:83–88.

Reid IR, Gallagher DJA, Bosworth J. Prophylaxis against vitamin D deficiency in the elderly by regular sunlight exposure. Age Ageing 1986;15:35–40.

Riggs B, Melton L. Involutional osteoporosis. New Engl J Med 1986;314:1676–1686.

Riggs B, Wahner H, Melton L, et al. Dietary calcium intake and rates of bone loss in women. J Clin Invest 1987;80:978–982.

Rosen CJ. Growth hormone, insulin-like growth factors, and the senescent skeleton: Ponce de Leon's fountain revisited? J Cell Biochem 1994;56:348–356.

Rossmanith WG, Liu CH, Laughlin GA, et al. Relative changes in LH pulsatility during the menstrual cycle: using data from hypogonadal women as a reference point. Clin Endocrinol Metabol 1990;32:667–680.

Rossmanith WG, Scherbaum WA, Lauritzen C. Gonadotropin secretion during aging in postmenopausal women. Neuroendocrinology 1991;54:211–218.

Rozenberg S, Bosson D, Peretz A, et al. Serum levels of gonadotrophins and steroid hormones in the postmenopause and later life. Maturitas 1988;10:215–224.

Rozenberg S, Ham H, Bosson D, et al. Age, steroids and bone mineral content. Maturitas 1990;12:137–143.

Rubin CT, Bain S, McLeod KJ. Suppression of the osteogenic response in the aging skeleton. Calcif Tissue Int 1992;50:306–313.

Rubin CT, Hawker GA, Peltekova VD, et al. Determinants of peak bone mass: clinical and genetic analyses in a young female Canadian cohort. J Bone Miner Res 1999;14:633–643.

Sabatier JP, Guaydiersouquieres G, Laroche D, et al. Bone mineral acquisition during adolescence and early adulthood: a study in 574 healthy females 10–24 years of age. Osteoporosis Int 1996;6:141–148.

Sandler R, Slemenda C, LaPorte R, et al. Postmenopausal bone density and milk consumption in childhood and adolescence. Am J Clin Nutr 1985;42:270–274.

Seeman E, Hopper J, Bach L, et al. Reduced bone mass in daughters of women with osteoporosis. New Engl J Med 1989;320:554–558.

Seeman E, Melton LJ, O'Fallon WM, Riggs BL. Risk factors for spinal osteoporosis in men. Am J Med 1983;75:977–983.

Shephard RJ. Exercise and aging. Med N Am 1989;1:75–79.

Shipman AJ, Guy GWG, Smith I, et al. Vertebral bone mineral density, content and area in 8,789 normal women aged 33–73 years who have never had hormone replacement therapy. Osteoporosis Int 1999;9:420–426.

Slemenda CW, Hui SL, Longcope C, et al. Predictors of bone mass in peri-menopausal women. Ann Intern Med 1990;112:96–101.

Smith RW, Walker RP. Femoral expansion in aging women: implications for osteoporosis and fractures. Science 1964;145:156–157.

Stevens DA, Williams GR. Hormone regulation of chondrocyte differentiation and endochondral bone formation. Mol Cell Endocrinol 1999;151:195–204.

Stevenson JC, Lees B, Devenport M, et al. Determinants of bone density in normal women: risk factors for future osteoporosis? BMJ 1989;298:924–928.

Stillman RJ, Lohman TG, Slaughter MH, et al. Physical activity and bone mineral content in women aged 30 to 85 years. Med Sci Sports Exerc 1986;18:576.

Torgerson DJ, Campbell MK, Reid DM. Lifestyle, environmental and medical factors influencing peak bone mass in women. Brit J Rheumatol 1995;34:620–624.

Tsai KS, Heath J III, Kumar R, Riggs BL. Impaired vitamin D metabolism with aging in women. Possible role in pathogenesis of senile osteoporosis. J Clin Invest 1984;73:1668–1772.

Twomey LT, Taylor J, Furniss B. Age changes in the bone density and structure of the lumbar vertebral column. J Anat 1983;136:15–25.

Twomey LT, Taylor JR. Factors Influencing Ranges of Movement in the Lumbar Spine. In GP Grieve (ed), Modern Manual Therapy of the Vertebral Column. Edinburgh, Scotland: Churchill Livingstone, 1986.

Twomey LT, Taylor JR. Age changes in the lumbar spine and intervertebral canals. Paraplegia 1988;26:238–249.

Twomey LT, Taylor JR. The lumbar spine: structure, function, age changes and physiotherapy. Aust J Physio 1994;40:19–30.

Tyan ML. Age-related osteopenia: evidence for an intrinsic defect of bone-resorbing cells and a possible treatment. Proc Soc Exp Biol Med 1985;179:240–247.

Vernon-Roberts B, Pirie CJ. Healing trabecular microfractures in the bodies of lumbar vertebrae. Ann Rheum Dis 1973;32:406–412.

Watson JB, Lee K, Klein R, et al. Epidemiologic evidence for the disruption of ionized calcium homeostasis in the elderly. J Clin Epidemiol 1997;50:845–849.

Weinstein RS, Hutson M. Decreased trabecular width and increased trabecular spacing contribute to bone loss with aging. Bone 1987;8:137–142.

Wémeau JL. Calciotropic hormones and ageing. Horm Res 1995;43:76–79.

Wishart JM, Need AG, Horowitz M, et al. Effect of age on bone density and bone turnover in men. Clin Endocrinol 1995;42:141–146.

Wooten R, Brereton P, Clarke M, et al. Fractured neck of femur in the elderly: an attempt to identify patients at risk. Clin Sci 1979;57:93–101.

Zioupos P, Currey JD. Changes in the stiffness, strength and toughness of human cortical bone with age. Bone 1998;22:57–66.

Chapter 6

Diagnostic Clinical Evaluation of Bone Metabolism and Structure

A wide variety of procedures exists for evaluating skeletal status, including radiologic and densitometric procedures, computer-assisted and magnetic resonance imaging (MRI), and an array of biochemical and immunochemical methods. Biochemical analysis and diagnostic imaging are complementary investigative procedures in the evaluation of skeletal disease.

Urine and Serum Biochemistry

Biochemical methods are of use in the diagnosis and evaluation of bone diseases, in population studies, and for monitoring responses to hormones and drugs in clinical studies. The measurement of bone proteins in blood is an important adjunct to diagnostic imaging evaluation of the skeleton (Deftos 1991). Markers of skeletal remodeling do not necessarily lead to formulating a diagnosis of disease, but rather may be interpreted as biochemical indicators of the degree of bone turnover, at any given time. Bone formation and resorption processes may be monitored in vivo by measuring specific enzymes and other protein products released by osteoblasts and osteoclasts. Biochemical markers of bone turnover can indicate a metabolic response of bone within 3–6 months of initiating therapy, which is far sooner than the 2 years required for bone density testing (Kress and Mizrahi 1999). In other words, although bone density measurement may be important clinically, efficacy of intervention may be less immediately evident using this technique than gauging biochemical markers of bone metabolism, a

process that allows for more real-time assessment of bone resorption, formation, and turnover.

The biochemical analysis of bone proteins is an important adjunct to imaging procedures for the clinical assessment of the skeleton (Table 6-1). The most routinely tested markers of bone formation are bone-specific alkaline phosphatase and osteocalcin; however, alternative biochemical markers for bone resorption and formation may be found in the use of alternate bone resorption markers (hydroxyproline, galactosyl-hydroxylysine, collagen pyridinium cross-links, tartrate-resistant acid phosphatase, and urinary calcium) and bone formation markers (bone sialoprotein and type I procollagen N- and C-terminal peptides) (Caulfield 1998).

Indicators of Bone Formation

Alkaline Phosphatase

The enzyme alkaline phosphatase is commonly measured in the serum and may reflect overall bone turnover when the bone resorption and formation processes are coupled (Kress 1998). It is derived from several tissues, but principally from bone and liver (Deftos 1991).

Osteocalcin (Bone Gla Protein)

Osteocalcin, also known as *bone Gla protein*, is the major noncollagenous protein of bone. As it is

Table 6-1. Biochemical Markers Indicative of Bone Formation and Resorption Processes

Process	Biochemical Markers
Bone formation	Alkaline phosphatase
	Osteocalcin (BGP = bone Gla protein)
	Propeptides derived from the N or C terminal ends of the type I procollagen molecule
Bone resorption	Breakdown products of type I collagen:
	Hydroxyproline in collagen peptides measured in urine but not specific to bone collagen
	Galactosyl hydroxylysine
	Collagen "pyridinium" cross-links: pyridinoline and deoxypyridinoline

almost exclusively produced by the osteoblast, the measurement of serum osteocalcin is uniquely valuable for assessment of skeletal metabolism. Osteocalcin is a Ca^{2+} binding protein found in the organic matrix of bone and dentin of teeth. Circulating osteocalcin is a highly specific osteoblastic marker; its role in the evaluation of bone turnover is elaborately described in other reports (Gundberg 1998). In general, plasma osteocalcin measurements have clinical potential in the management of patients with high turnover metabolic bone disorders (Power and Fottrell 1991).

Indicators of Bone Resorption: Collagen Products

Hydroxyproline

Because type I collagen is the major product of the osteoblast, the measurements of urinary and serum hydroxyproline are used to assess bone resorption. In general, urinary excretion of hydroxyproline is indicative of degradation of matrix collagen; however, hydroxyproline (measured in urine) is cumbersome to measure and is not specific to bone collagen.

Galactosyl Hydroxylysine and the Pyridinolines

Biochemical markers, such as galactosyl hydroxylysine and the pyridinolines, which are specific biochemical markers of bone resorption, are the focus of much attention (Colwell et al. 1993). The pyridi-

nolines and peptides derived from cross-linked regions (collectively referred to as *pyridinium cross-links*) in collagens appear to be the most promising markers of resorption. Their measurement enables quantitative evaluation of rates of bone resorption in humans (Russell 1997). Pyridinoline (PYR) and deoxypyridinoline (DPD) are the mature trivalent cross-links of collagen. Type I collagen prevails in bone and has a relatively high concentration of DPD. The measurement of PYR and DPD in urine accurately reflects bone resorption because of the skeletal mass and rate of bone collagen turnover, as compared to other collagen-containing tissues (Fraser 1998). In other words, the pyridinium cross-links are made only in extracellular collagen fibrils and their release comes only from the breakdown of a mature matrix and not from newly formed collagen, as occurs with new bone formation (Demers 1992). The main clinical application of PYR and DPD measurements is to establish baseline bone turnover, which may indicate the presence of bone disease, and to monitor the progress of therapeutic interventions applied for such conditions.

Imaging and Other Measurement Techniques

The noninvasive techniques used to evaluate bone include

1. MRI
2. Dual energy x-ray absorptiometry (DEXA)
3. Plain film radiography (x-ray)
4. Conventional tomography
5. Quantitative computed tomography (QCT)
6. Quantitative ultrasound (QUS)

The invasive measurement techniques used to evaluate bone include

1. Nuclear medicine bone scanning
2. Biopsy for histomorphometric analysis

Noninvasive Measurement Techniques

Magnetic Resonance Imaging

MRI provides noninvasive visualization of anatomic and physiologic information. The use of MRI for noninvasively evaluating orthopedic conditions is

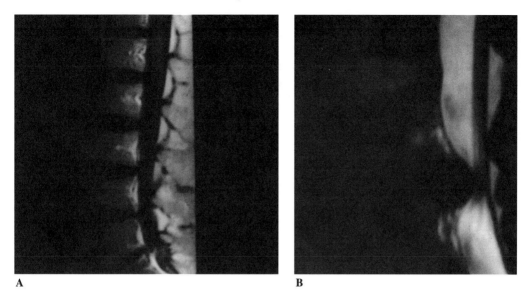

A   B

Figure 6-1. A. Magnetic resonance imaging (MRI): T1-weighted image of the lumbar spine. **B.** MRI: T2-weighted image of the lumbar spine. (Courtesy of Anthony Mascia, M.D., Toronto.)

rapidly emerging as the most popular imaging tool. MRI does not involve ionizing radiation but, rather, operates by the interaction of tissues with electromagnetic forces. The images created by distinct tissues are differentiated by their radio signal strength. Strong radio signals appear white; weak signals appear black. Every point in the image has a characteristic gray hue (Figure 6-1). Soft tissue and bony structures are well represented and are portrayed in every possible direction by MRI. MRI provides anatomic and physiologic information that is useful for identifying soft tissue trauma and tumors, fracture, and trauma to the growth plate in the young skeleton, and in evaluating neurovascular integrity after fracture. MRI can be used to evaluate acute extremity injuries, including physeal injuries, occult fractures, stress fractures, musculotendinous injuries, and ligamentous injuries (Ohashi et al. 1997). The role of MRI in joint evaluation is expanding because of its multiplanar capabilities. MRI is gradually replacing arthrography and arthroscopy in the evaluation of the knee joint (Nowicki-McKinnis 1994). MRI, as a three-dimensional imaging modality, offers the ability to separately examine different factors, including the density of the trabecular and cortical compartments and the pattern of trabecular microarchitecture, that may play independent and important roles in meta-

bolic bone diseases. High resolution MRI permits assessment of the trabecular texture at a range of peripheral sites, including the calcaneus, distal radius, and phalanges (Lang et al. 1998).

The presence of a pacemaker is an absolute contraindication for MRI, as they have the potential to be disrupted by the magnetic field. Ferrous metal prostheses or vessel clips that can be magnetic are considered a relative contraindication. Orthopedic fixation devices or total joint arthroplasty components are not made with ferrous metal and, therefore, are not contraindications.

Dual Energy X-Ray Absorptiometry

The determination of bone mineral density (BMD) is an integral part of the diagnosis, therapeutic planning, and monitoring of a patient with metabolic bone disease such as osteoporosis (Felsenberg and Gowin 1999; Seeger 1997). Its low cost and radiation dose, simplicity, and the ability to image several skeletal sites makes DEXA the most widely used technique for diagnostic and serial assessment of integral bone mass in osteoporosis and other metabolic bone diseases (Lang et al. 1998). Bone mass (mineral density) at the lumbar spine and femoral neck regions can be measured with good accuracy and considerable precision using DEXA

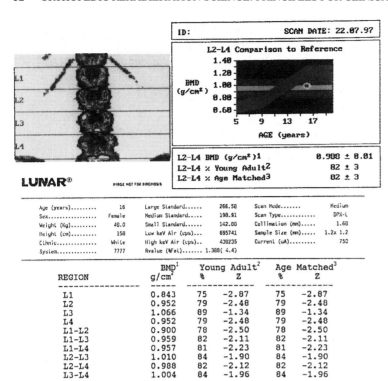

Figure 6-2. Dual energy x-ray absorptiometry scan for the measurement of bone mineral density in the lumbar spine region.

REGION	BMD[1] g/cm^2	Young Adult[2] %	Z	Age Matched[3] %	Z
L1	0.843	75	-2.87	75	-2.87
L2	0.952	79	-2.48	79	-2.48
L3	1.066	89	-1.34	89	-1.34
L4	0.952	79	-2.48	79	-2.48
L1-L2	0.900	78	-2.50	78	-2.50
L1-L3	0.959	82	-2.11	82	-2.11
L1-L4	0.957	81	-2.23	81	-2.23
L2-L3	1.010	84	-1.90	84	-1.90
L2-L4	0.988	82	-2.12	82	-2.12
L3-L4	1.004	84	-1.96	84	-1.96

1 - See appendix C on precision and accuracy. Statistically 68% of repeat scans will fall within 1 SD.
2 - USA AP Spine Reference Population, Ages 20-45.
3 - Matched for Age, Weight(males 25-100kg; females 25-100kg), Ethnic.

(Figure 6-2). In fact, assessing bone density by DEXA has an accuracy exceeding 95% and a precision in the range of 1% (Concensus Development Conference 1993). Minimal radiation exposure occurs with this technique. The value for the bone mineral content divided by the projected area of the bone is the BMD (measured in g/cm^2).

Plain Film Radiography

Plain film, or conventional, radiography is the fundamental imaging tool of the clinician involved in orthopedic radiology because plain film radiography is a time- and cost-effective technique to view bone and joint pathology, relative to other imaging techniques. Plain film radiology depicts the density of individual components of the human body (Figure 6-3). Plain film radiography involves taking x-ray films without the use of any contrast medium. X-ray (X-radiation) consists of a form of electromagnetic vibrations of short wavelength (1/10,000 the wavelength of visible light rays). X-rays operate by penetrating substances of various depths and densities and ionizing their components. The radiographic image results from the ionization of silver atoms on film. X-rays are absorbed by an object of relatively high density (e.g., cortical bone), and the corresponding image on the film appears radiopaque or more radiodense. The greater the atomic weight of a substance, the greater the attenuation of x-rays. When a structure only partially or minimally attenuates x-rays, a darker image is produced on the film; it is more radiolucent (e.g., tendon, ligament). The human body generally contains substances of four different densities: air, fat, water, and bone (Figure 6-4). Water has approximately the same density as blood, skin, and several of the soft, nonmineralized connective tissues, including muscle, cartilage, tendons, and ligaments. Bone is the most radiodense structure of the body, and dentin of the teeth is the most highly mineralized structure of the body. Prosthetic devices, such as total joint replacements or internal fixation devices, also appear solid white on radiographic film (Figure 6-5). Routine radiographs of bones and joints are most commonly taken in

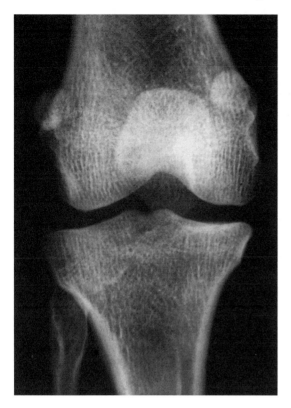

Figure 6-3. Plain film radiography. Note the different tissue densities.

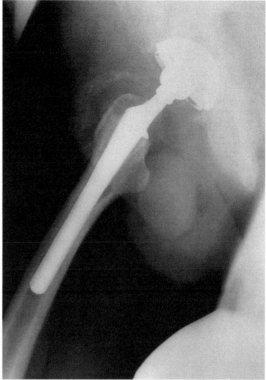

Figure 6-5. Plain film radiograph (anteroposterior view) of a hip prosthetic implant. Note the radiodensity of the prosthetic implant relative to other musculoskeletal structures.

anteroposterior (AP), lateral, and oblique projections. At least two of these projections are necessary to deliver sufficient information regarding the dimensions of the imaged structure. For further consideration of orthopedic radiography and its impact on the rehabilitation field, readers are referred to other sources (McKinnis 1997).

General musculoskeletal radiography entails the analysis of the "ABCs" (McKinnis 1997): *a*lignment, *b*one density, *c*artilage spaces, and *s*oft tissues. Radiography aids in the assessment of

1. General bony morphology
2. General bony contours

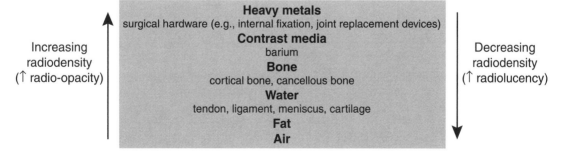

Increasing radiodensity
(↑ radio-opacity)

Heavy metals
surgical hardware (e.g., internal fixation, joint replacement devices)
Contrast media
barium
Bone
cortical bone, cancellous bone
Water
tendon, ligament, meniscus, cartilage
Fat
Air

Decreasing radiodensity
(↑ radiolucency)

Figure 6-4. Relationship of radiodensities of body tissues.

Clinical Note

Plain film radiography is a first-order diagnostic or screening tool for the majority of musculoskeletal diseases and dysfunctions. In addition, basic knowledge of its application and interpretation enhances clinical practice in physical rehabilitation by providing (1) a vehicle for education of patients and (2) a meaningful form of communication among other health professionals.

Once again, it is critical for the rehabilitation professional to have a knowledge base of pathology and related conditions that affect the musculoskeletal system to interpret and use radiographs for diagnostic and screening purposes.

3. Bone density (whole bone)
4. Focal changes in bone density
5. Joint articulation
6. Cortical outline and periosteal surface of bones
7. Articular cartilage (by joint space evaluation)
8. Subchondral bone
9. Joint capsules
10. Epiphyses
11. Marrow space
12. Soft tissues

Although plain film radiography is regarded as a first-order diagnostic and screening test in the assessment of the musculoskeletal system, many limitations in its application exist. Early diagnosis or recognition of several common musculoskeletal

Table 6-2. Limitations of Plain Film Radiography

Condition	Limiting Factors
Ectopic ossification	Soft tissue calcification is not generally detectable by x-ray until weeks after the process is initiated. The early calcification of specific structures, such as muscle, tendons, or bursae, cannot be seen on plain film radiographs.
Hairline stress fractures	Minute fractures may be obscured and easily missed.
Metastatic bone disease	Early stages of tumor growth may not be detectable.
Avascular necrosis	Early stages of avascular necrosis may not be detectable.
Soft tissue tears	Ligamentous laxity and tears may not be apparent on plain film radiographs.

conditions may not be possible with plain film radiographs (Table 6-2).

Conventional Tomography

Conventional tomography is an imaging technique that analyzes a specific, predetermined plane of the body. Structures lying in front of and behind this plane appear as contrasting, vague, or blurred images. One application of tomography is for the evaluation of obscure fractures that may not be clear using conventional radiography. Regions of the skeleton where tomography has an advantage revealing fractures include the tibial plateau, the cranium, and the cervical spine. These regions are typically difficult to visualize because of their depth in the body and the likelihood of interference from adjacent structures. Tomography may also be used to evaluate the state of healing at a fracture site. Soft tissue detail is limited in conventional tomography; the technique only works optimally in areas of high contrast, such as bone. Radiation levels are high.

Quantitative Computed Tomography

QCT is an "anatomic" imaging technique created by merging the technologies of x-rays and computers to form cross-sectional axial images of the body (Figure 6-6). QCT can determine the true volumetric bone density of cancellous bone and cortical bone separately and at any skeletal site (Prevrhal and Genant 1999). Integrating consecutive series of flat-plane images taken through the axial plane makes construction of a three-dimensional image possible. Tissues absorb levels of radiation relative to their densities. The information is then relayed to the computer for mathematical reconstruction of the imaged structure. Contrast of tissue densities and the general shape and position of structures is evaluated. Tissues undergoing a degenerative process, infection, hemorrhage, or some neoplasms appear with an increased tissue density by computed tomographic analysis. In contrast, infarctions, cysts, and benign tumors may appear with decreased tissue density.

The transverse anatomic sections afforded by QCT provide a three-dimensional image unobscured by overlying structures. The digital information derived from QCT provides quantitative diagnostic information (Gilsanz 1998). QCT also offers the ability to separately examine different factors that may play independent and important roles in metabolic bone conditions (e.g., osteoporosis), including the density of both the trabecular and cortical compartments and the pattern of trabecular microarchitecture. QCT also provides precise anatomic localization coupled with quantitative x-ray attenuation information that can be used to determine bone mineral content (Cann et al. 1980). The geography of structures imaged by QCT is more precise than that obtained by plain film radiography. New developments in QCT include volumetric approaches for precise compartmental assessment of the spine and proximal femur, and thin-slice tomography of the vertebral body for assessment of trabecular texture (Lang et al. 1998). Ultrahigh-resolution CT scanners have been developed for imaging of trabecular structure and, in some cases, the peripheral skeleton (Dambacher et al. 1998; Lang et al. 1998).

Information about musculoskeletal tissue metabolism or vascular perfusion may not be derived from CT scans. CT scanners are expensive in terms of purchase, maintenance, and operational training.

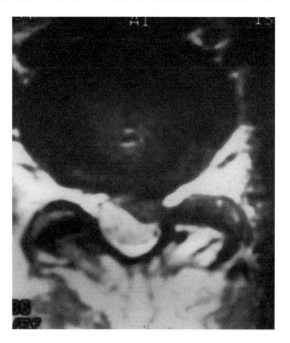

Figure 6-6. Computed tomographic scan of an intervertebral disk of the lumbar spine. Note the disk extrusion (herniation) with impingement on the thecal sac. (Courtesy of Anthony Mascia, M.D., Toronto.)

Quantitative Ultrasound

QUS is used to assess appendicular bone by measuring the changes that occur in the velocity and energy of ultrasound waves as they pass through bone tissue. QUS assessment of bone may permit an assessment of bone properties currently not available by bone densitometry techniques. Ultrasound attenuation associated with trabecular orientation is basically dominated by the mineral spread in a collagen framework (Wu et al. 1998). QUS is a relatively inexpensive, noninvasive instrument to measure bone integrity; it does not emit radiation and is used primarily in research settings. Although results from QUS have been correlated only loosely with BMD values, they may be as strong a predictor of osteoporotic fracture as BMD (Gregg et al. 1997). QUS may even predict fracture independently of BMD, because its measurements appear to be related to certain aspects of bone strength (Gilsanz 1998).

Invasive Measurement Techniques

Nuclear Medicine Bone Scanning

Nuclear medicine entails the diagnostic use of radioactive materials or isotopes to capture images of bone physiology rather than morphologic characteristics. A radionuclide bone scan, or scintigraphy, is a sensitivity test that operates by "hot spot" imaging—imaging after injection of

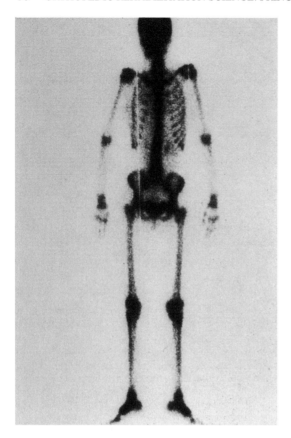

Figure 6-7. Nuclear medicine bone scan.

radiopharmaceuticals specific to bone tissue so that bone tissue areas of altered function may be identified (Figure 6-7). Darkened spots on a bone scan reveal regions of hyperfunction in bone tissue or changes in osteoblastic activity, such as in early bone disease and fracture healing. Healthy bone typically appears transparent and gray. Radionuclide bone scanning has retained its place in the evaluation of primary bone tumors and metastases as well as in screening patients with bone remodeling disorders.

The application of bone scans is indicated for diagnosis of Paget's disease, osteomyelitis, avascular necrosis, metastatic bone disease, and stress fractures, as well as for evaluating the state of fracture healing. Radionuclide bone scanning generally is used as an ancillary technique in conjunction with plain film radiography, conventional tomography, CT, and MRI. At times, it can be used as the primary modality for the early identification of skeletal lesions. It is also useful in diagnosing cases of unexplained bone pain

(Greenspan and Stadalnik 1997). In short, nuclear medicine bone scintigraphy provides unique information about local and regional bone metabolic properties that cannot be attained with other imaging techniques. Bone scintigraphy provides information about local osteoblastic activity that complements the information demonstrated on routine radiography, CT, or MRI. The high sensitivity of the study means that if no abnormality is detected, the search for osseous metastases can be ended (Donohoe 1998).

The lack of specificity in the differential diagnosis of disease is a limiting factor in the use and interpretation of bone scans.

Bone Histomorphometry

Bone histomorphometry is a technique based on systematic, unbiased counting and measuring of tissue constituents (Eriksen et al. 1989). Bone histomorphometry can yield important information on bone remodeling in a variety of metabolic bone diseases. Often the patient has received, at some prior time, tetracycline or some other fluorochrome label that deposits in the bone and enables the analysis of its dynamic turnover properties (Arnala 1991). Histomorphometric evaluation of tetracycline-labeled iliac crest biopsies is an accepted method for establishing the diagnosis and investigation of metabolic bone disease. Tetracycline antibiotics are deposited in vivo at sites of bone formation, as bone lends itself to incorporation of such a tissue time marker. When given to patients in two or more temporally distinct doses, tetracycline is deposited in separated bands or labels. These labels can be visualized under a microscope with fluorescent light (Podenphant 1990). Histomorphometric analysis may be performed on bone tissue biopsy that is obtained by taking a core sample of bone from, for example, the iliac crest. Altered quality and quantity of bone tissue can be identified using this technique. Histomorphometric analysis of both bone cell (osteoblast and osteoclast) and bone tissue morphology can reveal aberrant bone remodeling qualities. Trabecular connectivity also is recognized as an important measure of bone quality and architecture (Chappard et al. 1999). It may be evaluated using applications such as three-dimensional MRI microscopy on human cancellous bone biopsies (Wessels et al. 1997).

Although the diagnosis of skeletal diseases usually relies on noninvasive methods, bone histomorphometry is needed for the exclusive diagnosis of certain metabolic bone diseases and evaluation of related changes in cellular behavior.

Summary

Plain film radiography is a first-line, effective imaging technique to visualize an anatomic portion of the bones and joints of the musculoskeletal system. The radiodensity of a structure is determined by that structure's composition and thickness, based on whether its constituents are air, fat, water, and/or bone. Two projections taken perpendicular (AP, lateral, or oblique) to each other are necessary to attain a three-dimensional view of the structure. Although conventional radiography assumes a front-line position in the attempt to diagnose many musculoskeletal pathologies, many other diagnostic imaging tools, such as QCT, QUS, and MRI, are used to make a differential diagnosis of musculoskeletal pathology, because these are more sensitive to the detection of specific disorders. Invasive techniques in the diagnostic evaluation of bone tissue include radionuclide bone scanning and bone tissue histomorphometric analysis. Nuclear medicine offers unique information about the physiology of bone repair. The high sensitivity of the nuclear medicine scan and the specificity of radiographic imaging procedures provide complementary information to optimize accurate diagnosis and management of an array of orthopedic pathologies. The combination of serum/urine biochemical parameters, measurement of bone mineral density, and quantitative dynamic evaluation of bone histology is an ideal approach in evaluating and establishing a differential diagnosis of bone disease.

References

Arnala I. Use of histological methods in studies of osteoporosis. Calcif Tissue Int 1991;49(Suppl):S31–S32.

Cann CE, Genant HK, Ettinger B, Gordan GS. Spinal mineral loss in oophorectomized women: determination by quantitative computed tomography. JAMA 1980;244: 2056–2059.

Caulfield MP. Alternate markers for biochemical assessment of bone turnover. J Clin Ligand Assay 1998;21:149–158.

Chappard D, Legrand E, Pascaretti C, et al. Comparison of eight histomorphometric methods for measuring trabecular bone architecture by image analysis on histological sections. Microsc Res Technique 1999;45:303–312.

Colwell A, Russell RGG, Eastell R. Factors affecting the assay of urinary 3-hydroxy pyridinium crosslinks of collagen as markers of bone resorption. Eur J Clin Invest 1993;23:341–349.

Concensus Development Conference. Diagnosis, prophylaxis, and treatment of osteoporosis. Am J Med 1993;94:646–650.

Dambacher MA, Neff M, Kissling R, Qin L. Highly precise peripheral quantitative computed tomography for the evaluation of bone density, loss of bone density and structures: consequences for prophylaxis and treatment. Drugs Aging 1998;12(Suppl 1):15–24.

Deftos LJ. Bone protein and peptide assays in the diagnosis and management of skeletal disease. Clin Chem 1991;37:1143–1148.

Demers LM. A new biochemical marker for bone disease: is it a breakthrough? Clin Chem 1992;38:2169–2170.

Donohoe KJ. Selected topics in orthopedic nuclear medicine. Musculoskeletal Imag Update 1998;29:85–101.

Eriksen EF, Steiniche T, Mosekilde L, Melsen F. Histomorphometric analysis of bone in metabolic bone disease. Metab Bone Dis 1989;18:919–954.

Felsenberg D, Gowin W. Bone densitometry by dual energy methods. Radiologe 1999;39:186–193.

Fraser WD. The collagen cross-links pyridinoline and deoxypyridinoline: a review of their biochemistry, physiology, measurement, and clinical applications. J Clin Ligand Assay 1998;21:102–110.

Gilsanz V. Bone density in children: a review of the available techniques and indications. Eur J Radiol 1998;26: 177–182.

Greenspan A, Stadalnik RC. A musculoskeletal radiologist's view of nuclear medicine. Semin Nucl Med 1997;27: 372–385.

Gregg EW, Kriska AM, Alamone LM, et al. The epidemiology of quantitative ultrasound: a review of the relationships with bone mass, osteoporosis and fracture risk. Osteoporosis Int 1997;7:89–99.

Gundberg CM. Biology, physiology and clinical chemistry of osteocalcin. J Clin Ligand Assay 1998;21:128–138.

Kress BC. Bone alkaline phosphatase: methods of quantitation and clinical utility. J Clin Ligand Assay 1998;21:139–148.

Kress BC, Mizrahi IA. Monitoring antiosteoporotic treatment of postmenopausal women using biochemical markers of bone turnover. Drugs Today 1999;35:181–185.

Lang T, Augat P, Majumdar S, et al. Noninvasive assessment of bone density and structure using computed tomography and magnetic resonance. Bone 1998;22(Suppl 5):S149–S153.

McKinnis LN. Fundamentals of Orthopedic Radiology. Philadelphia: FA Davis Company, 1997.

Nowicki-McKinnis L. Fundamentals of Radiology for Physical Therapists. In JK Richardson, ZA Iglarsh (eds), Clinical Orthopaedic Physical Therapy. Philadelphia: WB Saunders, 1994;626–687.

Ohashi K, Brandser EA, el-Khoury GY. Role of MR imaging in acute injuries for the appendicular skeleton. Radiol Clin North Am 1997;35:591–613.

Podenphant J. Methodological problems in bone histomorphometry and its application in postmenopausal osteoporosis. Dan Med Bull 1990;32:424–433.

Power MJ, Fottrell PF. Osteocalcin: diagnostic methods and clinical applications. Clin Rev Clin Lab Sci 1991;28: 287–335.

Prevrhal S, Genant HK. Quantitative computed tomography. Radiologe 1999;39:194–202.

Russell RGG. The assessment of bone metabolism in vivo using biochemical approaches. Horm Metab Res 1997; 29:138–144.

Seeger LL. Bone density determination. Spine 1997;22(Suppl 24):S47–S57.

Wessels M, Mason RP, Antich PP, et al. Connectivity in human cancellous bone by 3-dimensional magnetic resonance microscopy. Med Phys 1997;24:1409–1420.

Wu C, Gluer C, Lu Y, et al. Ultrasound characterization of bone demineralization. Calcif Tissue Int 1998;62: 133–139.

Part II
Bone Biomechanics

Chapter 7

Basic Skeletal Biomechanics and Bone Tissue Response to Stress

The function of the skeletal system is diverse; it serves as a repository for calcium, protects organs, and permits weightbearing and movement. The dynamic strains engendered within bone tissue result from the variable degrees of load bearing that, in turn, provide the most functional influence on bone mass and architecture.

The functional requirements of weightbearing are viable as a result of three dynamic and tightly regulated processes: osteoclast resorption, fatigue damage of the inorganic matrix, and osteoblastic deposition of new bone. This system ensures that bone is optimally capable of responding to the range of loads it experiences. Equilibrium is achieved as a consequence of the communication between the cells involved in resorption and deposition of bone. In this way, the healthy, normally stressed skeleton is appropriately engineered for maximum mechanical effectiveness.

Mechanical Stress-Strain Relationship

A preliminary discussion of the relationship between stress and strain and the concept of bone modulus is warranted before addressing the effects of mechanical stress and strain on bone remodeling. The concepts of stress and strain that apply to inanimate materials also apply to bone; however, bone differs from engineering materials in that it can repair and remodel itself to adapt to its mechanical requirements. *Stress* is defined as force per unit area. Three types of stress exist that may be applied to bone: compressive, tensile, and shear (Figure 7-1). Compression results in a shortened material; tensile forces develop when the structure is lengthened; and shear stresses result when one region of a material slides relative to an adjacent region. Most often, a combination of these forces act on bone.

Strain is the percentage change in length or deformation of a structure in response to stress. It is unitless and usually reported in terms of a structure's relative deformation. Bone strains are expressed as microstrain (μE), and can be measured by special gauges. For instance, the application of 1,500 μE in compression shortens a bone to 99.85% of its original length, and normal bone fractures at about 25,000 μE in tension or compression (Frost 1992). If a material is stressed to 101% of its original length, it incurs a strain of 0.01, or 1%, deformation, also referred to as 10,000 μE. In any material structure, strain is the result of the load of the applied force against the mass, material properties, and geometry of the structure (Lanyon 1984). In the skeleton, it appears that strain regulation is primarily achieved by influencing the geometry of bone and adjusting the mass of its components while keeping material properties constant (Woo et al. 1981). The application of a mechanical load on bone tissue acts to deform or strain it, with the result that the tissue's intermolecular bonds stretch to resist the stress.

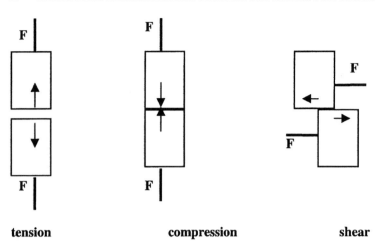

tension   **compression**   **shear**

Figure 7-1. The three basic types of stress applied to bone are tension, compression, and shear forces (F).

The relationship between stress and strain is presented as a stress-strain curve (Figure 7-2). The curve differs between, and is characteristic of, certain materials. The two regions of a stress-strain curve exhibit the two different material behavior patterns (Figure 7-3). The first region, the *elastic region*, is a linear zone representing the potential of the material that has been strained to regain its original shape (after the stress is removed). The slope of this linear segment is known as *Young's modulus* or the *elastic modulus*. The elastic region ends at the *yield point*, beyond which is the *plastic region*. At any point beyond the yield point, the material does not return to its original shape. As the end of the plastic region is reached, the material fails and

breaks. When a material is stressed continually, the elastic modulus slowly decreases as the material properties degrade or fatigue.

By sequentially demineralizing strips of cortical bone and subjecting them to bending loads, the mineral phase was shown to contribute extensively to the elastic properties (stiffness) of bone. The plastic region of the stress-strain curve, on the other hand, is solely a function of the matrix (Einhorn 1992). The ultimate yield strength of bone is therefore related to both its mineral content and to the way in which the mineral is distributed within the collagenous matrix. In other words, although studies have shown that approximately 75–80% of the variance in the ultimate strength of bone is

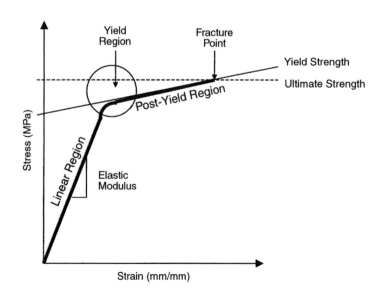

Figure 7-2. Typical stress-strain curve for cortical bone in tension, showing the linear, yield, and postyield regions.

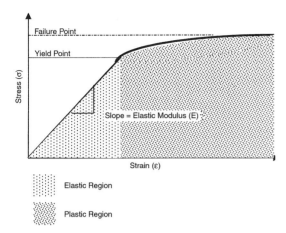

Figure 7-3. Stress-strain curve demonstrating two regions of material behaviors: elastic and plastic regions.

accounted for by bone density, a variety of changes in the material composition or structural geometry of the skeleton can offset the effects of altered bone mineral content.

Nature of the Mechanical Stimulus

Although local and systemic regulators are critical for bone formation and resorption, mechanical stimulation also is essential for bone growth. Mechanically, strain-related effects on the remodeling sequence are twofold: first, to inhibit resorption by decreasing the number of active remodeling units and, second, to be an osteogenic stimulus to increase bone formation (Lanyon 1993). Architectural modifications to achieve and maintain structural competence are made by the coordinated activity of osteoblasts and osteoclasts. Specific

Clinical Note

The following are selected pathologic bone conditions in which the material properties of bone are affected. These conditions are described in more detail in Chapters 12 and 13.

1. **Osteopenia:** Physiologic osteopenia is the state at which sufficiently reduced bone mineral density (BMD) (quantity and thus, in part, strength) exists, conducive to fracture with the occurrence of a fall or other significant trauma. Osteopenia may be transient in nature, may reflect the state of bone while a serious injury is healing, and it may resolve without intervention (Frost 1992).

2. **Osteoporosis (OP):** In OP, both reduced bone mineral quantity and altered quality of bone (distribution of mineral within existing matrix and bone tissue connectivity) exist. All mechanical properties of bone appear to be affected equally, and bone consequently fails under smaller loads. In true OP, bone fragility increases to such an extent that normal physical activity causes spontaneous fractures, bone pain, or both. A comparative study of the material properties of cancellous bone from femoral necks in patients with OP and normal controls identified that OP bone had the least apparent density and, thus, significantly lower stiffness (Li and Aspden 1997).

3. **Osteogenesis imperfecta:** Osteogenesis imperfecta is a condition in which the collagen component of bone is primarily affected. Stiffness and strength may be reduced proportionately, but the ability of the bone to deform under load (plasticity) is greatly compromised.

4. **Osteomalacia:** In osteomalacia, both stiffness and strength may be affected as the mineral phase becomes deficient in an otherwise normal collagenous matrix. Plastic deformation should be essentially normal.

5. **Osteoarthritis (OA):** A comparative study of the material properties of cancellous bone from femoral necks in patients with OA and normal controls identified differences in their composition and stiffness-to-density relationships. OA is, in part, a bone disease in which proliferation of defective bone results in an increase in bone stiffness (Li and Aspden 1997).

6. **Paget's disease:** The modulus of bone, a measure of stiffness, decreases in Paget's disease, which means that, compared to controls, the same levels of stress cause greater deformation (Frassica et al. 1997).

structure-function objectives at each location of the skeleton remain undefined; so too are the mechanisms by which tissue loading is transduced into cellular control.

A number of experiments have been performed in which bone strain is changed and a remodeling response observed (Hert et al. 1971; Lanyon et al. 1982; Lanyon and Rubin 1984; O'Connor et al. 1982; Rubin and Lanyon 1984). The basic science information provided by these studies is invaluable in substantiating clinical efforts in the physical rehabilitation of bone and bone disorders. Several key experiments, in particular those using the functionally isolated, externally loadable avian ulna preparations, have shown that changes in the parameters of a bone's mechanical strain environment are powerful determinants of its remodeling behavior (Lanyon and Rubin 1984; Lanyon et al. 1986; Rubin and Lanyon 1984; Rubin and Lanyon 1987). The structural variables of bone tissue, such as bone mass, material properties, and spatial organization, are all controlled by the bone cell population. The product of these variables and the load applied to the structures is the strain (proportional change in dimension) in the bone that the load engenders (Lanyon 1992a).

The influence of load-induced strain on bone may affect cells directly, by changing the cell shape, or indirectly, by its influence on variables such as fluid flow or intralacunar pressure. The relationship between cell morphology and cell metabolism and the role of mechanical load in bone remodeling is well recognized. Molecular mechanisms that relate osteoblast structure and gene expression is of interest in studies of bone extracellular matrix (ECM), integrins, the cytoskeleton, and the nucleoskeleton (nuclear matrix). Close examination of the nuclear matrix provides an understanding of the cell mechanics involved in the osteoblast's response to loading. Mechanical stimulation and altered focal contacts induce changes in the shape of osteoblasts, an adaptation that may, in part, be dependent on microtubule function (Guidnandon et al. 1997). In the tensegrity paradigm, a subcellular scaffolding— consisting of proteins from the ECM, the integrin receptors, and the cyto- and nucleoskeletons—is physically linked to the genes (Bidwell et al. 1998; Ingber 1993; Ingber 1997; Stamenovic et al. 1996). The study of the osteoblast nuclear matrix brings a

topography to the nuclear events that regulate bone cell biology and a molecular basis to osteoblast structure (Bidwell et al. 1998; Meazzini et al. 1998). The structural integrity of microfilaments appears to be necessary for the signal transduction of mechanical stimuli within osteoblasts. Disruption of the actin-cytoskeleton abolishes the response to stress, supporting the cytoskeletal involvement in cellular mechanotransduction (Burger and Kleinnulend 1998). Qualitative and quantitative changes within the cytoskeleton of osteoblasts are, therefore, crucial to the signal transduction processes of mechanical stimulation on these cells (Meazzini et al. 1998).

Mechanotransduction in bone may also occur via loading-dependent flow of interstitial fluid through the haversian canalicular network. The in vivo operating cell stress derived from bone loading is likely a result of interstitial fluid flowing along the surface of the osteocytes and lining cells. Osteoblasts, and osteocytes in culture, responded to pulsating fluid flow by releasing enhanced amounts of prostaglandin E_2 (PGE_2) (Ajubi et al. 1996) and reducing the release of transforming growth factor-beta (Sterck et al. 1998). The response of bone cells in culture to fluid flow includes prostaglandin synthesis, and expression of inducible cyclooxygenase (COX-2), an enzyme that mediates the induction of bone formation by mechanical loading in vivo (Burger and Kleinnulend 1998).

A dynamic mechanical strain environment affects the cellular network within bone. These strains arise from reaction forces associated with impact loads, mechanical resonances generated in the bone due to these impacts, and forces arising directly from the mechanics of muscular action (McLeod and Rubin 1990). In fact, the largest voluntary load applied to bone comes from muscle. It is thought that special ranges of strain thresholds determine where modeling adds and strengthens bone and where remodeling conserves or removes it (Schiessl et al. 1998). It is important to note that not all aspects of bone strain are equally influential on bone architecture. Unusual strain distributions, high strains, and high strain rates seem to be particularly osteogenic, and the osteogenic response consequent to such strains appears to saturate after only a few loading cycles (Lanyon 1996).

The architecture of cancellous bone is ultimately controlled by mechanosensitive bone cells and hormones. In pathologic bone states such as OP, the cells' response may be impeded by the altered hormonal levels, which alter the mechanical set point of the cells (Mullender et al. 1998). Estrogen may also contribute to the bone's adaptive response to loading by increasing its osteogenic and antiresorptive effect (Lanyon 1996). The osteoblast's proliferative response to strain may be associated with the estrogen receptor itself, lending reason to why bone may have a reduced ability to maintain structural strength after menopause, when estrogen is absent (Damien et al. 1998).

Animal Model Experiments

Number of Strain Cycles

The effect of the number of strain cycles necessary to influence bone remodeling was investigated in a functionally isolated avian (adult rooster) ulna (Rubin and Lanyon 1984). The application of 36 consecutive 0.5 Hz loading cycles, which are similar to peak strain levels induced by intact bone during vigorous wing flapping, saturated the osteogenic response to daily loading and caused a 33% increase in bone mineral content over a 6-week period. An increase in number of cycles per day did not induce further bone formation. Although as few as four cycles per day of this load regime were insufficient to stimulate formation of bone, they did prevent resorptive bone remodeling and a decline in bone mass on removal of the load (Rubin and Lanyon 1984). Intermittent loading was associated with a realignment of the proteoglycan protein cores, bringing them approximately 5 degrees closer to the direction of collagen fibrils in the matrix of cortical bone (Skerry et al. 1988; Skerry et al.

1990). In addition, intermittent loading on bone tissue produced rapid strain-related effects on the metabolism and increased synthetic activity of both osteocytes and periosteal cells (Skerry et al. 1989). As little as a single loading period per day was observed to stimulate transformation of a quiescent periosteum into one actively forming new bone within a 6-day period (Pead et al. 1988).

Peak Strain Magnitude

Using the ulna preparation from mature male turkeys, the number of cycles per day and the strain rate were kept constant at 100 cycles at 0.01 sec^{-1} while the peak strain magnitude was altered (Rubin and Lanyon 1983). Peak strains of 500 µE resulted in a reduction of cross-sectional area at the midshaft ulna, but when peak strain was increased to 1,000 µE, bone area was maintained. Strains above this level were associated with a proportional increase in new bone formation.

According to the mechanostat theory first proposed by Frost (1987), differing strain magnitudes alter the intensity of bone modeling unit activation. Zones of activation describe levels of microstrain that may induce bone formation in human bone (Martin and Burr 1989). The *trivial loading zone* corresponds to microstrains that do not provoke bone formation, falling below the physiologic lower limit. The *physiologic zone* represents the area of balance between the processes of bone resorption and deposition. Theoretically, strains above the physiologic range evoke a positive adaptive response, whereas strains below this range cause a negative adaptive response, measured as loss of bone. The skeleton is seldom subject to strains exceeding 3,000 µE (Rubin and Lanyon 1984). Two other zones exist that bone may encounter if bone strains are intolerably high

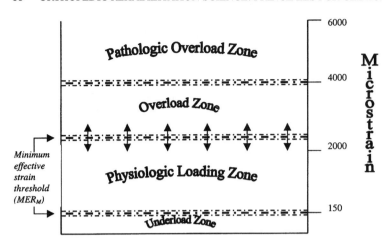

Figure 7-4. Adaptive reactions of bone in response to bone strain: microstrain and zones of activation. (Adapted from RB Martin, DB Burr. Structure, Function and Adaptation of Compact Bone. New York: Raven Press, 1989;143–185.)

or fatigue damage accumulates faster than it can be repaired: the *overload zone* and the *pathologic overload zone* (Figure 7-4).

Rate of Strain Change

The rate of change of strain to which a bone is subjected is an important determinant of the adaptive modeling response. Experimental evidence exists to support the idea that dynamic, but not static, loading provides the functional stimulus for bone remodeling (Hert et al. 1971; Lanyon and Rubin 1984). In fact, continuous static loading may affect bone remodeling activity in a manner similar to that associated with disuse (Lanyon and Rubin 1984). In the sheep radius model, peak strains imposed at high strain rates were associated with greater amounts of new bone formation; low strain rates were associated with either less osteogenesis or resorption (O'Connor et al. 1982). In summary, rate of strain change is a major determinant of the adaptive osteogenic and antiresorptive response to mechanical load. Therefore, across the physiologic range, a high rate of strain change provides a greater osteogenic stimulus than the same peak strain achieved more gradually (Mosley and Lanyon 1998).

Strain Distribution

Peak strain levels are deemed less responsible for stimulating the adaptive response than the concur-

rent change in strain distribution (Lanyon et al. 1982). This clinically important finding demonstrates the sensitivity of the remodeling response to a small strain change within the bone's customary (rather than its maximum attainable) strain range. In addition, different strain distributions produce different dose-response relationships between peak strain magnitude and change in bone cross-sectional area. For instance, in the avian ulna, peak principal strain levels produced by loading in torsion appeared less osteogenic than the same levels produced by loading in longitudinal compression (Pead and Lanyon 1990).

Wolff's Law: Influence of Loading on Bone Architecture

Wolff's law postulates that the form and function of bone is a result of changes in its internal architecture that is, in turn, created to best withstand the prevailing mechanical loads imposed on them. For example, the arrangement of the pattern of trabeculae in the proximal femur is created in response to trajectories of the principal dynamic compressive and tensile strains imposed at the site (Figure 7-5). The internal architecture of bone is, therefore, an important determinant of its strength and resistance to fracture.

Bone is continually adapting to its mechanical environment. Bone mass (quantity of bone mineral) and bone architecture (bone tissue quality) adjust according to the loads experienced; these changes are critical in order for the skeleton to withstand func-

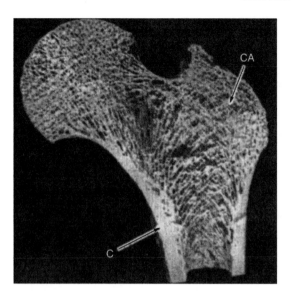

Figure 7-5. The relationship of form and function. Note the pattern of trabeculae in the proximal femur that has been created both in response to, and to best withstand, mechanical loads. (C = cortical; CA = cancellous.) (Courtesy of Dr. Marc Grynpas, Ph.D., Samuel Lunenfeld Research Institute, Mount Sinai Hospital, Toronto.)

tional loads without incurring damage. Functional strains transport information necessary for the feedback control of bone tissue architecture (Rubin 1984; Rubin and Hausman 1988; Rubin et al. 1990). In cortical bone, the degree of mineralization and porosity are considered the two most important determinants of its mechanical properties (Currey 1984a,b). Specifically, increased porosity and a higher prevalence of "giant" canals have a markedly negative influence on the ability of the cortical shell to withstand stresses associated with a fall (Bell et al. 1999). Modeling bone's mechanical properties requires detailed structural information on bone crystal shapes, sizes, and orientation, as well as information on the organization relative to the collagen framework and organization of lamellae into osteons or haversian systems (Wagner and Weiner 1992). Studies demonstrate that geometric changes in bone architecture in response to altered mechanical strain occur through the formation of woven bone (Burr et al. 1989). Woven bone can, in fact, be a normal adaptive response to an abnormal strain environment (intense mechanical challenge)—even in the absence of trauma or fatigue-induced damage—if the mechanical challenge is intense enough (Burr et al. 1989; Turner et al. 1991).

Signaling in Bone: Couriers and Interpreters of the Stress Message

The mechanisms involved in translating mechanical situations within the matrix into a stimulus recognizable by the cells are not fully recognized; strain, strain-induced release of matrix bound factors, intralacunar pressure, fluid flow, and streaming potentials all may contribute to the total osteogenic response. The dependence of coupling on mechanical stimuli in cancellous bone is acutely apparent in the case of immobilization, where rapid increases in bone resorption occur and bone formation processes are substantially decreased.

The nature of the signals controlling the response of bone to mechanical deformation (remodeling) has been a matter of conjecture for many years (Binderman et al. 1984; Bourret and Rodan 1976; Davidovitch et al. 1984; El Haj et al. 1990; Goodship 1992; Grimston 1993; Hirata and Axelbrod 1980; Lanyon 1987; Lanyon 1992b; Lanyon et al. 1979). Endogenously produced electric fields may participate in controlling bone cell activity. The electromechanical properties of dry bone can be explained in terms of its inherent piezoelectric response to loading (Fukada and Yasuda 1957). The discovery of piezoelectric potentials was instrumental in elucidating a plausible mechanism by which functional activity could intrinsically influence the tissue's cellular environment and, thus, affect skeletal mass and morphology (Rubin et al. 1993). Stress-generated potentials in bone in response to loading revealed that regions of compression are negative and regions of tension are positive (Bassett and Becker 1962). The interrelationship among collagen, other matrix components, and the inorganic mineral phase determines the nature of the electromechanical properties of bone and the bioelectric signals inherent to it (Guzelsu and Regimbal 1990).

Streaming Potentials

The magnitude of the signals observed in bent, wet bone is, however, larger than one would expect to be generated from a piezoelectric effect alone (Johnson et al. 1980). It is actually the streaming potential (which can be measured in wet materials, including structures such as bone) that acts as a quantity of electromechanical energy.

Clinical Note

The investigation into the effects of electrical fields applied to bone is of clinical interest, particularly as they relate to bone healing and repair. The application of low-level electric currents to bone in vivo, either directly (Bassett et al. 1964; Brighton et al. 1977; Lavine et al. 1972) or indirectly (Finkelson et al. 1983), results in cell activation and bone turnover. Regions of high bone formation activity have been reported to have a negative extracellular electrical potential, relative to less active regions (Rubinacci and Tessari 1983). The mechanisms that may be involved in natural remodeling, hormonal responsiveness, and the clinical application of electrical stimulation for bone healing may have some foundation in the observation that osteoclasts migrate, in an applied current, toward the anode of electric field applied to bone (Ferrier et al. 1986). The clinical application of electric fields in the treatment of delayed fracture union (see Chapter 9) is based on the premise that the external application of known signals, otherwise absent with the loss of loading, assist the repair process. Exposure to an extremely low frequency electric field stimulus appears to promote bone formation by affecting osteoblast differentiation rather than cell proliferation (McLeod et al. 1993).

A streaming potential is an electrical voltage generated across a region of porous material. When fluid flows through the pores of the structure, the mobile portion of an electrical double layer—located at the boundary between the solid and fluid—is transported (Otter et al. 1992). Alterations in properties of the fluid phase can modify the streaming and zeta potentials and may play a role in the biofeedback response of bone tissue (Walsh and Guzelsu 1993). Therefore, both piezoelectricity and streaming potentials appear to contribute to the response created by mechanical deformation in fully hydrated bone (Hastings and Mahmud 1988; Walsh and Guzelsu 1993).

Several theoretical models of bone remodeling mechanisms involve the behavior of the fluid in stressed bone. Among them are the following:

1. Fluid pressure, itself, may stimulate the cells (Rodan et al. 1975).
2. The stress-induced fluid flow causes mixing and aids in the transport of nutrients to the osteocytes (Piekarski 1977).
3. The streaming potentials produced by the stress-induced fluid flow stimulate the cells (Gross and Williams 1982).

However, experimental evidence concerning fluid behavior in stressed bone is fragmentary and often difficult to interpret (Johnson 1984).

Basic principles allow that, when a force is applied to a porous material, the solid matrix deforms, applying an initial pressure to the fluid in the pores. Fluid shear stress caused by mechanical load in bone tissue is important in both the bone structure and function, through its effects on osteocytes and osteoblasts (Gross and Williams 1982; Rodan et al. 1975; Sakai et al. 1998). The fluid pressure and the streaming potentials are thought to primarily affect osteocytes, cells in the interior of bone, and cells lining the vascular channels (Johnson 1984). What effect the fluid pressure or the streaming potentials have on the cells lining the periosteal or endosteal surfaces is not clear.

Summary of Potential Mechanisms for Bone Response

The search for potential mechanisms for how bone responds to loading leads to the following questions:

1. How does mechanical strain in the tissue matrix stimulate bone formation at the cellular or molecular level?
2. Which cells are sensitive to strain?
3. How is the mechanical signal transduced into a biochemical signal?

The following three explanations, either alone or in sum, are considered part of the interrelated mechanisms at play:

1. Effector cells are influenced directly by an extracellular consequence of loading, such as strain-generated electrical potentials. The effects of cytoskeletal changes and cell shape on cell replica-

Clinical Note

Site-Specific Response of Bone to Mechanical Stress

In one study, circumferential gradients of normal longitudinal strain were seen to be highly associated with specific sites of periosteal bone formation using an exogenous loading model (Judex et al. 1997). Such evidence indicates that when a specific mechanical stimulus is applied, bone activation at specific sites may be induced. This lends support for the prescription of exercise regimens that incorporate specific muscular loading at bony sites where increased fortification is most needed. The prescription of exercise designed to benefit bone architecture should incorporate the features and knowledge generated from basic science studies of adaptive remodeling bone responses to loading. Based on these study findings, exercise sessions for the specific benefit of bone health need not be lengthy in nature and should incorporate different strain distributions applied at high peak strain levels and rates. Such exercise sessions should be repeated every other day or daily. To maintain any exercise-induced level of bone mass, it is necessary to maintain the functional input; to sustain increasing levels of bone mass, the functional input must be of ever-increasing osteogenic potential (Lanyon 1996).

tion and phenotypic expression are well documented (Bidwell et al. 1998; Guidnandon et al. 1997; Sato et al. 1998). Each cell is attached to its surrounding matrix via specialized regions of the membrane that contain receptors for ECM proteins called *integrins*. These transmembrane receptors provide a direct link between the ECM and the cytoskeleton and, according to the tensegrity paradigm, mediate changes in matrix strain (Bidwell et al. 1998; Ingber 1993; Ingber 1997; Stamenovic et al. 1996).

2. Extensive communication is requisite between a widespread network of strain-sensitive cells that influence the activity of effector cells on the surfaces to be remodeled. Osteocytes and lining cells are strategically located to detect mechanical strain, as are the osteoblasts on any matrix surface. Loads transmitted to the framework of the skeleton are relayed to, and controlled by, the osteocyte (Lanyon 1993). The osteocyte and its neighbors are extensively networked and have been identified as critical players in perceiving strain throughout the matrix and, consequently, influencing adaptive modeling and remodeling in a strain-related manner. These cells communicate via gap junctions and can produce autocrine or paracrine factors. Osteocytes and surface osteoblasts have been observed to present an almost immediate response to strain change by increased production of prostacyclin (PGI_2). Surface osteoblasts also produce PGE. Only 5 minutes after a single period of loading, glucose-6-phosphate dehydrogenase activity in osteocytes was increased

in a local strain magnitude-related manner, and 24 hours later there was a sixfold increase in osteocyte RNA (Pead et al. 1988; Rawlinson et al. 1993).

3. The transduction of mechanical strain into a biochemical signal could occur via mechanosensitive or stretch-activated ion channels. Other known channel-activating substances are hormones, autocrine substances, and second messengers (Ypey et al. 1992). A study by Yellowley et al. (1998) supports the theory that a large proportion of the outward currents generated in the osteoclast is carried by K^+ ions through channels that may be sensitive to the internal Ca^{2+} ion concentration.

Regulation of Extracellular Matrix Synthesis

The ECM is responsible for providing mechanical support to tissues and is a substrate for cell adhesion and differentiation. As mentioned earlier (see The Nature of the Mechanical Stimulus), it is believed that intracellular signal transduction pathways are activated by the binding of cells to ECM via specific cell surface receptors that, in turn, behave as mechanochemical transducers. Although the exact mechanism is unknown, gene expression of certain ECM components themselves is modulated by this interaction. Ultimately, bone cells respond to mechanical strain by remodeling their matrix and re-orienting their bone trabeculae. Fibroblasts attached to a strained collagen matrix produce more of the ECM glycoprotein (tenascin) and type XII collagen than cells in a relaxed matrix. In vivo, these two proteins are specifically expressed in places where mechanical strain is high (Chiquet et al. 1996). It appears that connective tissue cells are capable of triggering the remodeling of their ECM by sensing "force vectors" within their environment and responding to any altered mechanical demands made of them by intracellular regulation of the transcription of specific genes for the ECM.

A study was made on the duration of changes in periosteal osteoblast cells in the tibia (rat model) after a single exposure of mechanical loading in four-point bending (Boppart et al. 1998). Cross sections from the loaded regions were examined for periosteal differences in bone lining cell surface length, osteoblast surface length, and alkaline phosphatase–positive cell surface length and width in the cellular layer. A single loading session increased osteoblast surface length by as early as day 2; however, 9 days after a single loading session, osteoblast surface length did not differ from nonloaded control levels. Therefore, an isolated loading session does not appear to exert any sustainable effect on osteoblast appearance or longevity (Boppart et al. 1998). This, of course, has practical implications on how the frequency of loading or muscular activity impacts on bone cells and modulates their genetic program for growth and differentiation.

Bone Response to Altered Patterns of Load Transmission

The metaphyses of long bones adapt to provide the largest possible weightbearing surface to decrease the unit load per surface area. Not only can bone adapt to its functional demands, but select sections of a given bone are responsive to, and responsible for, different tasks. Protection against joint unit overload occurs largely in the metaphyseal ends of bone, whereas the diaphyseal segments are more responsible for adaptation to the quantity and distribution of load or strain (Poss 1984).

Load transmission is accomplished within the physiologic range by any combination of the following mechanisms:

1. Force dissipation by the compliance of the transmitting hard tissues, such as articular cartilage and cancellous bone (Sledge 1981)
2. Transfer of a portion of the load into the soft tissues

3. Incongruity of joints, so that with increasing load the contact area increases (e.g., the humeral-ulnar joint) (Eckstein et al. 1999)

Unit Overload

The area available to transmit load may be dramatically diminished if the weightbearing surface of a joint is diminished. Additionally, a factor such as diminished range-of-motion of the joint limits the volume of surface that can participate in load transmission. Subchondral bone of concave joint partners encounters tension, leading to preferential direction of the collagen fibrils at a microstructural level (Vogt et al. 1999). Bone's adaptation to situations such as arthritis or total joint implants provides information about the limits of its tolerance to altered load or strain patterns. The consequence of excessive unit load over time is exemplified in congenital malalignment of the hip. In this condition, the individual does not have a well-centered hip, and radiographic changes demonstrate adaptive increases in bone density in response to the increased load—up to the point that such overload exceeds the adaptive capacity of bone and articular cartilage (Poss 1984). In cancellous bone, even occasional overloads may increase the risk of fracture by substantially degrading the mechanical properties of the underlying bone (Keaveny et al. 1999).

Adaptation to Bone Reconstruction, Prosthetic Implants, and Joint Arthroplasty

Osteotomy

The rationale for performing an osteotomy is that unit load can be reduced to fall within a physiologic range. This procedure has the dual effect of increasing contact area while reducing the forces of muscular contraction. By restoring the mechanical environment to a range compatible with bone and cartilage survival, any pathologic process caused by mechanical overload may not only be arrested, but even reversed (Poss 1984).

Distraction Osteogenesis

Distraction osteogenesis is a process of bone lengthening in which a bone separated by osteotomy is subjected to slow progressive distraction using an external fixation device. The application of appropriate mechanical tension and stress is believed to act therapeutically, to stimulate the process of osteogenesis. The purpose of distraction osteogenesis is to form a cartilaginous callus that is progressively replaced by bony callus via endochondral ossification processes; thereafter, new bone is formed directly by the process of intramembranous ossification.

Osseointegration of Bioimplants

Bone has the property of being osteoconductive. Osteoconduction occurs when living tissue for the host bed migrates into the cancellous structure, resulting in new bone formation and incorporation of that structure (Cornell and Lane 1998; Davies 1998). Cancellous bone, because of its porous and highly interconnected trabecular architecture, permits ingrowth of surrounding tissues with relative ease. Mineral and collagen are osteoconductive, as are fabricated materials with similar porosity to bone tissue. Examples of materials with optimized osteoconductive properties include certain ceramics, hydroxyapatite beads, porous metals, and biodegradable polymers. Incorporation of calcium salts and collagen by osteoconductive matrices leads to more comprehensive ingrowth with new bone formation (Cornell and Lane 1998).

Bone cement has been used extensively to stabilize joint arthroplasties within bone. Porous coated implants are used to stabilize the prosthesis. They depend on bone growth into small pores on the surface of the prosthesis. Porous coated prostheses must be implanted so as to obtain initial stability and close apposition between the porous coating and adjacent bone, making the anatomy, the design of the prosthesis, and surgical technique crucial variables (Goodman and Aspenberg 1993).

The surface of implantable biomaterials plays a critical role in determining biocompatibility because it is in direct contact with host tissue. To improve the integration of implants, it is desirable to control interfacial reactions such that nonspecific adsorption of proteins is minimized and tissue-healing phenomena can be controlled (Nanci et al. 1998). The widespread success of clinical implantology can be attributed to the bone's ability to form rigid, load-bearing connections to titanium and certain bioactive coatings. Adhesive biomolecules in

the ECM are presumed to be responsible for much of the strength and stability of these junctures (Klinger et al. 1998). The linking of selected molecules with known biological activity to oxidized titanium surfaces guides and promotes the tissue healing that occurs during implant integration in bone and soft tissues (Nanci et al. 1998). It has been suggested that proteoglycans permeate a thin, collagen-free zone at the most intimate contact points with implant surfaces. One model proposed that titanium surfaces accelerate osseointegration by causing the rapid degradation of a hyaluronan meshwork formed as part of the wound-healing response and further suggests that the adhesive strength of the thin, collagen-free zone is provided by a bilayer of decorin proteoglycans held in tight association by their overlapping glycosaminoglycan chains (Klinger et al. 1998).

Loosening of Endoprostheses and Implants

Loosening of internal fixation systems for bone may arise from overloading the bone-metal interface into bone's "pathologic loading window" (Frost 1992). "Load focusing," which represents stress foci, may induce this situation by concentrating loads normally spread over sizable areas and volumes of bone onto smaller ones touching and supporting the implant. If the prosthesis or implant is of poor design and fit, load focusing may occur, which can lead to loosening of fixation by screws, rods, pins, and wires, especially in the thin cortices and spongiosa typical of osteopenic patients (Frost 1992).

Total Joint Arthroplasty

The components of an artificial joint have two mechanically based functions: (1) to provide for adequate range of motion and (2) to transfer the joint load onto the bone. The implantation of metal and plastic components of joint arthroplasties induces altered strain distributions on joints that may render eventual loosening of components because of bone remodeling. Altered stress transmission imposed by the cemented metallic femoral component and the differences in torsional rigidity between cortical bone and the prosthesis are the most likely causes of bone resorption and prosthetic

Clinical Note

An evaluation of the interdependence between osseointegration, primary implant stability, relative micromotion of implant versus bone, and joint loading forces during postoperative mobilization was performed to determine the interaction between rehabilitative procedures and the periprosthetic phase of total hip arthroplasties (Wirtz et al. 1998). The purpose of this study was to develop guidelines for the rehabilitation of both cemented and uncemented hip arthroplasties to eliminate factors that disturb prosthetic integration and provide for the best long-term stability of the implanted prosthesis. From this study, it was determined that osseointegration of cementless implants was impossible if relative micromotions exceeded certain torsional stresses. Such activities included immediate climbing of stairs or rising from a seated position without arm supports, which act to destabilize uncemented femoral shaft implants. The recommendations from this study were as follows: (1) The cemented prosthesis may be loaded with full body weight postoperatively, (2) uncemented implants should be loaded only partially for at least 6 weeks, and (3) with uncemented implants, loading of the hip joint with more than twice the body weight (walking without crutches, physical exercise against high resistance or long levers) is to be avoided for 3 months postoperatively.

The most severe long-term complications of joint prostheses are associated with loosening of the implant-bone interface, the result of adverse reactions of bone and subsequent weakening of the association between the two materials. Hence, mechanical stresses caused by joint loading are believed to play a key dual-pronged role in the adaptation of the interface bone as well as in the process of its loosening. In short, variables such as the nature of the implant as well as patient-related variables must be considered in light of the altered biomechanical circumstances in the rehabilitation of patients after total hip arthroplasty.

loosening in these types of total hip arthroplasties (Radin et al. 1982). It is also generally regarded that, unless an implant allows the soft tissues to guide a joint through its functional range, the risk of loosening and failure is high.

Failure of a prosthetic component and its fixation material is definitely related to high stresses, and massive bone resorption and osteopenia have been attributed to the generation of these stress and strain patterns in bone (Huiskes and Nunamaker 1984). With prosthetic implants or total joint arthroplasty, bone remodeling occurs along the lines of load distribution. Once a stable link between bone and implant has been made, the prosthesis may be kept only partly loaded for a period, after which progressively increased loading may occur, because apposition patterns of bone are known to be enhanced by mechanical loading.

Complications associated with cemented arthroplasty and the presumption that a biological interface may confer improved long-term fixation of prosthesis to bone, have prompted widespread interest in total joint arthroplasty without the use of cement. Younger, active, heavier patients were observed to be at greater risk to failure of cemented implants; in one study, 57% of patients younger than 30 years of age

who had undergone total hip replacement had actual or potential loosening of at least one component (Chandler et al. 1981). The advances in a newer generation of arthroplasties (uncemented) aim to confer improved long-term results; it is recognized that certain biomaterials are more appropriate for particular applications. The overriding variables of success of arthroplasty are component strength, modulus, hardness, biological response, and use with or without cement (Rubash et al. 1998).

Osteolysis

Evidence exists that wear particle generation is a significant factor in stimulating periprosthetic inflammation and subsequent bone loss (Howie et al. 1996; Vernon-Roberts and Freeman 1977). Wear particles are generated after the implantation of a total joint replacement. Articulating and nonarticulating surfaces serve as the source of these particles that are generated by loss of material from these solid surfaces as a result of mechanical action (Lewis et al. 1998). Osteolysis may cause a critical loss of support for an implant and result in failure by actual sinkage of the implant (Lewis et al. 1998).

Osteolysis and aseptic loosening may actually represent common pathologic processes. The histologic appearance of tissues from both types of lesions depends on a number of factors, including the degree of loosening, the type of prosthetic material, the duration of the implant, and the amount and type of wear debris. In response to wear particles, many cell types appear to be involved in the pathogenesis of both aseptic loosening and osteolysis. Tissue macrophages, fibroblasts, foreign-body giant cells, and endothelial cells are frequently observed at the interface; lymphocytes, plasma cells, and polymorphonuclear leukocytes are only occasionally demonstrated (Rubash et al. 1998).

Pathogenesis of Bone Loss after Total Hip Arthroplasty

Loss of bone is a long-term complication after total hip arthroplasty (THA). Bone loss after THA can be problematic if revision surgery is needed; bone deficiencies may restrict reconstructive options, increase the difficulty of surgery, and necessitate autogenous or allogenic bone grafting (Rubash et al. 1998). Some of the possible reasons bone is lost after THA are as follows:

1. Bone loss occurs secondary to particulate wear debris (osteolysis). The main mechanism of bone loss after THA is thought to be secondary to the biological reaction to particle debris. Many cell populations are involved in the histopathology, the most important of which are activated macrophages. In response to the particle challenge, these cells secrete several proinflammatory mediators such as cytokines and growth factors, PGE_2, and proteolytic enzymes that can stimulate osteoclastic bone resorption (Rubash et al. 1998).
2. Adaptive bone remodeling and stress shielding may occur secondary to size, material properties, and surface characteristics of the prostheses. Specific design and material features of prostheses can affect the adaptive remodeling patterns.
3. Bone loss occurs as a consequence of natural aging. However, the aging process does not itself appear to threaten the mechanical stability of cemented femoral components (Jasty et al. 1990).

Pathogenesis of Bone Loss after Total Knee Arthroplasty

Failure of total knee arthroplasty (TKA) is closely associated with bone loss that may cause loosening of the arthroplasty, fracture of an unsupported portion of the implant, or periprosthetic fracture (Lewis et al. 1998). The nature of bone loss may be focal or widespread and may be associated with cemented or cementless fixation. Some of the possible reasons bone is lost after TKA are as follows:

1. Bone remodeling occurs in an effort to adapt to arthroplasty and may induce a diffuse loss of bone by stress shielding.
2. Osteolysis may cause focal or diffuse defects at the bone-prosthesis interface from a chronic inflammatory reaction to particulate debris.
3. An acute inflammatory reaction caused by infection may induce loss of bone.

Response of Bone to Postural Deviation and Altered Loading Patterns

Scoliosis

Structural scoliosis involves both a lateral curvature of the spine and rotation of the vertebrae. In addition to these changes in alignment, alterations occur in the structure and composition of hard and soft tissues of, and around, the scoliotic spine. Whether these changes are a cause or effect of the malalignment is uncertain. Bony changes include a shortening and thinning of the pedicles and laminae and narrowing of the vertebral canal on the concave side of the curve. Vertebral wedging and decreased disk height on the concave side of the curvature are remarkable with curves of four degrees or greater (Farkas 1954). These changes occur early and concurrently in scoliosis, implicating a possible extraskeletal cause, rather than growth disturbance of the vertebral body alone, in the early pathomechanism of scoliosis (Xiong et al. 1994). Other studies have identified a growth disturbance of the vertebral bodies due to injury or calcification of the cartilaginous endplate and the resultant malnutrition of areas in the disk (Roberts et al. 1993). Conditions of altered (decreased on the concave side) proteoglycan, water, and collagen distribution have been identified in affected disks and are likely due to the

---

Clinical Note

Shin splints is an all-encompassing term referring to a complex of symptoms commonly encountered in musculoskeletal practice. The condition, distinct from a stress fracture (see Chapter 9), results from periosteal irritation and superficial remodeling at the insertion of the soleus muscle and its fascia. Sharpey's fibers extend through the periosteum and beyond into the mineralized bone matrix where they can, if overloaded, put excessive stress on the periosteum and cortex. The affected bone remodels in an effort to adjust to the additional stress. Bone scintigraphy reveals an elongated, superficial site of increased bone tracer uptake posteromedial to the attachment of the soleus; it may resemble a stress fracture (Donohoe 1998).

---

asymmetrical forces imposed on them. Increased keratan sulphate, a molecule typically found in areas of poor nutrition, also has been identified in affected disks. Because the vertebral body usually receives nutrition via the endplate, calcification of the endplates may explain this state of malnutrition (Roberts et al. 1993).

The association between osteopenia and scoliotic parameters, such as pattern and magnitude of the scoliotic curve, has been explored. In one study, a lower BMD in young individuals (12–14 years of age) with idiopathic scoliosis was observed and compared to controls; however, the decreased BMD did not correlate with the scoliosis pattern or degree (Cheng and Guo 1997). These findings suggest that the osteopenia in idiopathic scoliosis may be related to the primary etiology of the disease rather than be secondary to the asymmetrical mechanical forces associated with the postural deformity.

Orthotic braces, such as the Boston Bracing System and Milwaukee Brace, aim to provide correction of scoliotic curvature by providing pelvic stabilization and a system of lateral corrective forces that promotes remodeling of the vertebral column. The overall goal of a bracing program is to prevent curve progression and to align the trunk over the sacrum (Cassella and Hall 1991). Correction of muscle imbalance inherent to scoliosis with postural exercises, which aim to elongate the spine by decreasing the lumbar and cervical lordosis, is also an important orthopedic measure in this population (Cailliet 1978).

Ankylosing Spondylitis

BMD was decreased in both the hip and spine in subjects with ankylosing spondylitis in spite of normal calcium homeostasis and bone remodeling indices (Bronson et al. 1998).

Adhesive Capsulitis

In the short term, adhesive capsulitis of the shoulder (i.e., frozen shoulder) results in significant bone loss in the humerus of the affected extremity but, in the long term, capsulitis-induced bone loss shows good recovery (Leppala et al. 1998).

Gait-Assistive Devices

Cane-assisted ambulation was not found to significantly lower strain magnitudes in the tibia; however, tibial strain rates were significantly lowered by both ipsilateral and contralateral cane use (Mendelson et al. 1998). Ipsilateral or contralateral cane use, therefore, may achieve a lower tibial strain rate. This may be of clinical benefit in the rehabilitation of, for example, a stress fracture at that site.

Tenoperiosteal Junction

Tendons, such as the Achilles tendon, insert into bone via a fibrocartilaginous zone. This zone consists of four regions: tendon proper, nonmineralized fibrocartilage, mineralized fibrocartilage, and bone (Fukuta et al. 1998). Type X collagen is found in the mineralized zone of the tendon-calcaneus junction and in the mineralized zone of the medial collateral femoral ligament insertion site. This suggests that type X is a resident of mineralized fibrocartilaginous zones of tendon or ligament-bone junctions and may participate in anchoring ligament or tendon to bone (Fukuta et al. 1998).

Unlike tendon fibers found elsewhere, the calcified fibrocartilage region of the quadriceps tendon is not crimped, and tendon fibers interdigitate among separate bone lamellar systems (osteons or marrow spaces) but do not merge with the collagen systems of individual lamellae (Clark and Stechschulte 1998). Traumatic avulsions of ligament or tendon insertions rarely occur at the actual interface with bone, suggesting that the attachment is strong, or otherwise protected from injury by the structure of the insertion complex (Clark and Stechschulte 1998).

Summary

To understand the mechanical properties of bone, a detailed knowledge of its structure and composition is required. External stimuli that induce an internal stress field in bone are known to play an important role in the structural adaptation of bone and its mechanical properties. The concept that molecular mechanisms link cell structure to gene expression is of current interest.

The mechanical behavior of bone is a result of its mineral content and geometric properties and architecture. If strains that are too high are generated within bone tissue, then damage and failure are likely. The application of mechanical force manifests the shape, structure, and form of adult bone, demonstrating an important structure-function relationship. The ability of the human skeleton to withstand functional loads without incurring damage relies on many factors, including an ability of bone cell populations to model and remodel bone architecture in relation to the strain magnitude and distribution incurred within the bone cell matrix. The osteocytes may relay and control how mechanical loads are perceived by the skeleton.

The capacity of bone tissue to adapt and organize its structure in response to altered mechanical demands imposed on it is well recognized. Bone, when subjected to routine mechanical use different from that to which it is accustomed, will adapt and alter its shape and structure to configure itself accordingly over time. Bone adapts during skeletal growth and development by adjusting its skeletal mass and architecture in relation to changing mechanical environments. Adaptive bone remodeling resulting in altered bone mass, tissue turnover, and replacement of tissue is responsive to alterations in magnitude, distribution, and rate of strain manifesting in bone tissue. It appears that only a minimal dynamic loading regime applied for relatively short periods of time is sufficient to maintain a quiescent remodeling state. Bone mass appears to be influenced by strain events induced by the application of short bursts of "osteogenic" activity involving altered patterns of muscle activity of vigorous nature. It is likely that human exercise regimens designed to increase or conserve bone mass should involve high strains imposed at high strain rates and present a range of diverse and unusual strain distributions. Specific strain-related responses to load bearing are not fully defined, although it is clear that they differ for cortical (within various regions of cortical bone) and cancellous bone. Radiographic changes demonstrate adaptive increases in bone density in response to overloading; ultimately, this overload exceeds the adaptive capacity of bone, and articular cartilage of joints and joint failure occurs. The goal of procedures such as osteotomy is to restore the mechanical environment to a range compatible with bone and cartilage survival. The advances in a new generation of joint arthroplasties aim to confer an optimal functional environment in the care of total joint failure. The overriding variables for success for arthroplasty are strength, modulus, hardness, biological response, and their application with or without cement. Wear particles are implicated in inducing bone loss adjacent to total joint arthroplasty; their generation is a significant factor in stimulating periprosthetic inflammation and subsequent bone loss referred to as *osteolysis*. The effects of bone overload in other musculoskeletal conditions manifest in postural deviations such as scoliosis and ankylosing spondylitis as well as at the tenoperiosteal junction with shin splints.

References

Ajubi NE, Klien-Nulend J, Nijweide PJ, et al. Pulsating fluid flow increases prostaglandin production by cultured chicken osteocytes: a cytoskeleton-dependent process. Biochem Biophys Res Commun 1996;225:62–68.

Bassett CAL, Becker RO. Generation of electric potentials by bone in response to mechanical stress. Science 1962;137:1063–1064.

Bassett CAL, Pawluk RJ, Becker RO. Effects of electric currents on bone in vivo. Nature 1964;204:652–654.

Bell KL, Loveridge N, Power J, et al. Regional differences in cortical porosity in the fractured femoral neck. Bone 1999;24:57–64.

Bidwell JP, Alvarez M, Feister H, et al. Nuclear matrix proteins and osteoblast gene expression. J Bone Miner Res 1998;13:155–167.

Binderman I, Shimshoni Z, Somjen D. Biochemical pathways involved in the translation of physical stimulus to biological message. Calcif Tissue Int 1984;36:S82–S85.

Boppart MD, Kimmel DB, Yee JA, Cullen DM. Time course of osteoblast appearance after in vivo mechanical loading. Bone 1998;23:409–415.

Bourret LA, Rodan GA. The role of calcium in the inhibition of cAMP accumulation in epiphyseal cartilage cells exposed to physiological pressure. J Cell Physiol 1976;88:353–362.

Brighton CT, Friedenberg ZB, Mitchell EI, Booth RE. Treatment of nonunion with constant direct current. Clin Orthop 1977;124:101–123.

Bronson WD, Walker SE, Hillman LS, et al. Bone mineral density and biochemical markers of bone metabolism in ankylosing spondylitis. J Rheumatol 1998;25:929–935.

Burger EH, Kleinnulend J. Microgravity and bone cell mechanosensitivity. Bone 1998;22(Suppl 5):127–130.

Burr DB, Schaffler MB, Yang KH, et al. Skeletal change in response to altered strain environments: is woven bone a response to elevated strain? Bone 1989;10:223–233.

Caillet R. Exercises for Scoliosis. In JV Basmajian, Therapeutic Exercise. Baltimore: Williams & Wilkins, 1978;430–449.

Cassella MC, Hall JE. Current treatment approaches in the nonoperative and operative management of adolescent idiopathic scoliosis. Phys Ther 1991;71:897–909.

Chandler HP, Reineck FT, Wixson RL, McCarthy JC. Total hip replacement in patients younger than thirty years old. J Bone Joint Surg 1981;63A:1426.

Cheng JCY, Guo X. Osteopenia in adolescent idiopathic scoliosis: a primary problem or secondary to the spinal deformity. Spine 1997;22:1716–1721.

Chiquet M, Matthisson M, Koch M, et al. Regulation of extracellular matrix by mechanical stress. Biochem Cell Biol 1996;74:737–744.

Clark J, Stechschulte DJ Jr. The interface between bone and tendon at an insertion site: a study of quadriceps tendon insertion. J Anat 1998;192:605–616.

Cornell CN, Lane JM. Current understanding of osteoconduction in bone regeneration. Clin Orthop 1998;355 (Suppl):267–273.

Currey JD. What should bones be designed to do? Calcif Tissue Int 1984a;36:S7–S10.

Currey JD. The Mechanical Adaptations of Bones. Princeton, NJ: Princeton University Press, 1984b.

Damien E, Price JS, Lanyon LE. The estrogen receptors' involvement in osteoblasts adaptive response to mechanical strain. J Bone Miner Res 1998;13:1275–1282.

Davidovitch Z, Shanfeld JL, Montgomery PC, et al. Biochemical mediators of the effects of mechanical forces and electric currents on mineralized tissues. Calcif Tissue Int 1984;36:S86–S97.

Davies JE. Mechanisms of endosseous integration. Int J Prosthodontics 1998;11:391–401.

Donohoe KJ. Selected topics in orthopaedic nuclear medicine. Orthop Clin North Am 1998;29:85–101.

Eckstein F, Merz B, Schon M, et al. Tension and bending, but not compression alone determine the functional adaptation of subchondral bone in incongruous joints. Anat Embryol 1999;199:85–97.

Einhorn TA. Bone strength: the bottom line. Calcif Tissue Int 1992;51:333–339.

El Haj AJ, Minter SL, Rawlinson SCF, et al. Cellular responses to mechanical loading in vitro. J Bone Miner Res 1990;5:923–932.

Farkas A. The pathogenesis of idiopathic scoliosis. J Bone Joint Surg 1954;36A:717–754.

Ferrier J, Ross SM, Kanehisa J, Aubin JE. Osteoclasts and osteoblasts migrate in opposite directions in response to a constant electrical field. J Cell Physiol 1986; 129:283–288.

Finkelson MD, Eymontt M, Shanfeld JL, et al. The increase in vivo by electric currents of the ^{99m}Tc–methylene diphosphonate uptake and cyclic AMP content of the bone of the cat mandible. Arch Oral Biol 1983;28:217–224.

Franssica FJ, Inoue N, Virolainen P, Chao EYS. Skeletal system: biomechanical concepts and relationships to normal and abnormal conditions. Semin Nucl Med 1997; 27:321–327.

Frost HM. The mechanostat: a proposed pathogenic mechanism of osteoporosis and the bone mass effects of mechanical and nonmechanical agents. Bone Miner 1987;2:73–85.

Frost HM. Perspectives: bone's mechanical usage windows. Bone Miner 1992;19:257–271.

Fukada E, Yasuda I. On the piezoelectric effect on bone. J Physiol Soc Jpn 1957;12:1158–1169.

Fukuta S, Oyama M, Kavalkovich K, et al. Identification of type II, type IX and type X collagens at the insertion site of the bovine achilles tendon. Matrix Biol 1998;17:65–73.

Goodman S, Aspenberg P. Effects of mechanical stimulation on the differentiation of hard tissues. Biomaterials 1993;14:563–568.

Goodship AE. Mechanical stimulus to bone. Ann Rheum Dis 1992;51:4–6.

Grimston SK. An application of mechanostat theory to research design: a theoretical model. Med Sci Sports Exer 1993;25:1293–1297.

Gross D, Williams WS. Streaming potentials and the electromechanical response of physiologically moist bone. J Biomech 1982;15:277.

Guignandon A, Usson Y, Laroche N, et al. Effects of intermittent or continuous gravitational stresses on cell-matrix adhesion: quantitative analysis of focal contacts in osteoblastic ros17/2.8 cells. Exp Cell Res 1997;236:66–75.

Guzelsu N, Regimbal RL. The origin of electrokinetic potentials in bone tissue: the organic phase. J Biomech 1990; 23:661–672.

Hastings G, Mahmud F. Electrical effects in bone. J Biomed Engl 1988;10:515–521.

Hert J, Liskova M, Landa J. Reaction of bone to mechanical stimuli. Part I. Continuous and intermittent loading of tibia in rabbit. Folia Morph (Praha) 1971;19:290–300.

Hirata F, Axelbrod J. Phospholipid methylation and biological signal transmission. Science 1980;209:1082–1090.

Howie DW, Rogers SD, McGee M, et al. Biological effects of cobalt chrome in cells and animal model. Clin Orthop 1996;329S:S217–S232.

Huiskes R, Nunamaker D. Local stresses and bone adaptation around orthopaedic implants. Calcif Tissue Int 1984;36:S110–S117.

Ingber DE. The riddle of morphogenesis: a question of solution chemistry or molecular cell engineering. Cell 1993;75:1249–1252.

Ingber DE. The architectural basis of cellular mechanotransduction. Ann Rev Physiol 1997;59:575–599.

Jasty M, Maloney WJ, Bragdon CR, et al. Histomorphological studies of the long-term skeletal response to well fixed cemented femoral components. J Bone Joint Surg 1990;72A:1220–1229.

Johnson MW. Behaviour of fluid in stressed bone and cellular stimulation. Calcif Tissue Int 1984;36:S72–S76.

Johnson MW, Chakkalakal DA, Harper RA, Katz JL. Comparison of the electromechanical effects in wet and dry bone. J Biomech 1980;13:437–442.

Judex S, Gross TS, Zernicke RI. Strain gradients correlate with sites of exercise-induced bone forming surfaces in the adult skeleton. J Bone Miner Res 1997;12:1737–1745.

Keaveny TM, Wachtel EF, Kopperdahl DL. Mechanical behavior of human trabecular bone after overloading. J Orthop Res 1999;17:346–353.

Klinger MM, Rahemtulla F, Prince CW, et al. Proteoglycans at the bone implant interface. Crit Rev Oral Biol Med 1998;9:449–463.

Krolner B, Toft B. Vertebral bone loss: an unheeded side effect of therapeutic bed rest. Clin Sci 1983;64:537–540.

Lanyon LE. Functional strain as a determinant for bone remodeling. Calcif Tissue Int 1984;36(Suppl 1):S56–S61.

Lanyon LE. Functional strain in bone tissue as an objective, and controlling stimulus for adaptive bone remodelling. J Biomech 1987;20:1083–1093.

Lanyon LE. The success and failure of the adaptive response to functional load-bearing in averting bone fracture. Bone 1992a;13:S17–S21.

Lanyon LE. Control of bone architecture by functional load bearing. J Bone Miner Res 1992b;7(Suppl 2):S369–S375.

Lanyon LE. Osteocytes, strain detection, bone modeling and remodeling. Calcif Tissue Int 1993;53(Suppl 1): S102–S107.

Lanyon LE. Using functional loading to influence bone mass and architecture: objectives, mechanisms, and relationship with estrogen of the mechanically adaptive process in bone. Bone 1996;18(Suppl 1):S37–S43.

Lanyon LE, Goodship AE, Pye CJ, MacFie H. Mechanically adaptive bone remodeling. A quantitative study on functional adaptation in the radius following ulna osteotomy in sheep. J Biomech 1982;15:767–781.

Lanyon LE, Magee PT, Baggott DG. The relationship of functional stress and strain to the processes of bone remodelling. An experimental study on the sheep radius. J Biomech 1979;12:593–600.

Lanyon LE, Rubin CT. Static versus dynamic loads as an influence on bone remodelling. J Biomech 1984;17:982–1005.

Lanyon LE, Rubin CT, Baust G. Modulation of bone loss during calcium insufficiency by controlled dynamic loading. Calcif Tissue Int 1986;38:209–216.

Lavine L, Lustrin S, Shamos MH, et al. Electrical enhancement of bone healing. Science 1972;175:1118–1121.

Leppala J, Kannus P, Sievanen H, et al. Adhesive capsulitis of the shoulder (frozen shoulder) produces bone loss in the affected humerus, but long term bone recovery is good. Bone 1998;22:691–694.

Lewis PL, Brewster NT, Graves SE. The pathogenesis of bone loss following total knee arthroplasty. Orthop Clin North Am 1998;29:187–197.

Li BH, Aspden RM. Composition and mechanical properties of cancellous bone from the femoral head of patients with osteoporosis or osteoarthritis. J Bone Miner Res 1997;12:641–651.

Martin P, Burr DB. Structure, Function, and Adaptation of Compact Bone. New York: Raven Press, 1989.

McLeod KJ, Donahue HJ, Levin PE, et al. Electric fields modulate bone cell function in a density-dependent manner. J Bone Miner Res 1993;8:977–984.

McLeod KJ, Rubin CT. Frequency specific modulation of bone adaptation by induced electric fields. J Theor Biol 1990;145:385–396.

Meazzini MC, Toma CD, Schaffer JL, et al. Osteoblast cytoskeletal modulation in response to mechanical strain in vitro. J Orthop Res 1998;16:170–180.

Mendelson S, Milgrom C, Finestone A, et al. Effect of cane use on tibial strain and strain rates. Am J Phys Med Rehabil 1998;77:333–338.

Mosley JR, Lanyon LE. Strain rate as a controlling influence on adaptive modeling in response to dynamic loading of the ulna in growing male rats. Bone 1998;23:313–318.

Mullender M, Vanrietbergen B, Ruegsegger P, Huiskes R. Effect of mechanical set-point of bone cells on mechanical control of trabecular bone architecture. Bone 1998;22:125–131.

Nanci A, Wuest JD, Peru L, et al. Chemical modification of titanium surfaces for covalent attachment of biological molecules. J Biomed Mater Res 1998;40:324–335.

Neidlinger-Wilke C, Stalla I, Claes L, et al. Human osteoblasts from younger normal and osteoporotic donors show differences in proliferation and TGFβ-release in response to cyclic strain. J Biomech 1995;28:1411–1418.

O'Connor JA, Lanyon LE, MacFie H. The influence of strain rate on adaptive bone remodeling. J Biomech 1982;15:767–781.

Otter MW, Palmieri VR, Wu DD, et al. A comparative analysis of streaming potentials in vivo and in vitro. J Orthop Res 1992;10:710–719.

Pead MJ, Lanyon LE. Adaptive remodeling in bone: torsion versus compression [Abstract]. Orthop Transact 1990; 14:340–341.

Pead M, Skerry TM, Lanyon LE. Direct transformation from quiescence to formation in the adult periosteum following a single brief period of loading. J Bone Miner Res 1988;3:647–656.

Piekarski K, Munro M. Transport mechanism operating between blood supply and osteocytes in long bones. Nature 1977;269:80–82.

Poss R. Functional adaptation of the human locomotor system to normal and abnormal loading patterns. Calcif Tissue Int 1984;36:S155–S161.

Radin EL, Rubin CT, Thrasher EL, et al. Changes in the bone-cement interface after total hip replacement: an in vivo animal study. J Bone Joint Surg 1982;64A: 1188–1200.

Rawlinson SCF, Mohan S, Baylink DJ, Lanyon LE. Exogenous prostacyclin, but not prostaglandin E_2, produces similar responses in both G6PD activity and RNA production as mechanical loading, and increases IGF–II release, in adult cancellous bone in culture. Calcif Tissue Int 1993;53:324–329.

Roberts S, Menage J, Eisenstein SM. The cartilage endplate and intervertebral disc in scoliosis: calcification and other sequelae. J Orthop Res 1993;11:747–757.

Rodan GA. Mechanical and Electrical Effects on Bone and Cartilage Cells: Translation of the Physical Signal into a Biological Message. In HG Barrer (ed), Orthodontics, The State of the Art. Philadelphia: University of Pennsylvania Press, 1981;315–322.

Rodan GA, Bourret LA, Harvey A, Mensi T. Cyclic AMP and cyclic GMP: mediators of mechanical effects on bone remodelling. Science 1975;189:467–468.

Rubash HE, Sinha RK, Shanbhag AS, Kim SY. Pathogenesis of bone loss after total hip arthroplasty. Orthop Clin North Am 1998;29:173–186.

Rubin CT. Skeletal strain and the functional significance of bone architecture. Calcif Tissue Int 1984;36: S11–S18.

Rubin CT, Donahue HJ, Rubin JE, McLeod KJ. Optimization of electric field parameters for the control of bone remodeling: exploitation of an indigenous mechanism for the prevention of osteopenia. J Bone Miner Res 1993;8(Suppl 2):S573–S581.

Rubin CT, Hausman MR. The cellular basis of Wolff's law: transduction of physical stimuli to skeletal adaptation. Orthop Surg Degen Arthritis 1988;14:503–517.

Rubin CT, Lanyon LE. Regulation of bone formation by applied dynamic loads. J Bone Joint Surg 1984;66A:397–402.

Rubin CT, Lanyon LE. Kappa Delta Award paper. Osteoregulatory nature of mechanical stimuli: function as a determinant for adaptive remodelling in bone. J Orthop Res 1987;5:300–310.

Rubin CT, McLeod KJ, Bain SD. Functional strains and cortical bone adaptation: epigenetic assurance of skeletal integrity. J Biomech 1990;23(Suppl 1):43–54.

Rubinacci A, Tessari L. A correlation analysis between bone formation rate and bioelectric potentials in rabbit tibia. Calcif Tissue Int 1983;35:728–731.

Sakai K, Mohtai M, Iwamoto Y. Fluid shear stress increases transforming growth factor-beta-1 expression in human osteoblast like cells: modulation by cation channel blockades. Calcif Tissue Int 1998;63:515–520.

Sato M, Yasui N, Nakase T, et al. Expression of bone-matrix proteins messenger RNA during distraction osteogenesis. J Bone Miner Res 1998;13:1221–1231.

Schiessl H, Frost HM, Jee WSS. Estrogen and bone-muscle strength and mass relationships. Bone 1998;22:1–6.

Skerry TM, Bitensky L, Chayen J, Lanyon LE. Loading-related reorientation of bone proteoglycans. A strain memory in bone tissue? J Orthop Res 1988;6:547–552.

Skerry TM, Bitensky L, Chayen J, Lanyon LE. Early strain-related changes in enzyme activity in osteocytes following bone loading in vivo. J Bone Miner Res 1989;4: 783–788.

Skerry TM, Suswillo R, El Haj AJ, et al. Load-induced proteoglycan orientation in bone tissue in vivo and in vitro. Calcif Tissue Int 1990;46:318–326.

Sledge CB. Developmental Anatomy of Joints. In D Resnick, G Niwayana (eds), Diagnosis of Bone and Joint Disorders. Philadelphia: WB Saunders 1981;2–20.

Stamenovic D, Fredberg JJ, Wang N, et al. A microstructural approach to cytoskeletal mechanics based tensegrity. J Theor Biol 1996;181:125–136.

Sterck JGH, Kleinnulend J, Lips P, Burger EH. Response of normal and osteoporotic human bone cells to mechanical stress in vitro. Am J Physiol Endocrinol Metab 1998;37:E1113–E1120.

Turner CH, Akhter MP, Raab DM, et al. A noninvasive, in vivo model for studying strain adaptive bone modeling. Bone 1991;12:73–79.

Vernon-Roberts B, Freeman MAR. The Tissue Response to Total Joint Replacement Prosthesis: The Scientific Basis of Joint Replacement. Kent, MA: Pitman Medical Publishing, 1977.

Vogt S, Eckstein F, Schon M, Putz R. Preferential direction of the collagen fibrils in the subchondral bone of the hip and shoulder joint. Ann Anat Anatomischer Anzeiger 1999;181:181–189.

Wagner HD, Weiner S. On the relationship between the microstructure of bone and its mechanical stiffness. J Biomech 1992;25:1311–1320.

Walsh WR, Guzelsu N. Ion concentration effects on bone streaming potentials and zeta potentials. Biomaterials 1993;14:331–336.

Wirtz DC, Heller KD, Niethard FU. Biomechanical aspects of the load-bearing capacity after total hip arthroplasty: an evaluation of the present knowledge in literature. Zeitschrift Orthop Grenzgebiete 1998;136:310–316.

Woo SLY, Kuei SC, Amiel D, et al. The effect of prolonged physical training on the properties of long bone. A study of Wolff's law. J Bone Joint Surg 1981;63A: 780–787.

Xiong B, Sevastik JA, Hedlund R, Sevastik B. Radiographic changes at the coronal plane in early scoliosis. Spine 1994;19:159–164.

Yellowley CE, Hancox JC, Skerry TM, Levi AJ. Whole cell membrane currents from human osteoblast-like cells. Calcif Tissue Int 1998;62:122–132.

Ypey DL, Weidema AF, Höld KM, et al. Voltage, calcium, and stretch activated ionic channels and intracellular calcium in bone cells. J Bone Miner Res 1992;7(Suppl 2): S377–S386.

Chapter 8
Physical Activity and Bone

Impact of Physical Activity on Bone

Physical activity is the functional application of mechanical stimuli to the skeleton; it plays a major role in the regulation of bone homeostasis. In partnership with genetically determined factors, local force-dependent transformation of bone is critical to the processes of building bone. Both hypodynamic and hyperdynamic states have been shown to affect bone mass, and increases or decreases in muscle contraction or weightbearing induce a corresponding gain or loss in bone mass (Smith et al. 1984).

The application of physical forces or stress on bone is functionally delivered by exercise training. Stress applied to the skeleton may be divided into those exercises involving ground-reaction forces (e.g., walking, jogging, stairs) and those involving joint-reaction forces (e.g., weight lifting, rowing). Femoral neck bone mineral density (BMD) in 39 women aged 60–74 years exercising over an 11-month period increased significantly with ground-reaction force exercise compared to joint-reaction force exercise; however, similar increases in BMD of the whole body were seen in both groups (Kohrt et al. 1997). Runners have greater BMD in their lower extremities than controls (Etherington et al. 1991), and both tennis and volleyball players have higher BMD in their dominant arm compared to their nondominant arm (Alfredson et al. 1998). These facts demonstrate that the response to loading may differ according to the type of physical activity and the level of exertion inherent to that activity

(Doyle et al. 1970). In one study of distal femoral bone mass in world-class athletes, weight lifters were reported to have the greatest bone mass, followed by throwers, runners, soccer players and, finally, swimmers (Nilsson and Westlin 1971), suggesting that the skeleton responds in a site-specific manner to mechanical loading, that the load magnitude is the salient factor in determining the degree of the skeletal response, and that bone responds more favorably to selective forms of mechanical loading (Lanyon 1996). Finally, nearly all cross-sectional studies of exercise and bone mass demonstrate strong relationships between bone hypertrophy in male and female athletes compared to sedentary controls, as measured by patterns of physical activity and other parameters of fitness and athletic status (Suominen 1993). An extensive review of such exercise and bone studies is, however, beyond the scope of this text, and the reader is directed to literature on this topic found elsewhere (Schoutens et al. 1989; Smith and Gilligan 1996). A meta-analysis of controlled exercise training programs on bone mass is found elsewhere (Wolff et al. 1999).

Limitations in the Interpretation of the Effects of Exercise Regimes on Bone Mass

Exercise programs designed for either research or clinical purposes are difficult to evaluate in randomized controlled trials because of dropouts, placebo group exercise, limited compliance, and lack of standardiza-

Clinical Note

The duration, level, and nature of exercise regimes, and the patient's physical condition and fitness, all must be considered when selecting an appropriate physical exercise program intended to improve bone health. Consideration of these parameters becomes even more critical for patients with a less than mechanically optimal skeleton (e.g., a patient with osteoporosis). Intervention during the early years (during skeletal growth and maturation, and premenopausal years in females) is of benefit as a preventive measure before physiologic bone loss occurs (Ulrich et al. 1999). It would be a prudent public health measure to make sure this information is applied before the periods of an individual's life when bone is sensitive to loss.

Many practical applications arise from the knowledge that functional adaptation in bone is responsive to local loading (Judex et al. 1999; Karlsson et al. 1995). Thus, it is logical that an osteogenic strain regime incorporates this knowledge by creating protocols that make the loading of specific muscles that have specific attachments at bony sites requisite where bone adaptation is needed and most likely to occur. Appropriate exercise by itself may modulate, or perhaps even partly reverse, bone loss in postmenopausal women (Simkin et al. 1987; Smith et al. 1989). Effective exercise prescription should incorporate the knowledge that the most osteogenic response to loading is produced by high strains, high strain rates, and strain distributions different from routine or regular patterns of loading.

The application of joint-reactive force exercise also has beneficial effects, such as increasing lean body mass and strength, which may be important in the associated aspects of preventing fracture, such as reducing the risk of falling. A commonsense approach to the design of beneficial therapeutic exercise programs, for the purpose of positively affecting bone mass, would thus entail the incorporation of both ground-reaction force and joint-reaction force exercise.

tion of the duration, specificity, and intensity of exercise practice. Much variability in the results of the effects of physical activity levels and bone mass may be owing to the type of activity, length of training, and exercise protocol, rather than the potential osteogenic effect of exercise (Blair et al. 1996; Ebrahim et al. 1997). In addition, many studies rely on recall of involvement in physical activity and, inherently, are not reliable. Both the dose and response relationship for exercise and bone in humans has been difficult, at best, to qualify and quantify. In fact, exercise quantification programs are often described so inadequately that they are neither quantitatively nor qualitatively reproducible (Hartard et al. 1996). In contrast to organ and cell cultures or animal models, direct measurement of the strain produced by exercise in humans and any resultant changes in bone strength has not been feasible (Smith and Gilligan 1996).

Parameters of Exercise

Physical activity sufficient to exert a positive effect on bone density is characterized by intensity of the exercise workload, duration of the exercise, frequency of training, length of the training period, and site affected by the activity (Hartard et al. 1996).

Intensity of Exercise Workload

Sufficient evidence exists that implies there may be a threshold intensity for the initiation of bone remodeling. For instance, a safe, reproducible, and adaptable strength training program, with the intensity of forces operating during exercise set at 70% of one maximal repetition, positively affected bone stability in a group of older women with osteoporosis (Hartard et al. 1996).

Duration (Number of Sets) and Frequency

Although the minimum duration of sufficiently intensive stimuli to maintain bone mass remains unqualified, it may be guided by methods of strength training whose premise is based on established biochemical, physiologic, and training effects

Table 8-1. Basic Concepts in the Application of Exercise on Bone

Concept	Clinical Application
Mechanical loading through physical exercise has a positive influence on bone mineral density.	Muscular contraction and gravity are the major mechanical forces influencing bone turnover.
A lack of physical activity has a negative influence on bone mineral density (see Response of Bone to Immobilization in Chapter 10).	Physical inactivity infers a reduction of necessary mechanical stress and has been implicated in bone loss. Extensive study of disuse osteoporosis shows that exercise without weightbearing cannot counteract the loss of bone mass provoked by bed rest or weightlessness (Schoutens et al. 1989).
Bone mass is maintained at appropriate levels to afford structural competence for functional loading.	Bone is a dynamic tissue that adapts to strain induced by applied loads on bone by adjusting its architecture and mass.
The positive influence of exercise on bone can be attenuated by environmental conditions, including an individual's hormonal and nutritional status.	The skeleton fulfills a dual role by maintaining mechanical support of the body and serving as a reservoir for serum calcium and systemic regulatory factors such as hormones, inflammation-mediated factors, and vitamins, which—aside from local mechanisms—affect bone turnover (Franck et al. 1991).

Adapted from GP Dalsky. Effect of exercise on bone: permissive influence of estrogen and calcium. Med Sci Sports Exerc 1990;22:281–285.

for improvement of maximum skeletal muscle strength.

Length of Training Periods

Bone density decreases after cessation of exercise training (Schoutens et al. 1989). Therefore, the adoption of exercise programs should be a lifelong endeavor. This concept is exemplified by a study of older, postmenopausal women that showed weight-bearing exercise leading to significant increases above the baseline in lumbar BMD that were maintained only with continued training (Dalsky et al. 1988).

Site of Activity

Much evidence demonstrates the local stimulatory effect on bone made by muscles exerting force on the skeleton during exercise (Beverly et al. 1989; Krolner et al. 1983; Lundon and Goode 1991; Simkin et al. 1987). After 1 year of strength training of the psoas muscle in postmenopausal women, lumbar bone loss was attenuated in the lumbar spine, demonstrating the site-specific effect of this type of exercise (Revel et al. 1993). A decrease in mean psoas muscle area was associated with low spine BMD loss in another study (Reeve et al. 1999).

Effects of Exercise and Physical Activity on Bone Mineral Density across the Lifespan

Considerable data supports a positive osteogenic reaction to increased levels of physical activity. Although the exact mechanism is unknown, the achievement of an osteogenic response is observed to occur via a hyperplastic response involving both proliferation of pre-differentiated osteoprogenitor cells and induced differentiation of mesenchymal stem cells, which may, in effect, be a limitless process (Lanyon 1984; Urist et al. 1983).

Contracting muscles are important determinants of the mass, geometry, and strength of bones to which they are attached (Sandler 1988). In a supportive and enabling metabolic environment, the skeleton can optimize its genetically determined bone mass through adaptive remodeling responses to dynamic loading patterns created by muscle contractions (Table 8-1). Muscle mass is considered an important determinant of bone mass in that the ash weight of the third lumbar vertebral body and the weight of the left psoas muscle were significantly correlated when body weight, age, and height were taken into account (Doyle et al. 1970).

Cross-sectional studies of athletes show that the highest BMD values are represented in strength-trained individuals, with a greater effect for training in men than in women (compared with age- and gender-matched sedentary controls). In a study in eumenor-rheic women that compared the effects of weight-training programs with endurance programs on bone density, bodybuilders were found to have greater bone mineral content than runners, swimmers, or controls. These findings illustrate the effectiveness of weight training in providing a stimulus for increasing bone mineral content (Bennell et al. 1997; Heinrich et al. 1990). These studies demonstrate that bone response to mechanical loading depends on the bone site, mode of exercise, and strain magnitude, which may, in sum, be more important in controlling bone adaptation to loading than the number of loading cycles.

Skeletal Growth and Modeling

Each individual's genetic program determines the form or the template on which functional and meta-bolic influences behave, as well as the sensitivity of this template's responsiveness to alterations in these factors. The determination of specific architectural fea-tures on which structural competence depends or that controls the remodeling activity necessary to maintain serum calcium components are influenced by contin-uous functional feedback mechanisms throughout life (Lanyon 1992). The overall design of each bone, the location of joint surfaces, and muscle attachments are all genetically determined skeletal features that develop regardless of functional load bearing. How-ever, the load-bearing capabilities of a bone are depen-dent on specific gross structural features, such as girth, cortical thickness, medullary cavity diameter, cross-sectional shape, and internal distribution of trabeculae in cancellous bone. These features of skeletal compe-tency are requisite for the success of bone in terms of bearing functional loads and are only developed and maintained in the presence of "normal" functional load bearing (Jaworski and Uhthoff 1986).

Skeletal Growth Periods

Young Adolescent Skeleton

Cross-sectional studies support the belief that high levels of physical activity (within the limits of a healthy lifestyle) appear to have a positive effect on BMD in both the adolescent and young skele-ton (Duppe et al. 1997). Experimental studies using young animal models give support to the positive

association of exercise and bone volume and mass (Goodship et al. 1979; Woo et al. 1981). Adoles-cent males involved in a 5-week program of endurance exercise demonstrated a substantial increase in markers of bone formation, underlining the rationale for school-based exercise training pro-grams for this age group (Eliakim et al. 1997). In a cross-sectional study of young eumenorrheic col-lege women, chronic muscle-building exercises augmented lumbar bone mass; the additive effect of such anaerobic exercise on bone density may be mediated by local weightbearing changes and pos-sible systemic factors (Davee et al. 1990). Young female athletes had significantly greater BMD and lean body mass than an age-matched, low body weight, sedentary group. In addition, lean body mass and weightbearing exercise were associated with enhanced BMD in eumenorrheic young adult women (Madsen et al. 1998).

During late puberty of adolescent males, the type of weightbearing activity may be an important determinant of bone density, whereas the bone area may be largely determined by parameters related to body size. Higher BMD values may be seen at the weightbearing sites in badminton players than in ice hockey players, despite less average weekly train-ing (Nordstrom et al. 1998; Pettersson et al 1999), indicating that physical activity that incorporates jumps in irregular patterns or directions has greater osteogenic potential in the growing skeleton. Fur-thermore, long-term intensive tennis playing, espe-cially if started in childhood or adolescence, clearly increases the humeral BMD and cortical wall thick-ness but seems to have only a minor effect on the overall width of this bone (Haapasalo et al. 1996; Kannus et al. 1995).

No association could be made between the femoral neck BMD of postmenopausal women and their participation in sports during adolescence (Teegarden et al. 1996). Results of a population-based study suggest, however, that intense recre-ational physical activity in adolescence could play some role in preventing axial (spinal) osteoporosis in females in later years (Puntila et al. 1997).

Adult Skeleton

Cortical Bone of Adult Animal Models. Increased osteoblast activation was evident in a his-tomorphometric study of the response of cortical bone to increased weightbearing exercise in adult

Clinical Note

Participation in functional load-bearing activities in both genders, and particularly during childhood and adolescent years (skeletal growth), is critical to optimizing the potential for developing the maximal BMD and architectural features of bone for that individual.

female swine (Raab et al. 1991). In addition, adaptation of diaphyseal structures (cortical bone) to increased mechanical usage in the adult rat (Jee et al. 1991) provide several findings useful for human extrapolation:

1. An inherent tendency for the marrow cavity to expand at the expense of the endocortical bone exists throughout life in all mammals.
2. Overloading inhibits bone marrow expansion.
3. Overloading increases periosteal expansion.
4. Overloading tends to increase net formation drifts (modeling in the formation model).
5. Overloading depresses bone remodeling and therefore the net losses of the subendocortical bone.

Premenopausal and Postmenopausal Adult Skeleton.   Muscle strength is considered an independent predictor of BMD, accounting for 15–20% of the total variance in BMD of young women. It appears that even muscle groups with attachments distant from the spine and hip may exert an important influence of BMD at these sites (Snow-Harter et al. 1990). In young to middle-aged men, muscle strength also makes important contributions to BMD, and the strength of back extensors more powerfully predicts lumbar BMD than age, body weight, or strength of other muscle groups (Snow-Harter et al. 1992). Regardless of menopausal status, long-term (4 years) exercise subjects show lower bone loss rates in their arms than control subjects (Smith et al. 1989). In active—but not athletic—premenopausal women (aged 30–40 years), additional moderate weight-lifting exercises involving loading and nonstrenuous strengthening exercises, performed over a period of 3 years, showed no significant effect on BMD at the spine, hip, or mid-radius, as compared to a "free physical activity group" (Sinaki et al. 1996). In contrast, strenuous, resistance exercise is associated with maintaining or increasing BMD in both premenopausal (Lohman et al. 1995) and post-

menopausal females (Aloia et al. 1978; Dalsky et al. 1988; Gleeson et al. 1990; Hartard et al. 1996; Kirk et al. 1989; Pruitt et al. 1992; Sinaki et al. 1989a). This effect may not only be limited to resistance exercise alone, and it may have age- and site-specific effects, as exemplified by an increase in femoral but not lumbar spine BMD in premenopausal women after high-impact exercise over a 1-year period (Bassey and Ramsdale 1994). For instance, the femoral BMD in premenopausal women increased slightly after brief, vertical jumping (50 vertical jumps, 6 days per week, for 5 months) exercise; however, the femoral BMD in postmenopausal women did not (Bassey et al. 1998). Therefore, an exercise regime that provided the weightbearing skeleton with repeated, regular, extra loads with a rapidly rising force profile—namely, jumping—may prove to be feasible and is associated with an increase in bone density in the femur in certain age groups (Bassey and Ramsdale 1994; Heinonen et al. 1999). A study of site specificity of BMD and muscle strength in premenopausal women concluded that the effect of muscle strength on bone mass may, in fact, be relatively more systemic than site specific (Sinaki et al. 1998).

Postmenopausal bone loss was unaffected by a modest exercise program for back extensor muscles despite an increase in muscle strength, leading to the conclusion that nonloading muscle exercises may be ineffective in retarding vertebral bone loss in ambulatory, healthy postmenopausal women (Sinaki et al. 1989b). Site-specific moderate physical exercises performed over the short term also appear to have very little effect on bone mass in the upper extremity (Adami et al. 1999). However, strong correlation between physical fitness (and, by implication, habitual physical activity) and bone mass can be witnessed in the femoral neck and lumbar spine in postmenopausal women (Pocock et al. 1986; Ryan et al. 1998). A meta-analysis of the effects of aerobic exercise on

Clinical Note

Normal forces encountered in daily activity effect a structural compression in the range of 200 to 2,500 microstrain (µE) (Frost 1993). An increase in bone density and remodeling processes requires higher intensities (>2,500 µE), a stimulus level to which older individuals may not routinely be exposed. Care should be taken to incorporate progressive, graduated strength training as part of a therapeutic exercise regimen for the older individual.

bone density at the hip in postmenopausal women suggest that site-specific aerobic exercise moderately increases bone density at this site (Kelley 1998).

Older Skeleton

Generally, physical activity is capable of stabilizing or even increasing adult bone mass; however, the specific osteogenic component of the mechanical stimulus is unknown. In cross-sectional studies of older women, physical activity is considered to have a strong association with bone mass (Suleiman et al. 1997) and has been attributed to attenuation of normal age-related bone loss of the vertebrae in groups of women in the early postmenopausal years (Pruitt et al. 1992) and in groups with a mean age of 61 years (Krolner et al. 1983) and 81 years (Smith et al. 1989). In the older skeleton, bone response to mechanical loading depends, as in other age groups, on the bone site and the mode of exercise (Bennell et al. 1997; Revel et al. 1993).

Physical Activity and Incidence of Fractures in the Adult Skeleton

In a study of physical activity and incidence of fractures in a middle-aged population of both men and women, the most physically active persons—among those 45 years or older—experienced fewer fractures in the weightbearing, but not in the nonweightbearing, components of the skeleton (Joakimsen et al. 1998). Participation in high levels of physical activity has been specifically associated with a lower incidence of hip fractures (Joakimsen et al. 1997). It is plausible that physical activity affects fracture incidence through mechanisms in addition to its effect on bone quantity and quality. In other words, physical activity may also play a substantive role in lowering fracture risk at weightbearing sites gained through properties of better balance and muscle strength that, in turn, prevent potentially injurious falls. Physical activity may have great potential to reduce the risk of fracture because at least three independent but interactive factors that contribute to this risk are positively affected. Three of the interactive factors that protect the skeleton from injury are bone strength, risk of falling, and the effectiveness of the neuromuscular response (Smith and Gilligan 1991).

Physical Activity, Calciotropic Hormones, and Bone

Muscle-building exercise is associated with increases in serum Gla-protein, serum $1,25 (OH)_2D_3$, and urinary cyclic adenosine monophosphate, which suggests that this form of exercise enhances bone formation (Bell et al. 1988).

Parathyroid Hormone

In a study by Zerath et al. (1997), they examined older men before physical training and found that a maximal exercise test induced a significant increase in parathyroid hormone (PTH) levels, accompanied by enhanced total calcium phosphate, alkaline phosphatase, and osteocalcin levels, when compared with resting values. This differs from the findings of another study in which a single bout of strenuous resistance exercise in men induced an immediate suppression in PTH levels and hypercalciuria (Ashizawa et al. 1997).

Growth Hormone

Although resistance training exercise of sufficient volume and intensity can markedly raise testosterone (Fahey et al. 1976), growth hormone (GH) (VanHelder et al. 1984), and both testosterone and GH levels (Craig et al. 1989) of young men, the long-term impact on bone is unknown. No significant changes in GH, insulin-like growth factor (IGF), testosterone, osteocalcin, or skeletal alkaline phosphatase occurred after a 16-week strength training program in older men, despite an increase in femoral neck, but not lumbar spine, BMD (Ryan et al. 1994). In a study of older men (aged 64–75 years) with normal bone density, short-term (4 months) resistance exercise training increased BMD, but the addition of daily GH administration did not enhance whole body or regional BMD, despite GH-induced increments in serum IGF-1 and osteocalcin (Yarasheski et al. 1997). These findings suggest that GH administration in this population undergoing short-term resistance exercise training may increase bone turnover without increasing bone mineral accumulation.

Physical Activity and Status of Nutrition and Minerals

Achieving adequate nutritional calcium requirements is of special concern for the athlete. An inadequate ingestion of certain minerals, such as calcium, may present a health risk for some athletes—particularly female gymnasts, long-distance runners, and ballet dancers—who restrict caloric intake to maintain low body weights and, as a side effect, risk amenorrhea (Clarkson and Haymes 1994). Calcium bioavailability impacts hormonal influences on bone remodeling processes; it is also interactive with physical activity in enhancing bone formation in young women (Kanders et al. 1988). An additive effect of calcium intake and physical activity on BMD occurs in both premenopausal (Recker et al. 1992) and postmenopausal (Prince et al. 1991) women. To support this, young women who consume high levels of calcium and perform high levels of physical activity have much higher BMD than women with low levels of both calcium and physical activity (Kanders et al. 1988). To

exemplify this, despite a common hormonal milieu, a loss of bone tissue during calcium insufficiency in bones not being subjected to functional loading was substantially greater than in those where functional loading continued (Lanyon and Rubin 1986). The loss of bone attributable to calcium insufficiency and that attributable to disuse, therefore, appear to be additive. In women, however, neither diet nor exercise, nor a combination of the two, can totally offset the negative effect of decreased sex steroid hormone levels experienced at menopause or in menstrual dysfunction on bone.

Acute Effects of Exercise on Bone

Exercise is known to have long-term benefits on bone mass, but little is known about the short-term effects of exercise on bone turnover. In one study, biochemical markers of bone resorption were elevated within 32 hours of moderate aerobic exercise (brisk treadmill walking), without a comparable effect on markers of bone formation (Welsh et al. 1997). In another study of the early response of bone to a single bout of resistance exercise in untrained young males, transient decreases in both bone formation and resorption indices were demonstrated within 5 days after exercise (Ashizawa et al. 1998). However, a study of young adult Asian males who followed a 4-month period of resistance training demonstrated increased markers of bone formation and a transient suppression of bone resorption parameters (Fujimura et al. 1997).

Skeletal Response to Intensive Physical Training

The long-term effects of intensive athletic training (e.g., dance and ballet training), particularly that accomplished during the years of the skeletal growth period, are not fully understood. More specifically, the contribution of the timing and duration of menstrual disruption on BMD remains an enigma (Keay et al. 1997). The adverse effects of hypoestrogenism in young women includes decreased acquisition of peak bone mass, decreased BMD, and increased stress fracture incidence, particularly among young athletes and ballet dancers.

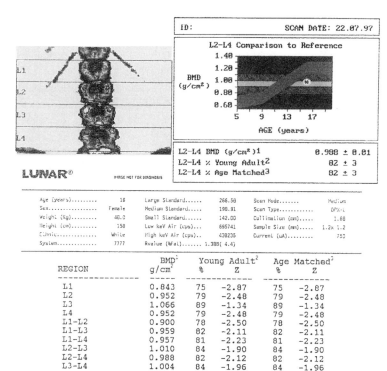

Figure 8-1. Dual energy x-ray absorptiometry scan of a young amenorrheic athlete (age 16 years). Note the significantly decreased bone mass in the lumbar spine relative to the normal, or expected, bone mass at this age. (Courtesy of S. Bibershtein, P.T., Osteoporosis Program, Women's College Hospital, Toronto.)

	ID:		SCAN DATE: 22.07.97

L2-L4 Comparison to Reference

REGION	BMD[1] g/cm²	Young Adult[2] %	Z	Age Matched[3] %	Z
L1	0.843	75	-2.87	75	-2.87
L2	0.952	79	-2.48	79	-2.48
L3	1.066	89	-1.34	89	-1.34
L4	0.952	79	-2.48	79	-2.48
L1-L2	0.900	78	-2.50	78	-2.50
L1-L3	0.959	82	-2.11	82	-2.11
L1-L4	0.957	81	-2.23	81	-2.23
L2-L3	1.010	84	-1.90	84	-1.90
L2-L4	0.988	82	-2.12	82	-2.12
L3-L4	1.004	84	-1.96	84	-1.96

L2-L4 BMD (g/cm²)[1]   0.988 ± 0.01
L2-L4 % Young Adult[2]   82 ± 3
L2-L4 % Age Matched[3]   82 ± 3

Age (years).........	16	Large Standard......	266.58	Scan Mode......	Medium
Sex.................	Female	Medium Standard.....	198.91	Scan Type..........	DPX-L
Weight (Kg).........	48.0	Small Standard......	142.00	Collimation (mm).....	1.68
Height (cm)........	158	Low keV Air (cps)...	695741	Sample Size (mm).....	1.2x 1.2
Ethnic.............	White	High keV Air (cps)..	430235	Current (uA)........	750
System.............	7777	Rvalue (%Fat)....... 1.388(4.4)			

1. See appendix E on precision and accuracy. Statistically 68% of repeat scans will fall within 1 SD.
2. USA AP Spine Reference Population, Ages 20-45.
3. Matched for Age, Weight(males 25-100kg; females 25-100kg), Ethnic.

Therefore, skeletal effects and clinical implications of menstrual disturbances exist in young female athletes. At the lumbar spine, menstrual disturbances are associated with premature bone loss or failure to reach peak bone mass (Prior et al. 1990), whereas appendicular sites are less affected (Bennell et al. 1997), suggesting that cancellous bone is more sensitive to hormonal stimuli and less responsive to mechanical loading than cortical bone during skeletal growth. Professional female dancers with a history of delayed menarche and amenorrhea (cessation of menstruation) were identified as a target group of premenopausal women potentially at risk of developing osteoporosis because of an associated decrease in BMD at the lumbar spine (Figure 8-1). The femoral neck in dancers with a history of amenorrhea was deemed partially protected from loss of BMD by virtue of its being the major weightbearing site in dance training. Age-matched, eumenorrheic (normally menstruating) dancers had significantly increased BMD at the femoral neck region compared to their amenorrheic counterparts, thus supporting the need for both normal menstrual function and weightbearing in promoting BMD during the skeletal growth period (Ramos and Warren 1995). Whether female athletes with menstrual disturbances are at a greater risk for osteoporosis later in life is not yet known; however, bone loss can be, at least partially, reversed with the spontaneous resumption of menses.

Female Athlete Triad

The female athlete triad is the classic triad of medical events that refers to the interrelationship of disordered eating habits (Figure 8-2), amenorrhea (cessation or absence of menses), and osteopenia. Athletic, or exercise-associated, amenorrhea is considered to be a subset of hypothalamic amenorrhea. The spectrum of menstrual disorders associated with the female athlete triad includes amenorrhea (primary [menstruation has never occurred] and secondary [menstruation has occurred before, but has since ceased]) and oligomenorrhea (infrequent menses). Amenorrhea is characterized by a decrease

Figure 8-2. Dual energy x-ray absorptiometry scan of a young female (age 15 years) with anorexia nervosa. Note the significantly decreased bone mass in the lumbar spine relative to the normal, or expected, bone mass at this age. (Courtesy of S. Bibershtein, P.T., Osteoporosis Program, Women's College Hospital, Toronto.)

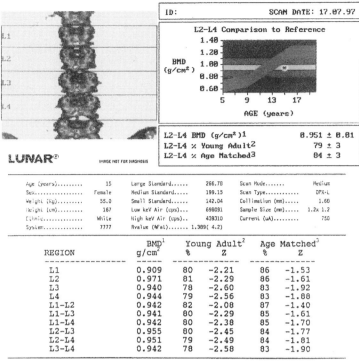

REGION	BMD[1] g/cm²	Young Adult[2] %	Z	Age Matched[3] %	Z
L1	0.909	80	-2.21	86	-1.53
L2	0.971	81	-2.29	86	-1.61
L3	0.940	78	-2.60	83	-1.92
L4	0.944	79	-2.56	83	-1.88
L1-L2	0.942	82	-2.08	87	-1.40
L1-L3	0.941	80	-2.29	85	-1.61
L1-L4	0.942	80	-2.38	85	-1.70
L2-L3	0.955	80	-2.45	84	-1.77
L2-L4	0.951	79	-2.49	84	-1.81
L3-L4	0.942	78	-2.58	83	-1.90

1 - See appendix C on precision and accuracy. Statistically 68% of repeat scans will fall within 1 SD.
2 - USA AP Spine Reference Population, Ages 20-45.
3 - Matched for Age, Weight(males 25-100kg; females 25-100kg), Ethnic.

in estrogen and progesterone levels, and strong evidence suggests a direct impact of athletic or secondary amenorrhea on bone mineral content and bone density (Drinkwater 1984; Miller et al. 1999). A growing body of evidence shows that female athletes undergoing intensive physical training are at risk for disturbances in menstrual function, which can have a negative effect on bone mineralization and may have short- and long-term consequences, including stress fractures, osteopenia, and osteoporosis (DiFiori 1995). Although it is definite that not all athletes with menstrual disturbances develop osteopenia, the risk of skeletal failure (e.g., stress fracture) is increased in athletes who also present with lower bone density; running-related fractures were more frequent in amenorrheic elite women distance runners than their eumenorrheic counterparts (Marcus et al. 1985). Female athletes who are amenorrheic or oligomenorrheic are known to have lower bone densities than eumenorrheic women despite their arduous training (Drinkwater et al. 1984; Moen et al. 1998). Studies indicate that bone mass in these women does not fully return to nor-

mal levels even after the resumption of normal menses; hence, early intervention to prevent irreversible bone loss in oligo- or amenorrheic athletes is essential (Cann et al. 1988; Drinkwater et al. 1990; Jonnavithula et al. 1993; Keen and Drinkwater 1997).

In young women aged 16–40 years, bone loss has been related to the duration and degree of estrogen deficiency associated with amenorrhea rather than to the underlying diagnosis (Davies et al. 1990). In one study, however, the BMD of the lumbar spine and femur was higher in college level gymnasts than age-, height-, and weight-matched nonathlete controls, despite the fact that gymnasts as a group had inadequate dietary calcium and a higher prevalence of menstrual irregularities (Kirchner et al. 1995). Also at this age, the impact on bone during gymnastics participation may benefit the spine and hip BMD, due to the weightbearing and resistance physical activity of the landing, swinging, and tumbling involved in the sport (Kirchner et al. 1995). Whether young athletes with intensive activity-induced menstrual disturbances are at

Clinical Note

Although the mechanism responsible for the detrimental effects of menstrual disturbances on bone is likely to be multifactorial, low circulating levels of estrogen and progesterone are thought to be the main causes. The clinical significance of menstrual disturbances depends on a number of factors, such as type of sport, genetic background, body composition, and dietary calcium intake. It is prudent, therefore, that the female athlete at risk for bone loss should be advised of the need for calcium supplementation, along with hormone therapy as medically indicated, to maintain bone density. Underlying causes of disordered eating, nutrition issues, and exploring psychosocial aspects, including the prescription of psychotherapy and possible antidepressant therapy, must all be addressed in the resolution of this condition (Joy et al. 1997).

greater risk for osteoporosis later in life is not yet known. Support exists for the concept that intense recreational activity that did not induce amenorrhea in adolescent females could play a role in preventing axial osteoporosis in later life (ages 48–58 years) (Puntila et al. 1997).

Summary

Current belief is that exercise affects bone remodeling by acting at a site-specific level where the maximal degree of mechanical loading occurs. Physical fitness and, by implication, habitual physical activity are considered major determinants of BMD across the skeleton. Much support exists for physical activity as a useful modality to increase or maintain bone mass and, in turn, prevent clinically important fractures at vulnerable sites, such as the femoral neck and vertebrae. Physical activity and exercise regimes have shown that bone loss may be reduced or mass increased in both men and women across a spectrum of ages. Physical activity increases skeletal competency to offer resistance to fracture. Physical activity accomplishes this in two ways: (1) maintaining, if not improving, BMD, and (2) enhancing neuromuscular competency. The benefits of physical activity include diminished skeletal fragility, reduced propensity to falls and, possibly, decreased overall impact of a fall. Therefore, exercise impacts on the risk of fracture by attenuating bone loss and decreasing the risk of falling and the force of impact by improving strength, balance, reaction time, and general flexibility.

In women, it appears that hypogonadism resulting from very intensive training and exercise is detrimental to the skeleton, affecting both cancellous and cortical bone compartments. Bone loss has been related to the duration and degree of estrogen and progesterone deficiency associated with amenorrhea. The long-term effects on the skeleton of menstrual disturbances associated with intensive physical training remains an area of intense research.

References

Adami S, Gatti D, Braga V, et al. Site specific effects of strength training on bone structure and geometry of ultradistal radius in postmenopausal women. J Bone Miner Res 1999;14:120–124.

Alfredson H, Nordstrom P, Pietila T, Lorentzon R. Long term loading and regional bone mass of the arm in female volleyball players. Calcif Tissue Int 1998;62:303–308.

Aloia JF, Cohn SH, Ostuni JA, et al. Prevention of involutional bone loss by exercise. Ann Intern Med 1978;89: 356–358.

Ashizawa N, Fujimura R, Tokuyama K, Suzuki M. A bout of resistance exercise increases urinary calcium independently of osteoclastic activation in men. J Appl Physiol 1997;83:1159–1163.

Ashizawa N, Ouchi G, Fujimura R, et al. Effects of a single bout of resistance exercise on calcium and bone metabolism in untrained young males. Calcif Tissue Int 1998;62:104–108.

Bassey EJ, Ramsdale SJ. Increase in femoral bone density in young women following high-impact exercise. Osteoporosis Int 1994;4:72–75.

Bassey EJ, Rothwell MC, Littlewood JJ, Pye DW. Pre- and postmenopausal women have different bone mineral density responses to same impact exercise. J Bone Miner Res 1998;13:1805–1813.

Bell NH, Godsen RN, Henry DP, et al. The effects of muscle-building exercise on vitamin D and mineral metabolism. J Bone Miner Res 1988;3:369–373.

Bennell KL, Malcolm SA, Wark JD, Brukner PD. Skeletal effects of menstrual disturbances in athletes. Scand J Med Sci Sports 1997;7:261–273.

Beverly MC, Rider TA, Evans MJ, Smith R. Local bone mineral response to brief exercise that stresses the skeleton. BMJ 1989;299:233–235.

Blair SN, Horton E, Leon AS, et al. Physical activity, nutrition and chronic disease. Med Sci Sports Med 1996;28:335–349.

Cann CE, Martin MC, Genant HK, Jaffe RB. Menstrual history is the primary determinant of trabecular bone density in women. Med Sci Sports Med 1988;20(Suppl 2):S59.

Clarkson PM, Haymes EM. Exercise and mineral status of athletes: calcium, magnesium, phosphorus and iron. Med Sci Sports Exerc 1995;27:831–843.

Craig BW, Brown R, Everhart J. Effects of progressive resistance training on growth hormone and testosterone levels in young and elderly subjects. Mech Ageing Dev 1989;49:159–169.

Dalsky GP. Effect of exercise on bone: permissive influence of estrogen and calcium. Med Sci Sports Exerc 1990;22:281–285.

Dalsky GP, Stocke KS, Ehsani AA, et al. Weight-bearing exercise training and lumbar bone mineral content in postmenopausal women. Ann Intern Med 1988;108:824–828.

Davee AM, Rosen CJ, Adler RA. Exercise patterns and trabecular bone density in college women. J Bone Miner Res 1990;5:245–250.

Davies MC, Hall ML, Jacobs HS. Bone mineral loss in young women with amenorrhoea. BMJ 1990;301:790–793.

Di Fiori JP. Menstrual dysfunction in athletes. Postgrad Med 1995;97:143–156.

Doyle F, Brown J, Lachance C. Relation between bone mass and muscle strength. Lancet 1970;1:391–393.

Drinkwater BL, Bruemmer B, Chesnut CH. Menstrual history as a determinant of current bone density in young athletes. JAMA 1990;263:545–548.

Drinkwater BL, Nilson K, Chesnut CH. Bone mineral content of amenorrheic and eumenorrheic athletes. New Engl J Med 1984;311:277–281.

Duppe H, Gardsell P, Johnell O, et al. Bone mineral density, muscle strength and physical activity: a population based study of 322 subjects aged 15–42. Acta Orthop Scand 1997;68:97–103.

Ebrahim S, Thompson PW, Baskaran V, Evans K. Randomized placebo-controlled trial of brisk walking in the prevention of postmenopausal osteoporosis. Age Ageing 1997;26:253–260.

Eliakim A, Raisz LG, Brasel JA, Cooper DM. Evidence for increased bone formation following a brief endurance type training intervention in adolescent males. J Bone Miner Res 1997;12:1708–1713.

Etherington J, Harris P, Nandra D, Hart D, Spector T. Bone mineral density and exercise: a comparison of female ex-elite athletes and age matched controls. Osteoporosis Imaging 1991;138:72.

Fahey TD, Rolph R, Moungmee P, et al. Serum testosterone, body composition and strength of young adults. Med Sci Sports Exerc 1976;8:31–34.

Franck H, Beuker F, Gurk S. The effect of physical activity on bone turnover in young adults. Exp Clin Endocrinol 1991;98:42–46.

Frost HM. Suggested fundamental concepts in skeletal physiology. Calcif Tissue Int 1993;52:1–4.

Fujimura R, Ashizawa N, Watanabe M, et al. Effect of resistance exercise training on bone formation and resorption in young male subjects assessed by biomarkers of bone metabolism. J Bone Miner Res 1997;12:656–662.

Gleeson PB, Protas EJ, LeBlanc AD, et al. Effects of weight lifting on bone mineral density in premenopausal women. J Bone Miner Res 1990;5:153–157.

Goodship AE, Lanyon LE, MacFie H. Functional adaptation of bone to increased stress. J Bone Joint Surg Am 1979;61:539–546.

Haapasalo H, Sievanen H, Kannus P, et al. Dimensions and estimated mechanical characteristics of the humerus after long term tennis loading. J Bone Miner Res 1996;11:864–872.

Hartard M, Haber P, Ilieva D, et al. Systematic strength training as a model of therapeutic intervention. Am J Phys Med Rehabil 1996;75:21–28.

Heinonen A, Kannus P, Sievanen H, et al. Good maintenance of high impact activity induced bone gain by voluntary, unsupervised exercises: an 8-month follow up of a randomized controlled trial. J Bone Miner Res 1999;14:125–128.

Heinrich CH, Going SB, Pamenter RW, et al. Bone mineral content of cyclically menstruating female resistance and endurance trained athletes. Med Sci Sports Exerc 1990;22:558–563.

Jaworski ZG, Uhthoff HK. Reversibility of nontraumatic disuse osteoporosis during its active phase. Bone 1986;7:431–439.

Jee WSS, Li X, Schaffler MT. Adaptation of diaphyseal structure with aging and increased mechanical usage in the adult rat: a histomorphometrical and biomechanical study. Anat Rec 1991;230:332–338.

Joakimsen RM, Fonnebo V, Magnus JH, et al. The Tromso study: physical activity and the incidence of fractures in a middle-aged population. J Bone Miner Res 1998;13:1149–1157.

Joakimsen RM, Magnus JH, Fonnebo V. Physical activity and predisposition for hip fractures: a review. Osteoporosis Int 1997;7:503–513.

Jonnavithula S, Warren MP, Fox RP, Lazaro MI. Bone density is compromised in amenorrheic women despite return of menses: a 2-year study. Obstet Gynecol 1993;81:669–674.

Joy E, Clark N, Ireland ML, et al. Team management of the female athlete triad (2): optimal treatment and prevention tactics. Round table. Physician Sports Med 1997;25:55.

Judex S, Whiting WC, Zernicke RF. Exercise induced bone adaptation: considerations for designing an osteogenically effective exercise program. Int J Indust Ergonom 1999;24:235–238.

Kanders B, Dempster DW, Lindsay R. Interaction of calcium nutrition and physical activity on bone mass in young women. J Bone Miner Res 1988;3:145–149.

Kannus P, Haapasalo H, Sankelo M, et al. Effect of starting age of physical activity on bone mass in the dominant arm of tennis and squash players. Ann Intern Med 1995;123:27–31.

Karlsson MK, Vergnaud P, Delmas PD, Obrant KJ. Indicators of bone formation in weight lifters. Calcif Tissue Int 1995;56:177–180.

Keay N, Fogelman I, Blake G. Bone mineral density in professional female dancers. Br J Sports Med 1997;31:143–147.

Keen AD, Drinkwater BL. Irreversible bone loss in former amenorrheic athletes. Osteoporosis Int 1997;7:311–315.

Kelley GA. Aerobic exercise and bone density at the hip in postmenopausal women: a meta analysis. Prev Med 1998;27:798–807.

Kirchner KM, Lewis RD, O'Connor PJ. Bone mineral density and dietary intake of female college gymnasts. Med Sci Sports Exerc 1995;27:543–549.

Kirk S, Sharp CF, Elbaum N, et al. Effect of long-distance running on bone mass in women. J Bone Miner Res 1989;4:515–522.

Kohrt WM, Ehsani AA, Birge SJ. Effects of exercise involving predominantly other joint reaction or ground reaction forces on bone mineral density in older women. J Bone Miner Res 1997;12:1253–1261.

Krolner B, Toft B, Nielsen SP, Tondevold E. Physical exercise as prophylaxis against involutional vertebral bone loss: a controlled trial. Clin Sci 1983;64:541–546.

Lanyon LE. Functional strain as a determinant for bone remodeling. Calcif Tissue Int 1984;36(Suppl 1):S56–S61.

Lanyon LE. Control of bone architecture by functional load bearing. J Bone Miner Res 1992;7(Suppl 2):S369–S375.

Lanyon LE. Using functional loading to influence bone mass and architecture: objectives, mechanisms and relationship with estrogen of the mechanically adaptive process in bone. Bone 1996;18(Suppl 1):37S–43S.

Lanyon LE, Rubin CT. Modulation of bone loss during calcium insufficiency by controlled dynamic loading. Calcif Tissue Int 1986;38:209–216.

Lohman T, Going S, Pamenter R, et al. Effects of resistance training on regional and total bone mineral density in premenopausal women: a randomized prospective study. J Bone Miner Res 1995;10:1015–1024.

Lundon K, Goode R. The effect of a five month muscle strength training program on the bone mass of postmenopausal women [Abstract]. Can J Physiol Pharmacol 1991;69:18.

Madsen KL, Adams WC, Vanloan MD. Effects of physical activity, body weight and composition, and muscular strength on bone density in young women. Med Sci Sports Exerc 1998;30:114–120.

Marcus R, Cann C, Madvig P, et al. Menstrual function and bone mass in elite women distance runners. Ann Intern Med 1985;102:158–163.

Miller KK, Klibanski A. Amenorrheic bone loss. J Clin Endocrin Metab 1999;84:1775–1783.

Moen SM, Sanborn CF, DiMarco NM, et al. Lumbar bone mineral density in adolescent female runners. J Sports Med Phys Fitness 1998;38:234–239.

Nilsson BE, Westlin NE. Bone density in athletes. Clin Orthop Rel Res 1971;77:179–182.

Nordstrom P, Pettersson U, Lorentzon R. Type of physical activity, muscle strength, and pubertal stage as determinants of bone mineral density and bone area in adolescent boys. J Bone Miner Res 1998;13:1141–1148.

Pettersson U, Nordstrom P, Lorentzon R. A comparison of bone mineral density and muscle strength in young male adults with different exercise level. Calcif Tissue Int 1999;64:490–498.

Pocock NA, Eisman JA, Yeates MG, et al. Physical fitness is a major determinant of femoral neck and lumbar spine bone mineral density. J Clin Invest 1986;78:618–621.

Prince RL, Smith M, Dick M, et al. Prevention of postmenopausal bone osteoporosis: a comparative study of exercise, calcium supplementation, and hormone replacement therapy. N Engl J Med 1991;325:1189–1195.

Prior JC, Vigna YM, Schechter MT, Burgess AE. Spinal bone loss and ovulatory disturbances. N Engl J Med 1990;323:1221–1227.

Pruitt LA, Jackson RD, Bartels RL, Lehnhard HJ. Weight-training effects on bone mineral density in early postmenopausal women. J Bone Miner Res 1992;7:179–185.

Puntila E, Kroger H, Lakka T, et al. Physical activity in adolescence and bone density in perimenopausal and postmenopausal women: a population based study. Bone 1997;21:363–367.

Raab DM, Crenshaw RD, Kimmel DB, Smith EL. A histomorphometric study of cortical bone activity during increased weight-bearing exercise. J Bone Miner Res 1991;6:741–749.

Ramos RH, Warren MP. The interrelationships of body fat, exercise, and hormonal status and their impact on reproduction and bone health. Semin Perinatol 1995;19:163–170.

Recker RR, Davies KM, Hinders SM, et al. Bone gain in young adult women. JAMA 1992;268:2403–2408.

Reeve J, Walton J, Russell LJ, et al. Determinants of the first decade of bone loss after menopause at spine, hip and radius. Q J Assoc Physicians 1999;92:261–273.

Revel M, Mayoux-Benhamou MA, Rabourdin JP, et al. One-year psoas training can prevent lumbar bone loss in postmenopausal women: a randomized controlled trial. Calcif Tissue Int 1993;53:307–311.

Ryan AS, Treuth MS, Hunter GR, Elahi D. Resistive training maintains bone mineral density in postmenopausal women. Calcif Tissue Int 1998;62:295–299.

Ryan AS, Treuth MS, Rubin MA, et al. Effects of strength training on bone mineral density: hormonal and bone turnover relationships. J Appl Physiol 1994;77:1678–1684.

Sandler RB. Muscle strength and skeletal competence: implications for early prophylaxis. Calcif Tissue Int 1988;42:281–283.

Schoutens A, Laurent E, Poortmans JR. Effects of inactivity and exercise on bone. Sports Med 1989;7:71–81.

Simkin A, Ayalon V, Leicher I. Increased trabecular bone density due to bone loading exercise in postmenopausal osteoporotic women. Calcif Tissue Int 1987;40:59–63.

Sinaki M, Fitzpatrick LA, Ritchie CK, et al. Site specificity of bone mineral density and muscle strength in women. Am J Phys Med Rehabil 1998;77:470–476.

Sinaki M, Wahner HW, Bergstralh EJ, et al. Three-year controlled, randomized trial of the effect of dose-specified loading and strengthening exercises on bone mineral density of spine and femur in nonathletic, physically active women. Bone 1996;19:233–244.

Sinaki M, Wahner HW, Offord KP. Relationship between grip strength and related regional bone mineral content. Arch Phys Med Rehabil 1989a;70:823–826.

Sinaki M, Wahner HW, Offord KP, Hodgson SF. Efficacy of nonloading exercises in prevention of vertebral bone loss in postmenopausal women: a controlled trial. Mayo Clin Proc 1989b;64:762–769.

Smith EL, Gilligan C. Dose-response relationship between physical loading and mechanical competence in bone. Bone 1996;18:45S–50S.

Smith EL, Gilligan C. Physical activity effects on bone metabolism. Calcif Tissue Int 1991;49(Suppl):S50–S54.

Smith EL, Gilligan C, McAdam M, et al. Deterring bone loss by exercise intervention in premenopausal and postmenopausal women. Calcif Tissue Int 1989;44:312–321.

Smith EL, Smith PE, Ensign CJ, Shea MM. Bone involution decrease in exercising middle-aged women. Calcif Tissue Int 1984;36:S129–S138.

Snow-Harter C, Bouxsein M, Lewis B, et al. Muscle strength as a predictor of bone mineral density in young women. J Bone Miner Res 1990;5:589–595.

Snow-Harter C, Whalen R, Myburgh K, et al. Bone mineral density, muscle strength and recreational exercise in men. J Bone Miner Res 1992;7:1291–1296.

Suleiman S, Nelson M, Li FM, et al. Effect of calcium intake and physical activity level on bone mass and turnover in healthy, white post-menopausal women. Am J Clin Nutr 1997;66:937–943.

Suominen H. Bone mineral density and long term exercise. An overview of cross-sectional athlete studies. Sports Med 1993;16:316–330.

Teegarden D, Proulx W, Kern M, et al. Previous physical activity relates to bone mineral measures in young women. Med Sci Sports Exerc 1996;28:105–116.

Ulrich CM, Georgiou CC, Gillis DE, Snow CM. Lifetime physical activity is associated with bone mineral density in premenopausal women. J Womens Health 1999;8:365–375.

Urist ME, DeLange RJ, Finerman GAM. Bone cell differentiation and growth factors. Science 1983;220:680–686.

VanHelder WP, Radomski MW, Goode RC. Growth hormone response during intermittent weightlifting exercise in men. Eur J Appl Physiol 1984;53:31–34.

Welsh L, Rutherford OM, James I, et al. The acute effects of exercise on bone turnover. Int J Sports Med 1997;18:247–251.

Wolff I, van Croonenborg JJ, Kemper HCG, et al. The effect of exercise training programs on bone mass: a meta-analysis of published controlled trials in pre- and postmenopausal women. Osteoporosis Int 1999;9:1–12.

Woo SLY, Kuei SC, Amiel D, et al. The effect of prolonged physical training on the properties of long bone. A study of Wolff's law. J Bone Joint Surg Am 1981;63:780–787.

Yarasheski KE, Campbell JA, Kohrt WM. Effect of resistance exercise and growth hormone on bone density of older men. Clin Endocrinol 1997;47:223–229.

Zerath E, Holy X, Guezennec CY, Chatard JC. Effect of endurance training on postexercise parathyroid hormone levels in elderly men. Med Sci Sports Exerc 1997;29:1139–1145.

Chapter 9
Injury, Regeneration, and Repair in Bone

Fractures of Long Bones: General Principles

Treatment of acute musculoskeletal trauma usually focuses on fractures and, therefore, on the restoration of bone structure and function. A fracture is a break in the continuity of bone or cartilage (Schultz 1990). Fractures can occur owing to low bone mass, altered internal orientation of bone tissue, and altered parameters of bone turnover; each factor plays a substantial role in the decline of bone integrity. However, even healthy bone has inherent structural properties that lend it to predictable patterns of injury equally dictated by the imposed external forces impacting on it. For instance, fractures may be influenced by extraskeletal factors such as falls, poor neuromuscular coordination, the amount of cushioning provided by soft tissues, and the physical environment (landing surface). In this way, the viscoelastic properties of bone, in concert with the load biomechanics, can be predictable determinants of the fracture pattern.

Five factors are involved in long-bone injury. Three of these factors relate to the nature of the load applied (type, magnitude, and rate of load). The other two factors (material and structural) are properties inherent to the long bone.

Nature of the Load

Type of Load

The application of force to bone results in biomechanical loading of its structure. Forces acting on long bone include tension, bending, compression, and torsion. Of all the forces impacting on bone, tension forces are well tolerated and, consequently, do not typically cause loading to induce fracture in any specific pattern. Rather, associated components of joints (e.g., ligaments) are most commonly affected by tension forces. Tension forces typically cause avulsion fractures where bone is torn at the site of ligamentous or musculotendinous attachment (e.g., quadriceps attachment to the patella). The clinically important ways in which long bones are loaded and fail are combinations of compression, bending, and torsion (Chaffin and Andersson 1991; Gozna and Harrington 1982). Several long-bone fracture patterns emerge as a result of the application of specific loads (Table 9-1). Cortical bone is generally stronger in compression than in tension, and stronger in tension than in shear.

Fractures in cancellous bone occur mainly from tensile and compression forces. Tensile forces are often produced by vigorous muscle contractions dislodging tendon and adjacent bone, whereas compression fractures often occur because of external loads.

Table 9-1. Summary of Long-Bone Fracture Biomechanics

Fracture Pattern	Appearance	Mechanism of Injury	Location of Soft Tissue Hinge	Energy
Transverse		Bending	Concavity	Low
Spiral		Torsion	Vertical segment	Low
Oblique transverse or butterfly		Compression and bending	Concavity or side of butterfly	Moderate
Oblique		Compression and bending and torsion	Concavity (often destroyed)	Moderate
Comminuted		Variable	Destroyed	High
Metaphyseal compression		Compression	Variable	Variable

Reprinted with permission from ER Gozna, IJ Harrington. Biomechanics of Musculoskeletal Injury. Baltimore: Williams & Wilkins, 1982;21.

Magnitude and Rate of Load

Not only is the type of force important, but the magnitude or energy that produces the fracture also bears impact on a long-bone fracture. Typically, a greater magnitude of force is related to higher energy content within bone and subsequent tissue destruction. The more complex pattern of fracture sustained is strongly related to the energy required to produce the fracture. The magnitude and rate of application of load is, thus, important in determining the amount of energy imparted to the bone. These factors, in turn, determine whether the force results in one of the simple fracture patterns (e.g., transverse or spiral), or whether it produces a severely comminuted fracture with extensive soft tissue destruction (Gozna and Harrington 1982).

Properties of Bone

Material properties of bone refers to the physical properties of bone. For instance, bone is heterogeneous and has both anisotropic and viscoelastic properties. The structural properties of bone refers to the size, shape, and configuration of the tissue, which are of importance in determining the overall strength of bone.

Healing and Repair of Long Bones after Fracture

Damage to cells and matrices plus the hemorrhage caused by acute traumatic injury initiates a tissue response that, in vascularized tissues such as bone, includes inflammation, repair, and remodeling processes. Inflammation, repair, and remodeling do not occur as discrete events; instead, tissue healing is a continuous sequence of cell, matrix, and vascular events initiated by injury that begins with the release of inflammatory mediators and ends when remodeling of the repair tissue ceases. With fracture healing in particular, a bone fracture initiates a sequence of inflammation, repair, and remodeling that can restore the injured bone remarkably close to its original state.

Inflammation

An injury that fractures bone not only damages the cells, blood vessels, and bone matrix, but also the surrounding soft tissues, including the periosteum and muscle. A hematoma accumulates within the medullary canal, between the fracture ends, and beneath elevated periosteum. The damage to the bone blood vessels deprives osteocytes of their nutrition, leaving the immediate ends of the bone fracture without living cells. Severely damaged periosteum, marrow, and other surrounding soft tissues may also contribute necrotic material to the fracture site. Inflammatory mediators released from platelets and from dead and injured cells cause blood vessels to dilate and exude plasma, leading to the acute edema seen in the region of a fresh fracture. Inflammatory cells, including polymorphonuclear leukocytes that are closely followed by macrophages and lymphocytes, migrate to the region.

Repair

Factors that stimulate repair include the chemotactic factors released during inflammation at the fracture site and bone matrix proteins exposed by disruption of the bone tissue. Although the inflammation caused by a fracture follows the same sequence for almost every fracture, the amount and composition of repair tissue may differ, depending on whether the fracture occurs through primarily cancellous bone in the metaphysis or through primarily cortical bone in the diaphysis. The amount and composition of repair tissue also depends on whether the fracture is stable or unstable during repair and the extent of soft tissue disruption surrounding the frac-

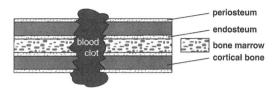

A. Post-fracture blood clot

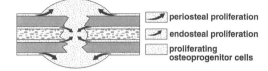

B. Proliferation of osteoprogenitor cells

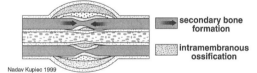

C. Formation of callus

D. Union of long bone fracture

Nadav Kupiec 1999

Figure 9-1. Healing and repair of a long-bone fracture. **A.** Disruption of blood vessels in the bone, marrow, periosteum, and surrounding tissue at the time of injury results in the extravasation of blood at the fracture site and the formation of a hematoma. **B.** Initiation and development of fracture callus. **C.** Note the simultaneous occurrence of chondrogenesis, endochondral ossification, and intramembranous bone formation in different regions of the fracture site. **D.** Union of a long-bone fracture.

ture. Disruption of blood vessels in the bone, marrow, periosteum, and surrounding tissue at the time of injury results in the extravasation of blood at the fracture site and the formation of a hematoma (Figure 9-1A). Organization of this hematoma is recognized as the first step in fracture repair. The fracture hematoma provides a fibrin scaffold that facilitates migration of repair cells. Growth factors and other proteins produced by cells in the fracture hematoma mediate the critical initial events in fracture repair, including cell migration, proliferation, and synthesis of a repair tissue matrix. Bone morphogenetic proteins are regulators of chemotaxis, mitosis, and differentiation, and that are recognized for their potential in initiating the fracture repair cascade (Reddi 1998).

At this stage, the microenvironment around the fracture is acidic, which may affect cell behavior during the early phases of repair. As repair progresses, the pH gradually returns to neutral and then to a slightly alkaline level. When an alkaline pH is attained, the activity of the alkaline phosphatase enzyme is optimal and an environment is created that is conducive to the mineralization of the fracture callus. Although the volume of the vascular bed of an extremity increases shortly after fracture, the osteogenic response is limited largely to the zones surrounding the fracture itself. It appears that, ordinarily, the periosteal vessels contribute the majority of capillary buds early in normal bone healing, with the nutrient medullary artery becoming more important later in the process. Pluripotential mesenchymal cells, probably of common origin, form the initial fibrous tissue and eventually bone at the fracture site (Yoo and Johnston 1998). The mesenchymal cells at the fracture site proliferate, differentiate, and produce the tissue known as *fracture callus*, which consists of fibrous tissue and woven bone (Figure 9-1B,C). The bone formed initially at the periphery of the inflammatory reaction by intramembranous bone formation is called the *hard callus*. The new tissue that arises in regions of low oxygen tension in the center of the inflammatory reaction is primarily cartilage and is called the *soft callus.*

Mineralized bone tissue gradually replaces the cartilage through the process of endochondral ossification, enlarging the hard callus and increasing the stability of the fracture fragments. The biochemical composition of the fracture callus matrix changes as repair progresses: The cells replace the fibrin clot with a loose fibrous matrix containing glycosaminoglycans, proteoglycans, and types I and III collagen. Analysis of fracture repair demonstrates a close correlation between the activation of genes for blood vessel, cartilage, and bone-specific proteins in the cells and the development of granulation tissue, cartilage, and bone, indicating that fracture repair depends on regulation of gene expression in the repair cells. Simultaneous occurrence of chondrogenesis, endochondral ossification, and intramembranous bone formation in different regions of the fracture callus (Figure 9-1C,D) suggest that local

mediators and small variations in the microenvironment, including mechanical stresses, determine what genes are expressed and, therefore, the type of tissue the repair cells form. Immunohistochemical studies show that expression of proliferating cell nuclear antigen is both time and space dependent and differentially expressed in the callus tissues formed by the intramembranous and endochondral processes (Einhorn 1998).

Nature and Effect of Mechanical Stress in Dense, Mineralized Connective Tissue Repair

Compressive forces discourage the formation of fibrous tissue. Intermittent cyclic strain produced by an externally applied and controlled cyclic load was observed as a more important stimulus to fracture healing than simple static compression, as demonstrated in animal models (Wolf et al. 1981). Tissue oxygen tension may help determine if bone or cartilage forms. For example, cartilage forms in regions with low oxygen tension (possibly because of the distance from blood vessels); bone seems to form directly in tissue that receives enough oxygen and is subject to the necessary mechanical or electrical stimuli. The fracture gap size and the amount of strain and hydrostatic pressure along the calcified surface of a fracture gap have been suggested to be the fundamental mechanical factors involved in bone healing (Claes et al. 1998).

Mineralization of fracture callus results from an ordered sequence of cellular activities (see Chapter 3). As mineralization proceeds, the fractured bone ends become enclosed in a mass of callus that contains increasing amounts of woven bone. An increasing mineral content correlates with an increasing hardness of the callus and can be visualized on x-ray. The internal and external callus formation contributes to the progressive increase in stability of the fracture site, and eventually clinical union occurs. However, the fracture callus remains immature because it is still weaker than normal bone, and it only gains strength during remodeling processes.

Remodeling

During the final stages of repair, remodeling of the repair tissue begins with replacement of woven bone by lamellar bone and resorption of unneeded

Clinical Note

The progression of fracture healing may be influenced by the application of mechanical load, with early weightbearing acting to accelerate the process of fracture healing. The premise for rehabilitation is that early functional weightbearing facilitates the maturation of the callus produced by endochondral ossification. After a period of protected loading, fractures stabilized with external fixation devices show an increased rate of healing with the application of controlled, cyclic loading. Variables such as the size of the initial gap, the stability of the bone-fixator construct, and the parameters of the applied motion (magnitude of the load, frequency, duration) appear to be extremely important in determining the quality of healing of a fracture (Goodman and Aspenberg 1993).

callus. According to radioisotope studies, fracture remodeling continues years after clinical union. Remodeling of fracture repair tissue after all woven bone has been replaced is achieved by osteoclastic resorption of excessive trabeculae and formation of new struts of bone along lines of force. Electrical fields influence fracture remodeling. Bone subjected to stress displays electropositivity and electronegativity on its convex and concave surfaces, respectively. The sequence of events across a 2-year course of healing of a long-bone fracture may be seen in Figure 9-2.

Variables That Influence Fracture Healing

Injury variables that affect fracture healing include severe soft tissue damage associated with open and comminuted, infected, segmental, and pathologic fractures. Fracture healing is influenced by tissue variables, such as poor local blood supply; patient variables, such as malnutrition and having other systemic diseases; and treatment variables, such as corticosteroids. The systemic status of an individual, the local limb status before injury, the nature of the traumatic injury, local host response to the injury, potential negative impact of orthopedic fracture, and pharmacologic variables all have an impact on bone fracture healing (Hayda et al. 1998).

Classification of Long-Bone Fractures

Bones may be classified as *long bones* (e.g., humerus, tibia, femur, phalanges) or *flat bones* (e.g., scapula, vertebrae, carpal bones). In health, the normal process of remodeling maintains resilient bone

by accommodating for wear and tear and even minor trauma via ongoing microrepair mechanisms, and by responding to altered patterns and magnitudes of load by realignment of its tissue. However, in any condition in which abnormal internal arrangement (internal architecture or geometry) of cortical bone exists, the bone is weakened.

Cortical Bone

Cortical bone is less able to withstand torsional stresses than tangential stresses. In other words, it is easier to fracture a long bone by twisting it, causing a spiral fracture that is usually a low-energy fracture and is associated with a lesser degree of soft tissue and skin damage. Tangential stresses, on the other hand, produce a transverse or short oblique fracture. A comminuted fracture is sustained (often with a butterfly fragment; see Figure 9-2E) with more severe violence. A comminuted fracture is usually a high-energy fracture and is often associated with a greater degree of soft tissue and skin damage.

Pathologic Fractures

Pathologic fracture refers to a fracture occurring through, and as a result of, previously diseased bone (Table 9-2). If the condition of the bone is significantly weakened, the fracture may occur spontaneously.

Classification of Fractures

Classification of fractures is necessary to ensure accurate communication among health profession-

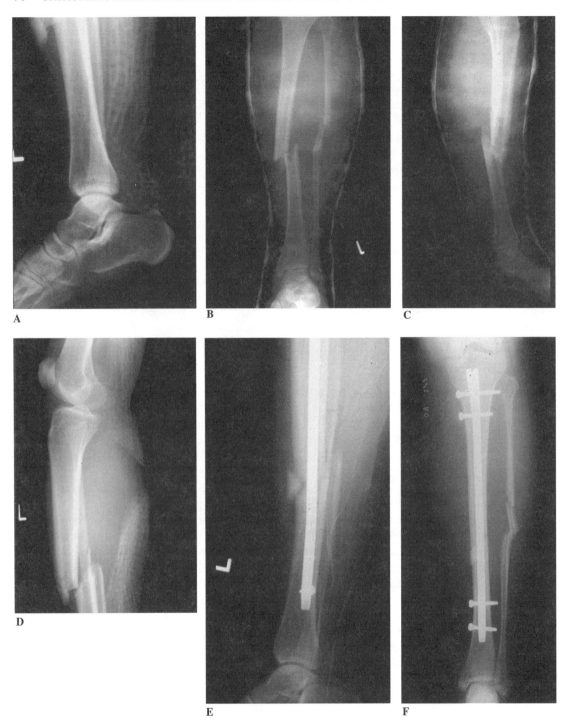

Figure 9-2. A–C. Day 0: The left tibia and fibula are seen through a cast. A comminuted fracture of the midshaft of the left tibia and fibula presents with dorsal angulation and foreshortening of the tibial fragments. **D.** Day 0: Comminuted fracture of the midshaft of tibia and fibula presents with overriding fracture fragments. **E,F.** Day 4: Surgery, post–open reduction and internal fixation of a comminuted fracture of the midtibial diaphysis with an anterior butterfly fragment and associated comminuted fracture of the midfibular diaphysis. An intramedullary nail has been inserted across the tibial fracture site. Anatomic alignment occurs across the fracture site.

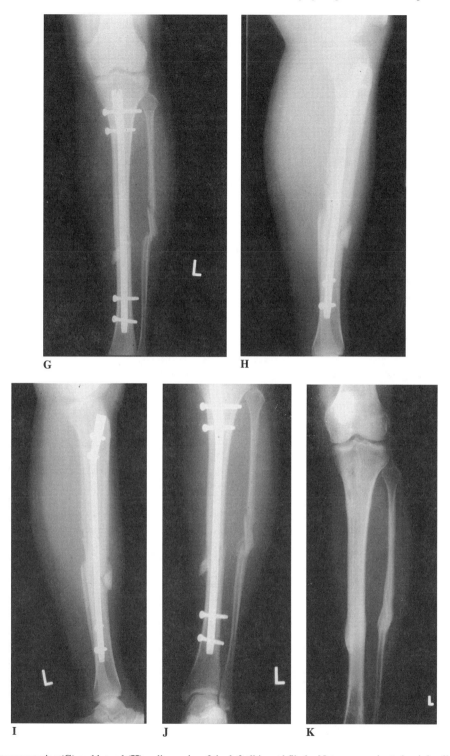

Day 17: Anteroposterior (**G**) and lateral (**H**) radiographs of the left tibia and fibula. Note a comminuted, minimally displaced fracture of the mid-diaphysis of the left fibula. No significant changes are seen in the bony alignment across the fractures, as compared to the previous examination. **I,J.** Day 62: An intramedullary rod is in place in the left tibia, with proximal and distal interlocking screws. Compared with previous examination, increased callus formation occurs around the fracture sites, demonstrating progress in the healing of both tibial and fibular fracture sites. **K.** Month 23: The intramedullary rod has been removed. (Courtesy of Dr. Harpul K. Gahunia, Ph.D.)

Table 9-2. Underlying Causes of Pathologic
Skeletal Fractures

Generalized bone disease
Osteoporosis
Osteogenesis imperfecta
Paget's disease
Tumors (secondary metastases)
Bone cysts and fibrous dysplasia
Other: avascular necrosis, chronic osteomyelitis

als and patients and to make informed decisions
regarding the management of the fracture (e.g., conservative versus open reduction internal fixation
[ORIF], prescription of weightbearing status). Clinicians involved in the physical management of
patients with bone fractures should understand the
basis of the decision-making process in order to foster good clinical judgment about bone and joint care
in the early stages of skeletal repair and across the
rehabilitative phase. For the purpose of fracture
classification, the general architecture of long or flat
bones are considered (Table 9-3). The classification
of long-bone fractures is presented in Figure 9-3.

A shaft (long-bone) fracture may be classified by
five characteristics:

1. *Site.* The site of a long-bone fracture may be
described at the shaft, proximal end, distal end, or
intra-articular or epiphyseal regions. Intra-articular
fractures may be further classified as linear, comminuted, impacted, or with bone loss (Figure 9-4).

2. *Extent.* A fracture may be either complete or
incomplete. A complete fracture occurs when all cortices of the long bone have been broken. An incom-

plete fracture occurs when only one portion of the
cortex is disrupted (e.g., crack or hairline fractures).
Incomplete fractures typically affect short bones and
flat bones in the adult. Green-stick, buckle, and bowing fractures are incomplete fractures that occur in the
pediatric population. In general, incomplete fractures
have inherent stability, relative to a complete fracture.

3. *Configuration.* A fracture has three types of
configurations: comminuted, linear, and segmental.
A comminuted fracture has more than two fragments with or without a butterfly wedge (see Figure 9.2E). A comminuted fracture does not always
display clear direction. Linear configurations can be
(1) transverse, manifesting at right angles to the
longitudinal axis or cortex of bone; (2) oblique, running in an oblique direction relative to the axis of
the long bone; or (3) spiral, usually occurring from
the application of torsional forces and presenting in
a similar manner to an oblique fracture except that it
affects a greater area of the shaft. In segmental configurations, various levels are affected and the bone
is segmented by more than one fracture line.

4. *Relationship of fracture fragments to each
other.* A fracture may be described as displaced or
undisplaced (Figure 9-5).

5. *Relationship to the external environment.* A
fracture is classified as closed or open, according to
whether the fracture site is exposed to the external
environment (Figure 9-6). The skin and soft tissue
overlying the area of a closed fracture are intact. In an
open fracture, the skin is perforated by the fracture
fragment or trauma. The open fracture site becomes
vulnerable to infection from the external environment.

General Management: Principles of Reduction and Fixation of Fractures

Reduction

After a fracture has been sustained, the fracture fragments are typically displaced. The restoration of normal anatomic alignment of the fractured bone is
accomplished by open or closed reduction. Open
reduction involves the surgical exposure of the fracture site, with or without the application of internal
fixation devices. Closed reduction involves the physical placement of bony fragments into normal alignment using traction or manipulation techniques.

Table 9-3. Classification of Fractures

Type of Bone	Fracture Region
Long bone	Intra-articular component
	Extra-articular component, made up of
	Proximal metaphyseal region
	Distal metaphyseal region
	Shaft region "in thirds" (proximal,
	middle, and distal)
Flat bone	Articular region
	Extra-articular region

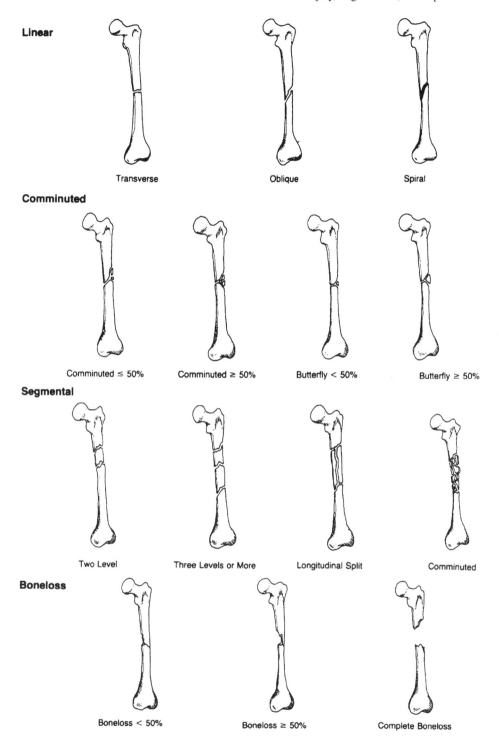

Linear

Transverse Oblique Spiral

Comminuted

Comminuted ≤ 50% Comminuted ≥ 50% Butterfly < 50% Butterfly ≥ 50%

Segmental

Two Level Three Levels or More Longitudinal Split Comminuted

Boneloss

Boneloss < 50% Boneloss ≥ 50% Complete Boneloss

Figure 9-3. Classification of long-bone fractures. (Reprinted with permission from RB Gustilo. The Fracture Classification Manual. St. Louis: Mosby–Year Book, 1991;12.)

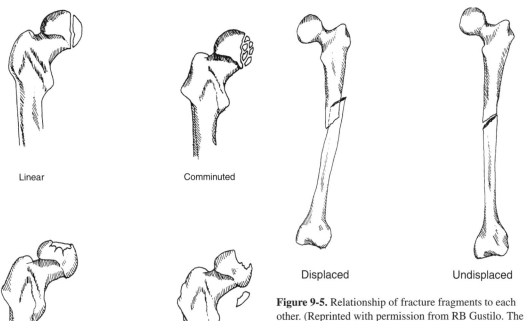

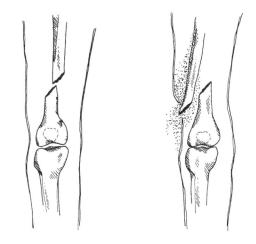

Linear

Comminuted

Impacted

Articular Boneless

Figure 9-4. Classification of intra-articular fractures. (Reprinted with permission from RB Gustilo. The Fracture Classification Manual. St. Louis: Mosby–Year Book, 1991;11.)

Displaced

Undisplaced

Figure 9-5. Relationship of fracture fragments to each other. (Reprinted with permission from RB Gustilo. The Fracture Classification Manual. St. Louis: Mosby–Year Book, 1991;13.)

Complications of Fractures

The complications of fractures can be classified in a temporal sequence as follows:

1. *Immediate complications* (occurring within days of fracture): fat emboli, deep vein thrombosis (DVT), nerve and/or vascular damage

Fixation

To support optimal bony healing, the fracture fragments may need to undergo fixation to maintain alignment after reduction. External fixation includes the use of plaster casts or splints. Internal fixation may involve the application of surgical hardware, including pins, wires, screws, rods, and plates (see Figure 9.2F).

Fracture Management Principles

The aim of general principles of fracture management is to (1) make accurate decisions (e.g., open or closed reduction) and (2) set goals to avoid infection, achieve union, avoid malunion, provide stability, prevent deformity, and allow for optimal function and mobility.

Figure 9-6. Relationship of the fracture to the external environment. (Reprinted with permission from RB Gustilo. The Fracture Classification Manual. St. Louis: Mosby–Year Book, 1991;14.)

Clinical Note

The signs and symptoms of vascular insufficiency may include the following:

- Pain that is persistent and, in some cases, becomes more acute with time
- Pain that may be more severe on passive movement, with the possible loss of the ability to perform active movements
- Color changes, such as duskiness, mottled pallor, and swelling
- Sensory changes, such as tingling and numbness
- Decreased temperature and absent pulses

2. *Delayed complications* (occurring within weeks or months of fracture): infection, joint stiffness, malunion
3. *Late complications* (occurring years after fracture): limb shortening, residual deformity, osteoarthritis, avascular necrosis, growth plate damage

Fat Emboli

Patients who sustain multiple fractures are particularly vulnerable to the development of fat emboli, which are caused by circulating fat globules and free fatty acids that aggregate and lodge themselves in the vascular system.

Deep Vein Thrombosis

DVT is common in patients who do not receive prophylactic treatment after certain, particularly long-bone, fractures. DVTs are thought to be initiated by endothelial vessel wall damage and further promoted by venous stasis. Anticoagulants and early mobilization are considered prophylactic treatments.

Avascular Necrosis

A compromised blood supply causes necrosis of bone fragments. Regions vulnerable to avascular necrosis are the head of the femur in a subcapital fracture; the body of the talus after a fracture dislocation or complete dislocation at the ankle; and the proximal pole of scaphoid, lunate, and capitate bones after fracture of the wrist (see Chapter 10).

Infection

Infection may be confined to open fractures and may manifest as secondary osteomyelitis. Osteomyelitis, once established, is very resistant to treatment and is associated with avascular necrosis and nonunion. The presence of foreign material, such as fixation devices, tends to potentiate infection (see Chapter 10).

Delayed Union

Delayed healing occurs when a fracture heals significantly more slowly than normal. Delayed healing is generally the result of a compromised blood supply, infection, pathology, or improper management. A compromised blood supply may be due to anatomic fragility (head of femur) or trauma. Excessively rigid external fixation is considered a contributing factor to fracture union problems, with inhibition of external callus formation, maintenance of a fracture gap aggravated by bone end resorption, and excessive protection of the healing bone from normal stresses producing adverse remodeling as possible causes (Aro et al. 1990). If the factors involved in this pathologic state of delayed union are not addressed, nonunion ensues.

Slow Union

Slow union may occur when, despite the presence of ideal circumstances, the rate of union appears slow, but it is actually normal for the prevailing conditions, such as patient age and fracture site.

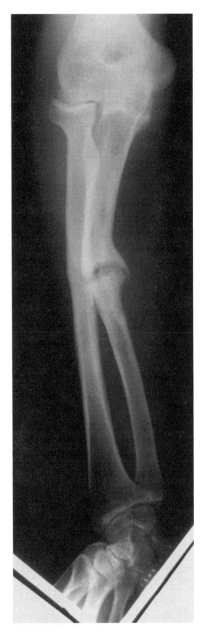

Figure 9-7. Nonunion of a fracture at the midradius. Note the sclerosis along opposing fracture surfaces. Bony proliferation at the margins and angular deformity are seen. (Courtesy of Dr. E. Becker, M.D., The Toronto Hospital, Toronto.)

Nonunion

Nonunion occurs when fracture fragments fail to unite and bony reparative processes have ceased. Unwanted movement at a healing site is the most common cause of nonunion. Bone grafting (autogenous) is often done in this situation. The fracture line and sclerosis persist with absent callus or bony healing efforts, which may be witnessed via radiograph (Figure 9-7).

Pseudoarthrosis

Pseudoarthrosis refers to the creation of a false joint where the fragmented bone ends do not normally connect with dense fibrous or fibrocartilaginous tissue. Instead, a false joint may be created between the ends that are surrounded by a bursal sac that contains synovial fluid. This condition is associated with nonunion.

Malunion

In malunion, union of fracture fragments occurs in an improper position, resulting in significant deformity. Corrective surgery may be indicated in certain cases of malunion, such as when loss of function or a notably disfiguring appearance has occurred.

Complex Regional Pain Syndrome Type I

In complex regional pain syndrome type I (formerly known as *reflex sympathetic dystrophy*) there is pain, hyperesthesia, and tenderness of the extremity. In the early stages, skin of the limb may assume a red, warm, and swollen appearance. Over time, the skin may display pallor and may be dry, shiny, and cool. The management principles in this case should focus on prevention, sympathetic blocks, pain management, gradual mobilization and, ultimately, stress loading through the limb.

Compartment Syndrome

Compartment syndrome may be due to excessively high pressures and bleeding in closed fascial compartments of an extremity, which may lead to muscle necrosis, fibrosis, and contracture. Ultimately, these symptoms must be relieved by compartment

Clinical Note

Determinants of Fracture Risk

Hip fracture: Hip fracture risk appears to be associated with bone fragility and its relation to geometric and physical factors or external forces such as a fall. Age, gait disorders, and falls present as interrelated variables in the manifestation of a hip fracture. Ninety percent of hip fractures occur after the age of 70. The incidence of hip fracture increases dramatically with age in both men and women (Jacobsen et al. 1990; Oden et al. 1999). Ninety percent of hip fractures are a consequence of a fall; approximately 80% of the falls occur due to pathologic balance and gait disorders (Runge 1997). Tall individuals sustain more hip fractures than shorter persons, and high body mass index is associated with fewer hip and forearm fractures (Joakimsen et al. 1999). Only a minority of those who sustain such falls regain their former level of locomotion.
Stroke: Fractures are a serious complication after stroke. Hip (femoral neck) fracture has been cited as the most frequent fracture after stroke, with its incidence 2–4 times higher in stroke patients compared with a reference population (Ramnemark et al. 1998). In addition, fractures after stroke usually are caused by falls and affect the paretic side.
Spinal cord injury: Low-energy fractures, especially of the lower extremities, are frequent in individuals with a spinal cord injury, especially among women (Vestergaard et al. 1998).

fasciotomy. The recognition of the onset of compartment syndrome at an early stage is of obvious importance.

Myositis Ossificans and Ectopic Ossification

(See Chapter 10 for information on myositis ossificans and ectopic ossification.)

Rupture of Tendons or Nerves

The nerve lesion is usually either a neuropraxia or axonotmesis. Recovery is usual after reduction of the fracture.

Bone Mineral Loss

Loss of bone mineral density (BMD) from the femoral necks of elderly patients (mean age, 77 years) in the year after an osteoporosis-related hip fracture was more than five times that reported in a nonfractured population (Dirschl et al. 1997). The phenomenon of bone mass loss after a hip fracture may persist at least a year after surgical repair

(Zerahn et al. 1998). This accelerated rate of bone loss may have drastic consequences in an elderly population already exhibiting osteopenia and propensity to sustain falls.

Skeletal Dimorphism

Fractures occur less commonly in men than in women (Vanderscheuren et al. 1998). Several reasons have been proposed for the sexual skeletal dimorphism and lower bone fragility in men (Seeman 1998):

1. Men have a higher peak bone mass and cross-sectional bone area than women.
2. The rate of bone loss in men may be lower than in women.
3. Cancellous bone loss by thinning may occur preferentially in men because of reduced bone formation. In contrast, perforation and loss of connectivity is commonly seen in women.
4. There may be relatively less endocortical resorption and greater periosteal bone formation in men than in women.
5. Men display less intracortical porosity than women.

Stress Fractures

Stress fractures present in two forms: *insufficiency fractures* and *fatigue fractures*. Insufficiency, or fragility, fractures manifest as a result of normal stress applied to bone that is affected by underlying pathology including osteoporosis, Paget's disease, osteomalacia, and osteogenesis imperfecta (Anderson and Greenspan 1996). However, for a fracture to occur, it is not always necessary for the ultimate stress to be exceeded. Repeated loading and unloading of the bone can cause it to fail, even if loads are below this level. This phenomenon is known as *fatigue failure*, and the fractures that result from this type of loading are hereafter referred to as *stress fractures*. Fatigue failure occurs when each loading cycle produces a minute amount of microdamage that accumulates with repetitive loads. The repair mechanisms inherent to bone deal with microdamage that accumulates with repetitive loading. In health, repair mechanisms inherent to bone cope with microdamage as it occurs and do not allow accumulation of these events. Biomechanically, stress fractures are most likely to occur when bone is loaded repeatedly in the *plastic region* (see Chapter 7). In addition, a possible pathogenetic role of local changes exists in bone remodeling at stress fracture sites.

Microfailure Theory

As mentioned before, stress fractures may also be referred to as *fatigue fractures*, fractures that occur in regions subjected to excessive and persistent mechanical stress. The neck of the second metatarsal is a common stress fracture (*march fracture*) site. Another common site, especially in runners and dancers, is the tibia. It has been postulated that accumulation of unrepaired microdamage in human bone increases bone fragility at any age (Frost 1960), and it is known that microdamage increases with age (Norman and Wang 1997). One of the theories of the mechanism of stress fracture is that, when a material such as bone is stressed continually, a slow decrease occurs in the elastic modulus of the stress strain curve as the material properties degrade or fatigue. Hence, the development of fatigue fractures is a gradual process and can be a real consequence of normal cyclic loading within the physiologic strain range after which brief periods of higher stress or strain loading occur (Schaffler et al. 1990). The reduction in mechanical properties may be attributed to small cracks within the bony structure. As these cracks grow and coalesce, the bone ultimately fails (Turner and Burr 1993). The ultimate effect of microcrack accumulation is to impair the mechanical properties of bone by reducing its elastic modulus (Burr et al. 1998). In fatigue of human compact bone, the principal mechanisms of matrix failure (e.g., linear microcracks, diffuse damage foci, and tearing damage) are strongly dependent on local strain type (Boyce et al. 1998). Although the mechanisms of fatigue damage accumulation are similar for both compression and tension failure of cortical bone, damage accumulates more rapidly in tensile cortices and crack growth is greater in compressive cortices (Burr et al. 1998). They may be difficult to see because often only a minute crack can be visualized on x-ray.

Etiology: Predisposing Factors for Stress Fractures

It is unclear the extent to which muscular, gravitational, or compressive forces contribute, or are interdependent to, stress fracture incidence. High intensity physical training has been associated with the occurrence of stress fractures (Bennell et al. 1997a; Bennell et al. 1998). Physical training refers repetitive loads to the skeleton from external sources (e.g., weightbearing and foot impact), internal sources (e.g., muscle action or strength), or a combination of the two (muscle fatigue and decreased shock-absorbing capacity of muscle on protecting bone).

Internal Shearing of Bone

Forces generated within cortical bone by musculature during nonweightbearing activities (e.g., the forces generated within the humerus by the muscles used while playing tennis) represent internal stresses on bone. Muscles are capable of transmitting significant forces to the skeletal system and, after repetitive cycles, have initiated stress fractures (Matheson et al. 1987a).

Clinical Note

Muscles lower the bending stress on bone and attenuate the dynamic load on the human musculoskeletal system. Fatigue may diminish the ability of skeletal muscle to dissipate and attenuate loading on the system (Voloshin et al. 1998). Weakness of musculature surrounding a bone can result in increased distribution of stress to that bone, increasing its responsibility for bearing and dissipating the forces (Matheson et al. 1987a). This altered pattern of shock absorption causes a redistribution of forces onto the bone, yielding focal areas of concentrated stress. These particular areas are susceptible to stress fractures. During athletic training, terrain and choice of footwear dictate the amount of auxiliary shock absorption available to the weightbearing bones. Hence, these variables have an influence on bone injury.

Biomechanical Alignment

Altered biomechanical alignment of the lower extremity has been documented in cases of stress fractures (Reid 1992). Athletes with stress fractures were more likely to have pronated feet than cavus foot alignment (Matheson et al. 1987a). Metatarsal stress fractures were more common in dancers, rendering them unable to work in true vertical and ankle alignment during demi-pointe and pointe work (Khan et al. 1995). Dancers who presented with longer second metatarsals and who were, consequently, required to balance on the third, fourth, and fifth rays displayed a tendency to "sickle in" and develop stress fractures in these areas (Khan et al. 1995).

Low Bone Density

Decreased bone density appears to increase vulnerability to the detrimental impact of repetitive strain on bone (Young 1994). Decreased BMD levels, altered menstrual function, decreased calcium intake, and lower oral contraceptive use are consid-

Clinical Note

Signs of stress fracture include point tenderness of bone, soft tissue swelling, warmth, alteration of gait, muscular atrophy, full and pain-free range of motion of adjacent joints, pain-free resisted active movement of joints, and palpation of callus over time (Reid 1992). A positive "hop test"—when hopping on one leg elicits pain at the site of a lower extremity stress fracture—has been included as a final criterion in the clinical diagnosis of lower extremity stress fractures (Matheson et al. 1987a). Percussion of the bone may produce pain at a distant site (Anderson and Greenspan 1996); groin pain elicited with the hop test suggests a pelvic stress fracture (Sallis and Jones 1991).

A differential diagnosis of a stress fracture must be established to exclude

- Primary or metastatic neoplasms
- Infections (e.g., periostitis)
- Musculoskeletal soft tissue injuries (tendonitis, sprain, strain, compartment syndromes, shin splints, medial tibial stress syndrome)
- Nerve compression syndromes
- Intermittent claudication
- Joint diseases

ered predisposing risk factors to stress fracture development in athletes (Bennell et al. 1997b; Myburgh 1990).

Clinical Diagnosis

In one study of 320 stress fractures, cases diagnosed on the basis of clinical presentation alone did not differ from those confirmed by bone scan in terms of the time taken to diagnose, time to recover, tenderness and swelling, demographic features, or biomechanical abnormalities (Matheson et al. 1987b). Stress fractures of the axial and appendicular skeleton typically present with localized pain that develops without a history of specific acute injury. The typical clinical presentation is insidious onset of localized pain that is activity-related and abates with rest. If activity continues and microdamage accumulates, the pain may progress and become constant.

Imaging

Radiographs, bone scans, ultrasound, computer-assisted thermography, and computed tomography (CT), along with clinical evaluation of presenting signs and symptoms, are useful in establishing a diagnosis of stress fracture. Plain film radiographs may demonstrate changes consistent with a fracture, such as a fracture line or callus (Figure 9-8). In many cases, however, radiographs may be normal, especially when they are obtained soon after the onset of symptoms (before a fracture line or evidence of new bone formation appears). When the fracture involves areas of the skeleton that are difficult to evaluate by plain films, such as the spine and pelvis, a stress fracture may escape diagnosis. In addition, detection of a stress fracture becomes difficult with patients who are osteopenic; a fracture line and callus may be obscured in these cases. Therefore, the use of radiographs in detection of stress fractures often has been considered an unreliable source when used independently of other investigative methods. When plain films are normal, other tests, such as bone scans, CT, and magnetic resonance imaging (MRI), are useful to demonstrate the fracture. A triple phase bone scan involves the focal uptake of technetium-99 polyphosphonate at the site of pain (Matheson et al. 1987b). CT and MRI are considered the best diagnostic tools in the detection of longitudinal (e.g., tibial) stress fractures in terms of timely and efficient diagnosis. Although sensitive, the bone scan has lower specificity than either CT or MRI (Shearman et al. 1998).

Incidence

In a review of 3,198 stress fractures, a sport-specific trend emerged in correlation with the site of stress fracture (Reid 1992). Eighty-two percent of these cases involved the lower extremity and all were associated with weightbearing activities, such as jogging, running, ballet, basketball, soccer, and aerobic dance (Reid 1992). It has been hypothesized that both compression and tension forces act on weightbearing bone (compared to only tension forces occurring in nonweightbearing bone); this may account for the high rate of fracture occurrence in the lower extremities (Alonso-Bartolome et al. 1999). Dance was the activity that most commonly caused metatarsal stress fractures; the usual location of this fracture being the proximal metaphyseal-diaphyseal junction (Lundon et al. 1998; O'Malley et al. 1996). Tibial stress fractures were most commonly sustained in distance running and track; some track athletes were additionally vulnerable to navicular stress fractures (Bruckner et al. 1996). Stress fractures comprise nearly 25% of all musculoskeletal injuries in runners (Fredericson 1996), with the tibia accounting for nearly one-half of these, followed by the tarsal navicular, fibula, metatarsals, and sesamoids (Matheson et al. 1987a). In another study of incidence and distribution of stress fractures of track and field athletes, foot fractures were associated with sprinters, hurdlers, and jumpers, whereas long-bone and pelvic fractures were associated with middle- and long-distance runners (Bennell et al. 1996).

Lower extremity injuries are commonly associated with jogging, running, ballet, basketball, soccer, and aerobic dance.

- Track and field
  Site of stress lesion or fracture commonly associated with sprinting, hurdling, jumping: foot fractures (navicular, pars interarticularis, metatarsal)

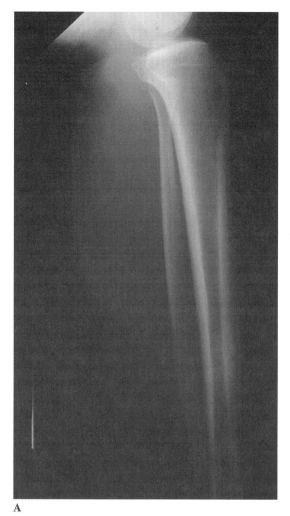
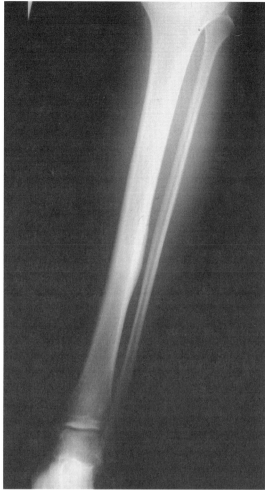

A

B

Figures 9-8. A,B. Stress fracture of the tibia in a young adolescent female involved in intensive ballet training. (Courtesy of Sarah McCutcheon, P.T., National Ballet School, Toronto.)

Site of stress lesion or fracture commonly associated with long-distance running: long bone (tibia, fibula), pelvis
- Ballet
  Site of stress lesion or fracture: base of second metatarsal (proximal metaphyseal-diaphyseal junction or extension into tarsometatarsal joint), tibia, fibula
  Contributing factors: over-training, delayed menarche, poor nutrition

Although stress fractures are most commonly found in the lower limb, they also occur in the upper limb in particular association with upper limb–dominated sports (e.g., tennis, swimming, and those involving throwing activities) (Bruckner 1998; Cervoni et al. 1997).

Upper extremity injuries are commonly associated with baseball, gymnastics, weight lifting, javelin throwing, racket sports, and sports of the wheelchair-bound.

- All are susceptible to stress lesions in the bones of the upper extremities (ulna, humerus, radius, scapula).
- Injuries range from periostitis to bone spurs to stress fractures.
- Injuries in adolescents typically involve the growth plates, whereas midshaft injuries at the

Clinical Note

Other Management Strategies

Conservative: Depending on the stress fracture site involved, casting may be required. For example, in the case of a fracture of the second metatarsal, a short walking cast may be applied in the acute phase.
Surgical: In extreme cases, bone grafting may be indicated to resolve persistent symptoms.
Prevention: In a study of stress fracture occurrence in military recruits, the rate of stress fracture development was reduced from 4.8% to 1.6% with the addition of intermittent rest periods during training (Scully and Besterman 1982). Reduced march speed, running on soft surfaces, individual march step instead of marching in step, and interval-running training were preventive strategies successfully used to reduce pelvic stress fractures in military recruits (Pope 1999). In one prospective study, the use of custom-made biomechanical shoe orthoses reduced the incidence of metatarsal stress fractures in military recruits (Finestone et al. 1999).

area of muscle insertion are more common in adults.

Trunk and spine injuries (vertebrae, pelvis, ribs) are associated with weight lifting, football, gymnastics, wrestling, diving, running, and rowing.

- Similarities between stress fractures of the rib in elite rowers and fractures caused by cough have yielded thoughts that actions of the serratus anterior and external oblique muscles on the rib may cause stress fractures because of the repetitive bending forces common to both rowing and coughing (Karlson 1998).

Rehabilitation of Stress Fracture

Early diagnosis is of great importance in the treatment of stress fractures because it allows earlier resolution to injury and minimum interruption of activity. The necessity of obtaining a detailed activity history, physical examination, and biomechanical assessment has been emphasized for successful efforts at rehabilitation (Reid 1992). Modified rest and alternative non-weightbearing activities or a program involving cross-training (e.g., cycling, swimming, resistance running in water) are advocated for the acute treatment of stress fractures (Matheson et al. 1987a; Reid 1992). In addition, local muscle strengthening and retraining are critical during the first phase of rehabilitation for stress fractures (Matheson et al. 1987a). The treatment of stress fractures also includes appropriate choice of footwear and an orthotic prescription.

The gradual reintroduction of sport-specific training is a critical process for the complete repair of a stress fracture. This introduction should begin once the individual has remained pain-free for 10–14 days (Matheson et al. 1987a). The gradual resumption of activity must occur with a prescribed progression of exercise starting at levels of frequency, duration, and intensity well below normal (Reid 1992). During re-entry to the activity or sport, the treatment shifts from alleviation to prevention, with a focus on assessment, correction, and prevention of recurrence of the problem. Correction of training errors, modification of training surfaces, and orthotics assessment are all components of this second phase of rehabilitation (Matheson et al. 1987a).

In cases of repetitive injuries, as those commonly associated with ballet dancers, an approximate activity modification period of 4–8 weeks is recommended to allow for the repair of fracture sites at the base of the metatarsal, shaft of the metatarsal, tibia, and fibula (Khan et al. 1995). In cases involving the metatarsal, dancers may be required to use crutches for the first 4 weeks post-injury in an attempt to decrease the loads on the metatarsal. Rest and supervised restricted weightbearing is the recommended course in the successful management of the fractured metatarsal shaft (Khan et al. 1995).

Cancellous Bone Fractures

Repetitive, low-intensity loading from normal daily activities can generate fatigue damage in cancellous bone and in turn act as a potential cause of spontaneous fractures at the hip and spine (Bowman et al. 1998). "Crushing" of the trabeculae in cancellous bone is common. Because cancellous bone is extremely vascular, it typically heals rapidly, albeit often incompletely. The vertebral crush fracture is a typical cancellous bone fracture that may become wedge-shaped (Figure 9-9). There is minimal or no callus formation during the healing of cancellous bone fractures. The healing processes occur directly by osteoblastic activity at the fracture site (creeping substitution) with the success of healing lying in the close apposition of fracture fragments to one another. Vertebral fractures associated with osteoporosis (see Chapter 12) involve the vertebral body and include some combination of compression (collapse of the entire vertebral body), concavity (collapse of the vertebral endplates), or wedging (relative loss of anterior height). The prevalence of one or more vertebral fractures increased with age independently of declining bone mass, reaching 42% in women with spinal BMD less than 0.6 g/cm^2 as measured by dual photon absorptiometry (Melton et al. 1989). Bone mass and age contribute independently to the risk of vertebral fracture. Vertebral deformities (including wedge, midbody, and crush fractures) are prevalent in older men and also occur in the presence of reduced BMD (Mann et al. 1992; Melton et al. 1998).

Spinal osteoporosis is linked with a loss of stature because of the shortening of the trunk, which is partly due to the loss of bone substance and also to changes in vertebral body shapes that proceed to vertebral body wedging and collapse (Buchanan et al. 1987). Resistance to fracture depends less on the total amount of bone than on the adequate spatial arrangement and form of each structural element. To exemplify this, an equivalent amount of bone distributed as widely spaced, disconnected thick trabeculae is biomechanically less competent than when distributed as numerous, connected thin plates (Kleerekoper et al. 1985). These structural changes are more severe in patients with compression fractures, in whom the additional deficit in trabecular bone volume is the result mainly of a further reduction in trabecular plate density and further increase in trabecular plate separation (Parfitt et al. 1983). In addition, creep plays a fundamental role in the fatigue of cancellous bone (Bowman et al. 1998).

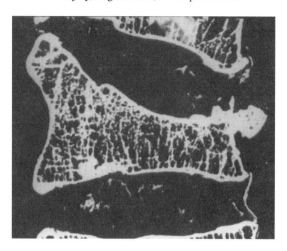

Figure 9-9. Wedge fracture of cancellous bone in the vertebral body. (Courtesy of Dr. M. D. Grynpas, Ph.D., Samuel Lunenfeld Research Institute, Mount Sinai Hospital, Toronto.)

Compression Fractures

Removal of the horizontal trabeculae or lateral support crossties can alter the architectural arrangement and lead to reduced load-bearing capacity (Mosekilde et al. 1985). As a result, the vertical trabeculae begin to behave as columns that, if subjected to loads, collapse. For example, it is known that a 50% reduction in cross-sectional area contributed to by these horizontal trabeculae is associated with a 75% reduction in load-bearing capacity of the vertebral body (Yamada 1970).

Burst Fractures

An array of trabeculae are present in the thoracolumbar vertebrae that extend from the medial corner of the base of the pedicles and reach in a radial array throughout the vertebral body (Heggeness and Doherty 1997). The cortex of the vertebral canal thins abruptly near the base of the pedicle, creating the semblance of a stress concentration at this site. In axial load type burst fractures, the bony fragments, which are typically trapezoidal in shape, may be retropulsed into the spinal canal and are considered to be a result of the presence of this stress concentration.

Summary

All basic fracture patterns are the result of the combination of bending, torsion, and/or compression loads, and they are further influenced by the magnitude and rate of application of the load and inherent characteristics of the bone. The five factors which influence how a long bone will fracture include the type, magnitude, and rate of load in concert with the influences supplied by material and structural properties of bone. Healing and repair of the long bones involves inflammation, repair, and remodeling processes. Mechanical stress of an intermittent cyclic nature is an important stimulus to optimize fracture healing processes. Classification of long-bone fractures is by site, extent, configuration, and relationship of fracture fragments to each other and their relationship to the external environment. Complications of fractures include fat emboli; DVT; avascular necrosis; infection; delayed, slow, mal-, or nonunion; pseudoarthrosis; complex regional pain syndrome type I; compartment syndrome; ectopic ossification; and bone mineral loss.

Normal physiologic loading of bone is cyclic in nature and occurs at both stresses and strains well below forces that cause bone to fracture in isolated episodes. A stress fracture is the clinical failure of bone that results from cyclic loading through a progressive process referred to as *fatigue failure*. Spontaneous fractures of cancellous bone at the hip and spine may also occur with repetitive, low-intensity loading. Vertebral body fractures present with compression, concavity, or wedging appearances, resulting in loss of stature. The loss of horizontal trabeculae, in particular, is associated with substantive losses in the load-bearing capacity of the vertebral body, resulting in compression fractures.

References

Alonso-Bartolome P, Martinez-Taboada VM, Blanco R, Rodriguez-Valverde V. Insufficiency fractures of the tibia and fibula. Semin Arthritis Rheum 1999;28:413–420.

Anderson MW, Greenspan A. Stress fractures. Radiology 1996;199:1–12.

Aro HT, Kelly PJ, Lewallen DG, Chao EYS. The effects of physiologic dynamic compression on bone healing under external fixation. Clin Orthop 1990;256:260–273.

Bennell KL, Malcolm SA, Brukner PD, et al. A 12-month prospective study of the relationship between stress fractures and bone turnover in athletes. Calcif Tissue Int 1998;63:80–85.

Bennell KL, Malcolm SA, Khan KM, et al. Bone mass and turnover in power athletes, endurance athletes and controls: a 12 month longitudinal study. Bone 1997a;20:477–484.

Bennell KL, Malcolm SA, Thomas SA, et al. The incidence and distribution of stress fractures in competitive track and field athletes: a 12-month prospective study. Am J Sports Med 1996;24:211–217.

Bennell KL, Malcolm SA, Wark JD, Brukner PD. Skeletal effects of menstrual disturbances in athletes. Scand J Med Sci Sports 1997b;7:261–273.

Bowman SM, Guo XE, Cheng DW, et al. Creep contributes to the fatigue behavior of bovine trabecular bone. J Biomech Engl 1998;120:647–654.

Boyce TM, Fyhrie DP, Glotkowski MC, et al. Damage type and strain mode associations in human compact bone bending fatigue. J Orthop Res 1998;16:322–329.

Bruckner P. Stress fractures of the upper limb. Sports Med 1998;26:415–424.

Bruckner P, Bradshaw C, Khan KM, et al. Stress fractures: a review of 180 cases. Clin J Sport Med 1996;6:85–89.

Buchanan JR, Myers C, Greer RB, et al. Assessment of the risk of vertebral fracture in menopausal women. J Bone Joint Surg Am 1987;69:212–218.

Burr DB, Turner CH, Naick P, et al. Does microdamage accumulation affect the mechanical properties of bone? J Biomech 1998;31:337–345.

Cervoni TD, Martire JR, Curl LA, McFarland EG. Recognizing upper extremity stress lesions. Physician Sports Med 1997;25:69.

Chaffin DB, Andersson GBJ. The Structure and Function of the Musculo-Skeletal System. In Occupational Biomechanics (2nd ed). Toronto: Wiley, 1991;27–29.

Claes LE, Heigele CA, Neidlingerwilke C, et al. Effects of mechanical factors on the fracture healing process. Clin Orthop Rel Res 1998;335(Suppl):132–147.

Dirschl DR, Henderson RC, Oakley WC. Accelerated bone mineral loss following a hip fracture: a prospective longitudinal study. Bone 1997;21:79–82.

Einhorn TA. The cell and molecular biology of fracture healing. Clin Orthop 1998;355S:S7–S21.

Finestone A, Giladi M, Elad H, et al. Prevention of stress fractures using custom biomechanical shoe orthoses. Clin Orthop Rel Res 1999;Mar:182–190.

Fredericson M. Common injuries in runners. Diagnosis, rehabilitation and prevention. Sports Med 1996;21:49–72.

Frost HM. Presence of microscopic cracks in vivo in bone. Bull Henry Ford Hospital 1960;8:25–35.

Goodman S, Aspenberg P. Effects of mechanical stimulation on the differentiation of hard tissues. Biomaterials 1993;14:563–568.

Gozna ER, Harrington IJ. Biomechanics of Musculoskeletal Injury. Baltimore: Williams & Wilkins, 1982.

Gustilo RB. The Fracture Classification Manual. St. Louis: Mosby–Year Book, 1991.

Hayda RA, Brighton CT, Esterhai JL. Pathophysiology of delayed healing. Clin Orthop 1998;355(Suppl):31–40.

Heggeness MH, Doherty BJ. The trabecular anatomy of thoracolumbar vertebrae: implications for burst fractures. J Anat 1997;191:309–312.

Jacobsen SJ, Goldberg J, Miles TP, et al. Hip fracture incidence among the old and very old: a population-based study of 475,435 cases. Am J Public Health 1990;80:871–873.

Joakimsen RM, Fonnebo V, Magnus JH, et al. The Tromso Study: body height, body mass index and fractures. Osteoporosis Int 1998;8:436–442.

Karlson KA. Rib stress fractures in elite rowers: a case series and proposed mechanisms. Am J Sports Med 1998;26:516–519.

Khan K, Brown J, Way S, et al. Overuse injuries in classical ballet. Sports Med 1995;19:341–357.

Kleerekoper M, Villanueva AR, Stanciu J, et al. The role of three-dimensional trabecular microstructure in the pathogenesis of vertebral compression fractures. Calcif Tissue Int 1985;37:594–597.

Lundon K, Bray K, Melcher L. Stress fracture incidence in students involved in intensive ballet training. Momentum-Sports Physiother Can 1998;22:18–22.

Mann T, Oviatt SK, Wilson D, et al. Vertebral deformity in men. J Bone Miner Res 1992;7:1259–1265.

Matheson G, Clement DB, McKenzie DC, et al. Stress fractures in athletes. Am J Sports Med 1987a;15:46–58.

Matheson G, Clement DB, McKenzie DC, et al. Scintigraphic uptake of 99-Tc at nonpainful sites in athletes with stress fractures: the concept of due strain. Sports Med 1987b;4:65.

Melton LJ, Atkinson EJ, O'Connor MK, et al. Bone density and fracture risk in men. J Bone Miner Res 1998;13:1915–1923.

Melton LJ, Kan SH, Frye MA, et al. Epidemiology of vertebral fractures in women. Am J Epidemiol 1989;129:1000–1011.

Mosekilde L, Viidik A, Modekilde LE. Correlation between the compressive strength of iliac and vertebral trabecular bone in normal individuals. Bone 1985;6:292–295.

Myburgh MH, Hutchins J, Fataar AB, et al. Low bone density as an etiologic factor for stress fractures in athletes. Ann Intern Med 1990;113:754–759.

Norman TL, Wang Z. Microdamage of human cortical bone: incidence and morphology in long bones. Bone 1997;20:375–379.

Oden A, Dawson A, Dere W, et al. Lifetime risk of hip fractures is underestimated. Osteoporos Int 1998;8:599–603.

O'Malley MJ, Hamilton WG, Munyak J, Defranco MJ. Stress fractures at the base of the 2nd metatarsal in ballet dancers. Foot Ankle Int 17:89–94.

Parfitt AM, Mathews CH, Villanueva AR, et al. Relationships between surface, volume and thickness of iliac trabecular bone in aging and in osteoporosis. Implications for the microanatomic and cellular mechanisms of bone loss. J Clin Invest 1983;72:1396–1409.

Pope RP. Prevention of pelvic stress fractures in female army recruits. Mil Med 1999;164:370–373.

Ramnemark A, Nyberg L, Borssen B, et al. Fractures after stroke. Osteoporosis Int 1998;8:92–95.

Reddi AH. Initiation of fracture repair by bone morphogenetic proteins. Clin Orthop 1998;355(Suppl):66–72.

Reid DC. Sports Injury Assessment and Rehabilitation. New York: Churchill Livingstone, 1992.

Runge M. The multifactorial etiology of gait disorders, falls, and hip fractures in the elderly. Zeitschrift fur Gerontologie Geriatrie 1997;30:267–275.

Sallis RE, Jones K. Stress fractures in athletes. How to spot this underdiagnosed injury. Postgrad Med 1991;89:185–188,191–192.

Schaffler MB, Radin EL, Burr DB. Long term fatigue behavior of compact bone at low strain magnitude and rate. Bone 1990;11:321–326.

Schultz RJ. The Language of Fractures (2nd ed). Baltimore: Williams & Wilkins, 1990;4.

Scully TJ, Besterman G. Stress fracture: a preventable training injury. J Mil Med 1982;147:285–287.

Seeman E. Advances in the Study of Osteoporosis in Men. In PJ Meunier (ed). Osteoporosis: Diagnosis and Management. London: Dunitz 1998;211–232.

Shearman CM, Brandser EA, Parman LM, et al. Longitudinal tibial stress fractures: a report of 8 cases and review of the literature. J Comput Assist Tomogr 1998;22:265–269.

Turner CH, Burr DB. Basic biomechanical measurements of bone: a tutorial. Bone 1993;14:595–608.

Vandershueren D, Boonen S, Bouillon R. Action of androgens versus estrogens in male skeletal homeostasis. Bone 1998;23:391–394.

Vestergaard P, Krogh K, Rejnmark L, Mosekilde L. Fracture rates and risk factors for fractures in patients with spinal cord injury. Spinal Cord 1998;36:790–796.

Voloshin AS, Mizrahi J, Verbitsky O, Isakov E. Dynamic loading on the human musculoskeletal system: effect of fatigue. Clin Biomech 1998;13:515–520.

Wolf JW, White AA, Panjabi MM, Southwick WO. Comparison of cyclic loading versus constant compression in the treatment of long-bone fractures in rabbits. J Bone Joint Surg 1981;63:805–810.

Yamada H. Strength of Biological Materials. In FG Evans (ed), Baltimore: Williams & Wilkins, 1970.

Yoo JU, Johnstone B. The role of osteochondral progenitor cells in fracture repair. Clin Orthop Rel Res 1998;355 (Suppl):73–81.

Young N, Formica C, Szmukler G, et al. Bone density at weightbearing and non-weightbearing sites in ballet dancers: the effects of exercise hypogonadism and body weight. J Clin Endocrinol Metab 1994;78:449–454.

Zerahn B, Olsen C, Stephensen S, et al. Bone loss after hip fracture is correlated to the postoperative degree of mobilization. Arch Orthop Trauma Surg 1998;117:453–456.

Part III
Pathophysiology of Mineralized Connective Tissue

Chapter 10
Acquired Disorders of Bone

Response of Bone to Immobilization

The maintenance of an optimal level of bone mass relies on the sustained application of mechanical stimuli. This concept is exemplified by the immediate activation of bone remodeling units and loss of bone tissue that occurs when functional loading is reduced. Conditions that lead to accelerated bone resorption and hypercalcemia, particularly in individuals whose underlying rate of bone turnover is already high, include bed rest (Krolner and Toft 1983), limb immobilization (Uhthoff and Jaworski 1978), stress protection adjacent to internal fixation devices (Woo et al. 1976), or weightlessness during space flight (Smith et al. 1977; Tilton et al. 1980).

The classic clinical scenario of bone atrophy and corresponding hypercalciuria is witnessed in the patient convalescing from a bone fracture that may necessitate a degree of immobilization for varying periods of time. Regardless of the cause, immobilization in plaster, bed rest, and the weightless state all result in derangements in phosphorus, nitrogen, and calcium metabolism and muscle atrophy. Immobilization, if continued for an extended period of time, results in detectable demineralization, particularly in the load-bearing extremities. In cases of severe paralysis, notable demineralization manifests at a much slower rate in the upper extremities compared to the lower extremities, indicating a difference in the response of weightbearing and nonweightbearing bones to immobilization. Decreased muscle pull on the periosteum, diminished direct physical forces on the bone, and corresponding circulatory and systemic changes associated with disuse contribute to the overall effect of bone loss under these conditions (Figure 10-1). The mechanism by which unloading of the skeleton results in rapid mobilization of calcium stores from the skeleton and bone resorption remains speculative, and the changes in metabolism under conditions of weightlessness are complex. This mechanism may be related to down regulation in parathyroid hormone (PTH) and 1,25-dihydroxyvitamin D_3 ($1,25[OH]_2D_3$) production (Horlick 1998). An increased resorption of bone is indicated by an increase in both urinary hydroxyproline and calcium excretion. In addition, evidence of interruption of bone *formation* processes exists in space flight (Carmeliet and Bouillon 1999; Morey and Baylink 1978), in patients with recent paralysis from poliomyelitis (Whedon and Shorr 1957), and in the immobilized (suspended) femora from growing animal models (Chen et al. 1992; Li et al. 1990). Therefore, both increases in resorption and decreases in bone formation occur under conditions of disuse. In cancellous bone, the combination of elevated bone resorption and depressed bone formation processes creates a negative bone balance, with the overall effect of reduced number and connectivity of the trabeculae (Chen et al. 1992).

Effect of Immobilization on the Organic Matrix of Bone

In one study of bone matrix, mature, stable cross-link concentrations and their molecular loci remained constant under conditions of both limb immobilization

Clinical Note

Clinical Hallmarks of Bone Loss

1. Hypercalcemia, which develops within days to weeks of the onset of bed rest, is associated with:
   (a) uncoupling of bone cell activity (e.g., increased osteoclastic bone resorption, decreased osteoblastic bone formation) and (b) hypercalciuria leading to both upper and lower urinary tract nephrolithiasis.
2. Increased urinary hydroxyproline excretion, indicating an increased resorption of bone matrix.
3. Osteopenia.

and subsequent re-ambulation. Covalent intermolecular cross-links between collagen molecules are essential in providing connective tissue matrices with stability and tensile strength. Long-term recovery of bone is likely based on new collagen formation processes (Yamauchi et al. 1988) and the eventual return of the rate of collagen synthesis to the levels seen in control bone. Long-term disuse also has been associated with decreased proteoglycan synthesis and altered orientation in bone tissue (Dodds et al. 1990).

In a clinical study, significant loss in both cortical and cancellous bone regions was observed after 17 weeks of continuous bed rest in normal males; however, skeletal recovery within 6 months of re-ambulation was varied (LeBlanc et al. 1990). In this study, select bones, such as the calcaneus, demonstrated complete recovery of bone mass in comparison to significant, but incomplete, recovery at the pelvis and trunk regions. This finding suggests that bone loss from certain regions is differentially reversible.

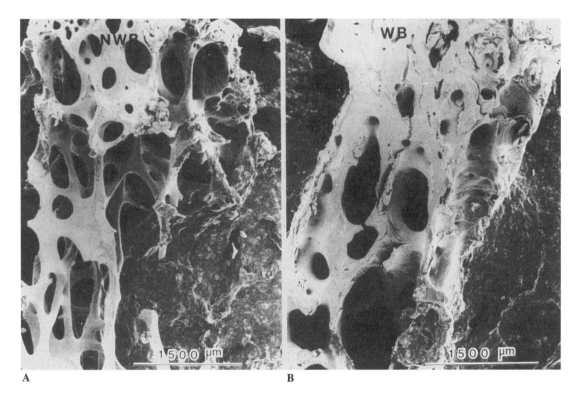

A   B

Figure 10-1. Cancellous bone loss under (**A**) nonweightbearing (NWB) and (**B**) weightbearing (WB) conditions in mature age-matched bone. (Courtesy of Marc Grynpas, Ph.D., Samuel Lunenfeld Research Institute, Mount Sinai Hospital, Toronto.)

Clinical Note

Bed rest may be advocated when it is requisite to diminish the functional demands on the body; however, it is associated with many rapidly occurring adverse effects on skeletal integrity that begin at all ages and continue for an extended period. The immobilized patient recovering from a bone fracture presents the classic scenario for atrophy of bone and hypercalciuria. Care must be taken when prescribing bed rest for other conditions. For instance, a significant decrease in bone mineral of the lumbar spine was demonstrated in patients placed on prolonged bed rest in the management of low back pain. The overall change in bone mineral density (BMD) during this period of bed rest was a decrease of 3.6% (±1.2%) or an average of 0.9% per week. Although bone mass was restored at a rate of 1% per month on re-ambulation (Krolner and Toft 1983), recovery of bone with re-ambulation may not occur as rapidly as the bone loss over the period of disuse.

Apparently, for some areas, the bone that is lost during bed rest is recoverable, but the rates of recovery are site-dependent and possibly vary among individuals. Large regions of the total body appear to regain bone, whereas some regions (the spine and hip, in particular) show recovery rates significantly less than the initial rates of loss (LeBlanc et al. 1990). In patients immobilized for injuries other than fracture, the rate of bone loss from the spine can be up to 4–8 times greater than in bed rest alone (Hansson et al. 1975; Krolner and Toft 1983; Mazess and Whedon 1983). This pattern of bone loss under conditions of immobilization is selectively reversible, and bone can be restored, at least partially, by re-introducing load-bearing activity (Krolner and Toft 1983).

Spinal Cord Injury, Paraplegia, and Bone Loss

A significant increase in markers of bone resorption and modest changes in bone formation were observed 10–16 weeks after acute spinal cord injury (SCI), with marginally elevated levels in markers of bone resorption in quadriplegia compared to paraplegia (Roberts et al. 1998). Significantly greater differences in loss of BMD in the lumbar spine, trochanteric region, and upper extremities were observed in quadriplegic compared to paraplegic patients (Tsuzuku et al. 1999).

Stroke and Bone Loss

Hemiplegia is associated with excessive bone loss in the paralyzed arm. In one study of bone loss in a normal versus hemiplegic extremity, the bone at both cancellous and cortical sites was positively correlated with the duration of stroke and negatively correlated with a reduction in forearm function (Prince et al. 1988). In other words, a reduction in function is associated with significant bone loss occurring over prolonged periods that may, at least in part, account for the significant bone loss seen in persons with conditions resulting in reduced mobility, such as neurologic and obstructive airways diseases. Good functional status and absence of spasticity appear to protect against bone loss in regions of cancellous bone; good functional status appears to be most protective in regions of cortical bone affected by hemiparesis (Prince et al. 1988). Two studies have shown an increased incidence of hip fracture of the hemiparetic limb compared to the normal limb after stroke (Mulley and Espley 1979; Peszczynski 1957), underlining the clinical ramifications of bone loss induced by the paretic or immobilized state.

Space Flight and Bone Loss

Strength testing before and after space flight indicates the partial success of exercise countermeasures during the in-flight period. An in-flight exercise program may be effective in protecting the muscles during space flight–induced weightlessness (Thornton and Rummel 1977); however, bone loss may continue, although to a lesser degree, in comparison to ground-based bed rest studies (Smith et al. 1977).

Management of Immobilization-Induced Bone Loss

Weightbearing

Osteoclastic bone resorption, hypercalciuria, and hypercalcemia are all associated with immobilization and may reverse with the resumption of normal weightbearing. In those for whom ambulation is impossible, the simple act of standing each day may be adequate to prevent bone loss resulting from immobilization. In fact, in a study of healthy immobilized persons (Krolner and Toft 1983), excessive bone loss was attenuated by quiet standing for short periods. Calcium excretion induced by immobilization was lessened by maintaining subjects on an oscillating bed for 8 hours per day during 5 weeks of bed rest (Dietrick et al. 1948).

Exercise

The purpose of performing active muscle contraction is to stimulate the sites where muscles attach to bone. Isometric exercise is at least partly protective against excessive bone loss under conditions of weightlessness. An isometric exercise regime may be effective in preventing full muscle atrophy in immobilized humans for other reasons (Donaldson et al. 1970) and additionally simulates partial loading on bone in situations in which standing is not possible. Passive range of motion (ROM) exercises are essentially ineffective in inducing an osteogenic response.

Pharmacology

Pharmacologic treatment includes the use of bisphosphonates, which may reverse or diminish immobilization-induced hypercalcemia and osteopenia. The general effect of these drugs is to attenuate osteoclastic activity and specifically decrease levels of circulating PTH, $1,25(OH)_2D_3$, and urinary cyclic adenosine monophosphate excretion.

Osteopathy Associated with Organ Transplantation

Organ transplantation is the end-stage treatment for renal, hepatic, cardiac, and pulmonary disease. Phar- macologic regimens to prevent rejection after organ transplantation commonly include high-dose glucocorticoids and calcineurin-calmodulin phosphatase inhibitors (the cyclosporines and tacrolimus). These drugs are detrimental to bone and mineral homeostasis because they are associated with rapid bone loss that is often superimposed on an already compromised skeleton (Rodino and Shane 1998). Routine assessment of skeletal status of organ transplant recipients is now a consideration both before and after organ transplantation (Seibel 1997). The purpose of this is, first, to detect existing or pre-transplantation bone disease and, second, to ensure vigilance for signs of osteopathy that may develop after organ transplantation.

Pretransplantation Osteopathy

Specific and broad clinical evaluation, including biochemical tests, are selected according to the underlying disease and type of organ failure. At this point, biochemical markers (e.g., alkaline phosphatase levels) may be helpful in providing information about imbalances in bone remodeling processes. However, biochemical markers of bone metabolism have inherent limitations in that complex metabolic perturbations typical of chronic organ failure may obscure meaningful and accurate interpretation of these findings as they relate to skeletal dynamics. Low pretransplant BMD appears to increase the risk of fracture after organ transplant; however, patients may sustain fractures posttransplant despite normal pretransplant BMD values (Rodino and Shane 1998).

Post-Transplantation Osteopathy

Osteopenia is a frequent and severe complication of organ transplantation that substantially reduces the recipient's quality of life should fracture occur. Incidence of fracture may range from 8% to 65% during the first year post-transplantation, with fracture and the greatest bone mineral loss occurring during the first 6–12 months after organ transplantation. Fracture rates appear to be lowest in renal transplant recipients and highest in patients who receive a liver transplant for primary biliary cirrhosis (Rodino and Shane 1998). Biochemical markers of bone turnover may assist in monitoring skeletal response after organ transplantation. Pre– and post–organ transplantation measurement of bone mass using dual energy x-ray absorptiometry may be obtained to assess the individual's risk of fracture. Because osteopenia and osteoporosis may be induced with the use of corticosteroids alone in the preventive management of acute rejection of the transplant, it is considered prudent to use prophylactic measures to prevent this bone loss whenever possible. If osteoporosis ensues after organ transplantation, a triple therapy approach, consisting of calcium, vitamin D, and either calcitonin or bisphosphonates, may be used without negative effects on graft function (Grotz et al. 1997). Most pharmacologic agents available for therapy of osteoporosis have not been subject to prospective controlled studies in organ transplant recipients; however, antiresorptive drugs, such as the bisphosphonates, do appear to hold therapeutic promise (Rodino and Shane 1998).

Osteopathy Associated with Specific Organ Transplantation

Gastrectomy

Osteopenia and enhanced risk of fracture have been reported after partial gastrectomy (Liedman et al. 1997). In gastrectomy, altered calcium and bone metabolism results in a high prevalence of bone disorders. Postgastrectomy bone disease is hypothesized to result from a calcium deficit, which increases calcium release from bone and impairs calcification of newly built bone matrix (Zittel el al. 1997b). It has been suggested that because of the impaired calcium absorption that follows gastrectomy, serum calcium is decreased, resulting in counter-regulation by PTH release and $1,25(OH)_2D_3$ formation. Both PTH and $1,25(OH)_2D_3$ are known to release calcium from bone, and loss of bone mass and increased fracture risk results in many gastrectomized patients (Zittel et al. 1997a). In fact, one study demonstrated a sixfold increase in the risk of sustaining a vertebral fracture and deformity after gastrectomy (Zittel et al. 1997a).

Renal Transplantation

Osteopenia and osteoporosis are frequent complications after kidney transplantation (Coleman 1998). Immunosuppressive agents and a persistence of hyperparathyroidism have been implicated in its etiology (Dissanayake and Epstein 1998). In addition, renal transplantation patients are unique in that the bone changes may occur superimposed on preexisting renal osteodystrophy. Cyclical therapy with antiresorptive agents did, however, effect gains in BMD at the lumbar spine in patients with low bone mass after kidney transplantation (Grotz et al. 1998).

Cardiac Transplantation

Bone loss occurs at an impressive rate in the first postoperative year after cardiac transplantation; however, prophylactic administration of calcium carbonate and vitamin D supplements are considered useful agents to reduce the related bone loss and the potential complications of osteopenia in this population (Vancleemput et al. 1996).

Lung Transplantation

Recipients of lung transplants are also at risk for osteopenia. In one study, 42% of lung transplant recipients sustained vertebral fractures, with symptomatic bone disease attributed to high turnover bone loss and hypovitaminosis D associated with this condition (Aringer et al. 1998).

Osteopathy Associated with Systemic Disease

The risk of osteopenia and osteoporosis is increased in patients with conditions such as inflammatory bowel disease (Schoon et al. 1999; Tirpitz et al. 1999), especially if additional risk factors such as glucocorticoid therapy, hypogonadism, or malnutrition coexist (Compston 1997; Schulte et al. 1998). Clinical and immunologic studies support an important etiopathogenetic link between intestinal and articular inflammation, and there is increasing evidence of a negative relationship between bone mass and intestinal inflammation (Devos et al. 1998). Bone disorders also are associated with cirrhosis; females with this condition are the most likely to lose bone mass (Masaki 1998). Chronic renal failure is often associated with bone disorders, including secondary hyperparathyroidism, aluminum-related low turnover bone disease, and osteomalacia (Urena 1998). Decreased bone density and increased risk of fractures are typical in patients with cystic fibrosis. Suboptimal vitamin D levels, nutrition problems, hypogonadism,

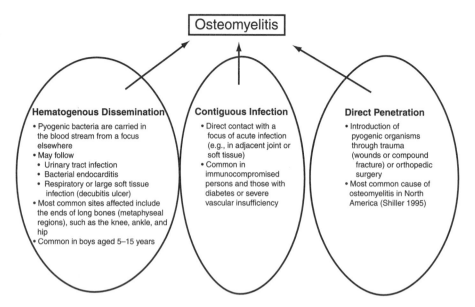

Figure 10-2. Osteomyelitis: routes by which bone may become infected.

inactivity, corticosteroid use, and altered cytokines all may potentially contribute to the low bone mass seen in these patients (Ott and Aitken 1998). Osteopenia is also a well recognized medical complication of anorexia nervosa (Lennkh et al. 1999).

Infectious Diseases of Bone

Osteomyelitis

Osteomyelitis is the invasion of bone and marrow cavities by infectious, pyogenic organisms, leading to inflammation of the bone. Immunosuppressed or chronically debilitated persons (e.g., persons with diabetes and alcoholism) are at great risk for developing osteomyelitis.

Etiology

Three routes exist by which infection of bone may occur (Figure 10-2). In 60–70% of cases, hemolytic *Staphylococcus aureus* is the organism that causes osteomyelitis. Other organisms, such as group B streptococcus, pneumococcus, *Escherichia coli*, *Neisseria gonorrhoeae*, *Haemophilus influenzae*, and salmonella, or any bacterial or fungal agent may also be involved. Sources of bony infections include vascular prosthesis, heart valves, sutures,

catheters, and allografts, to name a few. In the orthopedic population, bone and joint infections may develop after the surgical insertion of prostheses or implantation of fixation devices (Felten et al. 1998). Although the metaphyseal region is the most common site of infection in children, any region of the bone may be infected in adults.

Pathogenesis

With proliferation of the invading virulent organism, pressure on adjacent thin-walled vessels is created. Trauma may also increase the likelihood of infection by impeding blood flow. This encroachment results in compromised blood supply to the area and induces bone necrosis within a few days. The point of entry for these organisms is through the nutrient or metaphyseal vessels, with subsequent movement into the medullary canal (Figure 10-3). An inflammatory process is triggered, with an accumulation of polymorphonuclear leukocytes at the site of bacterial invasion and an increase in vascularity and edema. With time (2–6 weeks), portions of affected bone die as a result of ischemia caused by the thrombosis of local blood vessels. Necrotic areas merge to create an avascular zone, which allows even more extensive bacterial proliferation. Increased pressure on the confined area causes the pus to be extruded through Volkmann's

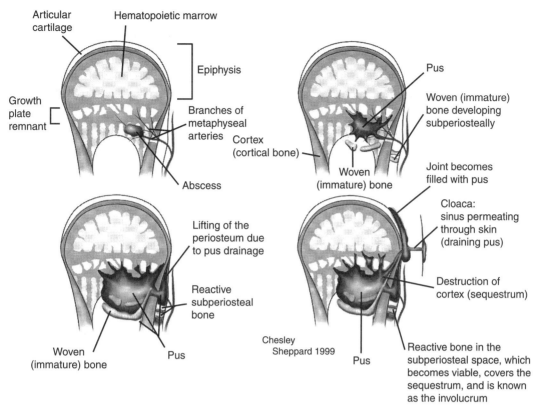

Figure 10-3. Pathogenesis of hematogenous osteomyelitis.

canals and haversian canals of the cortex to the surface of the bone where it may then spread subperiosteally to enter the bone at another site or may burst out into surrounding tissues (Figure 10-4). When the periosteum becomes detached, a subperiosteal abscess is created, disrupting the blood supply to the bone and resulting in further ischemic necrosis of the bone. At this point, the infection may spread to the epiphysis and joint capsule. After approximately 6 weeks, this necrosis may stimulate the periosteal osteoblasts to form a sheath of bone (involucrum) that surrounds the necrotic bone (sequestrum) (Figure 10-5) and separates it from viable bone tissue. Bone lesions may be the result of either osteolytic or osteoblastic activity. Osteolytic activity involves bone destruction; osteoblastic activity involves the reparative or reactive bone formation. Osteolytic bone lesions may be one of three different destructive bone processes. The first, referred to as *geographic destruction*, occurs when large patches of bone become destroyed and in turn

are reflected in radiolucent areas by radiographic analysis. When several small holes appear through the bone, it is referred to as *moth-eaten destruction*. The final type of destruction of bone, *permeative destruction*, occurs across the haversian systems. Because the periosteum is firmly attached to the articular margins in adults, extension of infection to joints is limited; however, pathologic fractures may ensue because of the weakened bone cortex (Mourad 1994). Over time, pus may penetrate the periosteum and the skin to create a sinus draining pus, bone, and bacteria from the *cloaca* (the hole created during formation of a draining sinus) to the skin (Figure 10-6).

Tuberculous Osteomyelitis

Mycobacterial infection of bone complicates an estimated 1–3% of cases of pulmonary tuberculosis (TB). This condition is problematic in developing

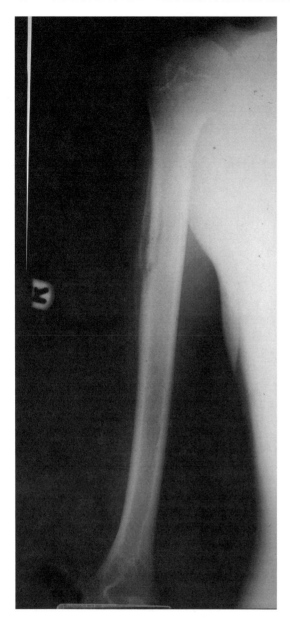

Figure 10-4. Sixteen-year-old male presenting with *Staphylococcus aureus* osteomyelitis affecting the humerus. (Courtesy of Dr. Edna Becker, M.D., Toronto Hospital, Toronto.)

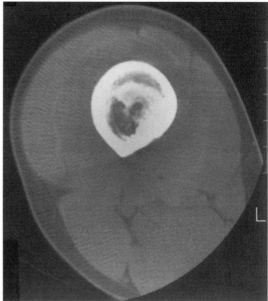

Figure 10-5. Computed tomographic scan demonstrating the involucrum and sequestrum typical of osteomyelitis (at approximately 6 weeks post-infection). (Courtesy of Dr. Edna Becker, M.D., Toronto Hospital, Toronto.)

countries and is becoming increasingly prevalent in industrialized countries with the resurgence of TB (Burns and Kumar 1997). The mycobacterium may reach the bone via hematogenous spread targeting the long bones and vertebrae. TB of the vertebral bodies is referred to as *Pott's disease*, a condition that manifests as vertebral deformity and collapse. A "cold abscess" may be witnessed in the psoas muscle, representing an extension of the tuberculous osteomyelitis infection of the spine.

The investigation of osteomyelitis may begin with routine radiography. Laboratory values and radiographs are typically negative in the early stages of osteomyelitis. Normal, healthy periosteum is indistinct in plain film radiography; when radiographic changes are noted in the early investigation of osteomyelitis, many findings are nonspecific. Although significant bony destruction may have ensued, bone changes in acute osteomyelitis may not be detectable on routine radiographs until more than 1 week after systemic signs and symptoms occur. A subperiosteal abscess that becomes apparent as lifting or thickening of the periosteum occurs away from bone cortex may be seen on plain film radiographs at this time. Other signs of bone destruction may be apparent. Radiologic evidence is typically noted after approximately 10 days. The three-phase bone scintigram is sensitive and specific in the study and diagnosis of osteomyelitis when routine radiographs demonstrate no other evidence for bone remodeling. In acute osteomyelitis, the blood-flow phase demonstrates increased perfusion at the site of inflammation. The second phase demonstrates increased blood-pool activity, and the third shows bone remodeling (Dono-

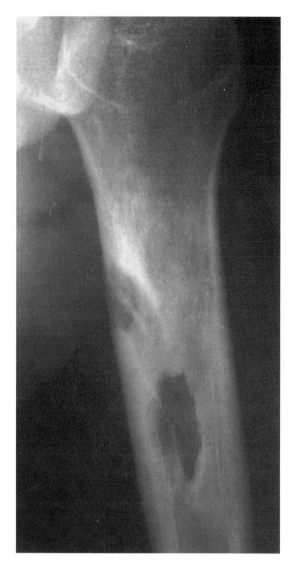

Figure 10-6. Osteomyelitis. Penetration of the periosteum as well as the skin creates a sinus that drains pus, bone, and bacteria from the cloaca to the skin. (Courtesy of Dr. Edna Becker, M.D., Toronto Hospital, Toronto.)

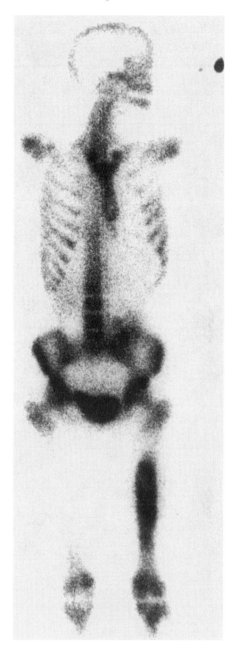

Figure 10-7. Osteomyelitis. Radionuclide bone scans are useful in locating the infection and identifying multiple sites of involvement. (Courtesy of Dr. Edna Becker, M.D., Toronto Hospital, Toronto.)

hoe 1998). Therefore, radionuclide bone scans are used to locate the infection site in the early stages of osteomyelitis and are useful in detecting and identifying multiple sites of involvement (Figure 10-7).

Acute Osteomyelitis

In the initial stages, osteomyelitis induced by pyogenic organisms causes systemic signs and symptoms typical of any acute infection, including fever, chills, an acutely ill appearance, malaise, degrees of leukocytosis, an extremely painful limb ("throbbing" pain), redness and swelling, diminished joint function, and hypersensitivity to touch. Infections related to the insertion of a joint prosthesis may manifest within a few days along the postoperative course.

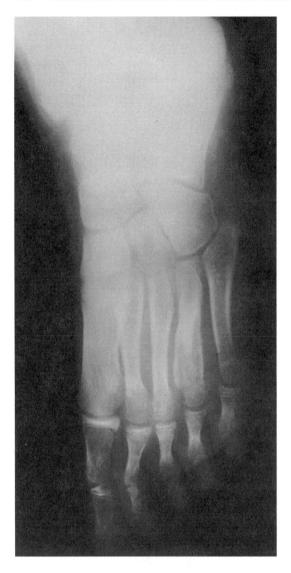

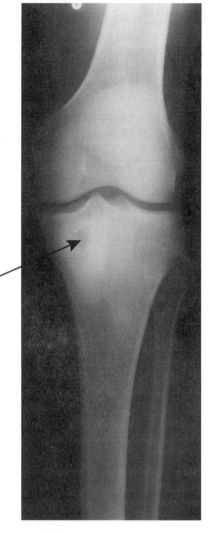

Brodie's abscess

Figure 10-9. Chronic osteomyelitis in a 30-year-old man with a 12-year history of periodic swelling in the proximal right tibia. The culture was positive for *Staphylococcus aureus*. Note the Brodie's abscess. (Courtesy of Dr. Edna Becker, M.D., Toronto Hospital, Toronto.)

Figure 10-8. Young male who presented with a recent history of pneumonia. Within a few weeks, subsequent bone pain was reported in the fourth metatarsal region. The diagnosis was osteomyelitis. (Courtesy of Dr. Edna Becker, M.D., Toronto Hospital, Toronto.)

Osteomyelitis may commence in cancellous bone that lacks pain sensory fibers so that pain may not present in the early acute phase. A deep, constant pain exacerbated by weightbearing may be experienced once the infection reaches the highly innervated periosteum (Figure 10.8). In the case of vertebral osteomyelitis, back pain may be intermittent or constant. The pain may throb at rest and worsen with movement. There may be spinal tenderness and rigidity. If the pain radiates, it may present with a radicular distribution. Characteristics of sacroiliac osteomyelitis include extreme localized pain that may radiate to the buttocks or abdomen, tenderness, swelling, and antalgic gait. Erythema, localized pain, and draining sinuses occur, regardless of whether osteomyelitis is induced by a hematogenous or post-traumatic route. Osteomyelitis is typically associated with the loosening of prostheses for joint arthroplasty or fixation devices for fracture stabilization. Post-traumatic osteomyelitis that continues to spread may manifest as local pain and draining sinuses. Although the delineation between acute and chronic osteomyelitis is not

Clinical Note

Osteomyelitis and Implications for Physical Rehabilitation

By current standards, the use of biomaterials, implants, fixation devices, and prostheses is common, and a large portion of physical rehabilitation is devoted to the postoperative care of these applications in the clinical setting. Clinicians involved in the physical management of musculoskeletal disorders are likely to encounter patients with osteomyelitis and can play an important role in its diagnosis and rehabilitation. Cognizance of the pathobiology underlying musculoskeletal infections enables the clinician to contribute to both establishing a diagnosis and initiating its management. When prostheses or internal fixation devices are used, special attention should be paid to monitor the drainage from surgical incisions, local signs of redness and swelling, increased body temperature, and unusual pain with routine exercise and weightbearing. Extreme discomfort with movement is felt in the acute phases of osteomyelitis, and it is prudent to rest the affected part so that infection is not spread further by mechanical means. Active, active-assisted, or passive exercise to maintain ROM at adjacent and unaffected joints is indicated as appropriate.

always clear, the transition can occur when treatment is delayed or inadequate in the early phases.

Chronic Osteomyelitis

Chronic osteomyelitis is essentially incurable, especially when it involves the entire bone; necrotic bone or sequestra may become scar tissue, which in turn forms an enclosed bony area around the infection that is impenetrable to antibiotics known as *Brodie's abscess* (Figure 10-9). Organisms resistant to antibiotic therapy fill these chronically draining sinuses. The management of chronic osteomyelitis includes surgical débridement and a lifelong course of antibiotics. Chronic osteomyelitis may result as a complication of the treatment of open fractures. Great pain may be experienced in chronic osteomyelitis, and prolonged hospitalization may be required in its management.

Vertebral Osteomyelitis

Osteomyelitis may involve vertebral bodies in adults and typically is spread hematogenously from pelvic or urinary tract infections. The infectious organism may invade vertebral bodies, traversing and destroying the intervertebral disk as it progresses. Vertebral osteomyelitis is caused by *S. aureus* in the majority of cases; however, *E. coli* and other enteric organisms are also culprits in this condition. The lumbar

spine is the most commonly involved area (Patzakis et al. 1991). Severe cases of vertebral osteomyelitis may progress to vertebral collapse and cord compression, resulting in related neurologic deficits. Hip pain may be the result of a paravertebral abscess that extends to the psoas muscle.

Complications

Osteomyelitis may be further complicated by septicemia (bacteremia), acute bacterial arthritis, pathologic fracture, and endocarditis. Much less common complications are reactive systemic amyloidosis and squamous cell carcinomas within chronic sinus tracts (Burns and Kumar 1997).

Prevention and Treatment

When open fractures are being treated, best efforts to prevent osteomyelitis include thorough débridement, irrigation of the wound, and leaving it open for delayed closure. Massive and sometimes prolonged antibiotic therapy typically arrests the infection. Infection that follows total joint arthroplasty may require removal of the hardware and surgical débridement for joint sepsis (Gristina et al. 1991). Because blood cultures may or may not indicate the presence of the causative organism, needle biopsy of the infected bone may be necessary in some cases (e.g., vertebral osteomyelitis). The infectious microorganism may be identified by aspiration, needle biopsy, or swab so that

Table 10-1. Risk Factors Associated with Acquired Ectopic Ossification (EO) Development in Various Populations

Condition	Risk Factor
Myositis ossificans traumatica	Male, early adult (20–30 yrs), contact with high velocity objects (Paterson, 1970)
Burns	Skin grafting (Elledge et al. 1988)
	Deep burn (Elledge et al. 1988)
	Type of joint affected (Elledge et al. 1988)
	Large body surface area burn, upper extremity burn, delayed grafting, excision
Total hip arthroplasty	Osteoarthritis with extensive osteophytes (Ritter and Vaughan 1977)
	Ankylosing spondylitis (HLA-B27-positive) (Ritter and Vaughan 1977)
	Previous hip surgery and EO development increases the likelihood of EO with surgery for contralateral hip (Coventry and Scanlon 1981; Ritter and Vaughan 1977)
	Reduced preoperative hip movement (Ritter and Vaughan 1977)
	Postoperative course without use of nonsteroidal anti-inflammatory agents (Pedersen et al. 1989)
	Previous preoperative hip joint dislocation (Vicar and Coleman 1984)
Spinal cord injury	Complete lesions, cervical lesions, midthoracic lesions and, less often, thoracolumbar lesions, lumbar lesions (Lal et al. 1989)
	Pressure sores (Lal et al. 1989)
	Spasticity (Lal et al. 1989)
	Age <30 yrs
	Male
	? Urinary/respiratory infections (Wittenberg et al. 1992)
Traumatic brain injury	Older than 11 years of age (Hurvitz et al. 1992)
	Associated musculoskeletal trauma and spasticity (Garland 1988; Mital et al. 1987)
	Coma >7 days (Hurvitz et al. 1992; Mital et al. 1987)

Source: Reprinted with permission from K Lundon and D Hampson. Acquired ectopic ossification of soft tissues: implications for physical therapy. Can J Rehab 1997;10:231–246.

appropriate medication and antibiotic care may be prescribed. Surgical removal of the foreign material may be required when possible (Felten et al. 1998). If the infection has disseminated to the joints, surgical intervention becomes necessary. Because articular cartilage may become damaged within hours, it becomes necessary to expedite the drainage of exudate or pus from the bone or joint. Débridement of both bone and surrounding soft tissue and reconstructive procedures may be required once the infection is controlled. The treatment of chronic osteomyelitis is more difficult than acute osteomyelitis because of the nature of the condition, and its prognosis is poor. Antibiotics and radical surgery to remove infected tissue may be performed; however, these efforts may not fully eradicate the infectious organism with any certainty.

Ectopic Ossification

Ectopic ossification (EO) is a biological process whereby new bone is formed, due to metaplasia of connective tissue, in areas which normally do not ossify. Although frequently benign, the development of EO may become painful, restrict motion, and require surgical intervention. The development of EO follows lesions of the central nervous system, such as traumatic brain injury (TBI) and spinal cord injury (Garland 1988; Wittenberg et al. 1992) and is a common complication after total hip arthroplasty (THA) (Brooker et al. 1973) and severe burns (Elledge et al. 1988). The risk factors for the development of EO in each population affected are summarized in Table 10-1. Immobilization, prolonged pressure transferred to periarticular structures, microtrauma, vascular stasis, lesions of the autonomic nervous system, hypoxia, hyperthermia, mobilization of the calcium pool, and genetic predisposition may all, or in part, be contributing factors to the prevailing conditions (Béthoux et al. 1995). In fact, bleeding alone, independent of skeletal trauma, may evoke a systemic osteogenic response by activating osteoprogenitor cells in the bone marrow (Lucas et al. 1997). EO is one of three main types of extraskeletal ossification involving induction and mineralization of bone matrix with osteoblasts and osteoclasts present. The other two types of extraskeletal ossification include metastatic calcification, which is calcification due to hypercalcemia or hyperphosphatemia, and dystrophic calcification, which involves amorphous calcium deposition due to abnormalities in tissue and in the absence of any osteoblastic activity (Russell and Kanis 1984).

EO may be acquired or congenital. The congenital form, *fibrodysplasia* (*myositis*) *ossificans progressiva* (MOP) is a rare, primary disorder of connective tissue with secondary involvement of muscle fibers involving the deposition of bone in the large striated muscles of the limb girdle and the paravertebral muscles of the back (Garland 1988; Smith 1998). Ultimately, large groups of muscles become ossified, leading to an early death from terminal asphyxia due to the restricting effect of the ectopic bone on joint mobility and respiratory movement. EO that is *acquired* as a result of traumatic injury to muscle tissue is herein referred to as *myositis ossificans traumatica* (MOT). The term *heterotopic ossification* encompasses all other forms of acquired EO that may occur in the burn, THA, and TBI populations.

Although it is recognized that EO is a process of abnormally located bone growth, the etiology and pathophysiology of acquired EO are unknown (Hinck 1994). The triggering mechanism by which undifferentiated connective tissue cells develop into osteoblasts rather than other connective tissue types or muscle has been under intense investigation (Grigoriadis et al. 1988; Grigoriadis et al. 1990). Perivascular mesenchymal connective tissue cells have been implicated as a source of fibroblasts and osteoblasts (Buring 1975). Other factors include antigen-antibody interaction, metabolic disorders, mechanical stimulation (including trauma) (Jowsey et al. 1977), neural influences (Goodman et al. 1997), and a naturally occurring chemical stimulant that appears in the area of ectopic bone formation (Hinck 1994).

Two distinct cell populations have been implicated in the formation of ectopic bone: (1) cells present in periosteal, endosteal, and stromal connective tissue that may have osteogenic potential derived from previous contact with bone tissue and (2) a more slowly reacting cell population present in mesenchymal cells of endomysium that, under the influence of some triggering mechanism, pro-

liferate and show an ability to differentiate into osteoblasts and produce osseous matrix (Kewalramani 1977). The condition *rhabdomyolysis* occurs when there is lysis of striated muscle cells that release their content into the extracellular space, and it has been associated with the development of EO (Béthoux et al. 1995). Chantraine and Minaire (1981) claim that factors such as immobilization, edema, and infection are associated with the latent development of EO. Although the triggering factor is unknown, mesenchymal cells have been observed to undergo metaplastic changes to embryonic osteoblasts that then have the potential to develop into ectopic bone (Kewalramani 1977). A genetic predisposition is another possible etiologic factor in the development of EO, because those with ankylosing spondylitis (many of whom develop EO around the hip after THA) are positive for the HLA-B27 antigen. One study observed differential expression of bone- and cartilage-related genes in cell lines of MOT lesions in humans that may identify a molecular pathogenesis regulated by specific sets of genes that contribute to skeletal formation and repair (Shafritz and Kaplan 1998). In this study, cells derived from various osteogenic disorders, one of which was MOT, expressed different repertoires of bone morphogenetic proteins. In fact, retention of levels of bone morphogenetic protein-2 (BMP-2) was seen to induce bone formation under experimental conditions (Yamamoto et al. 1998).

Ectopic bone grows at triple the normal bone formation rate, displaying high cellular activity (Elmstedt et al. 1985) and a progression toward mature organized bone matrix over a 2-month to 2-year period (Hinck 1994). Cells derived from EO lesions have been shown to produce high levels of osteocalcin (bone Gla-protein), type I collagen, and alkaline phosphatase activity with increased rates of collagen synthesis and cell proliferation compared with normal osteoblasts (Kaysinger et al. 1997). As ectopic bone is being actively formed, an associated rise in local temperature and edema occurs. Once established, hard bone masses can be palpated in the deeper adjacent tissues. The spectrum of tissues that can be affected by EO includes muscle, tendon, ligament, menisci, and/or even the abdominal wall (Hinck 1994). EO presenting with neurologic lesions never involves either the periosteum or articular surfaces (Kewalramani 1977).

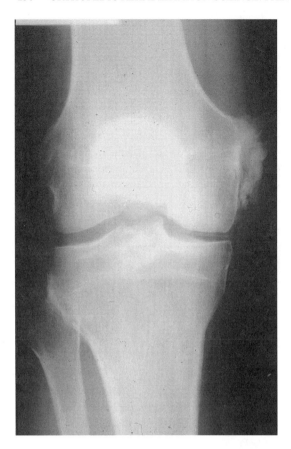

Figure 10-10. Ectopic ossification is established along the distal medial femoral condyle.

ing in hematoma. Despite evidence to suggest a causative role for trauma, the precise etiology in isolated cases of MOT remains unknown (Cvitanic and Sedlak 1995). It has been hypothesized that trauma acts to release osteogenic cells from the damaged periosteum, either as a flap or as free tissue that survives within the hemorrhagic tissues to form bone, and/or that osteoblasts form within repair tissue by metaplasia of cells indigenous to scar tissue (Walton and Rothwell 1983).

Plain film radiographs usually show soft tissue calcification in the muscle groups adjacent to the trauma (El-Khoury et al. 1996; Sud et al. 1992) within 3 weeks of injury (acute phase), reaching maturity within 6 months (Figure 10-10). Early lesions are characterized by degeneration of muscle cells, organization of the hemorrhage, and proliferation of connective tissue and, occasionally, cartilage (Ackerman 1958; Cushner and Morwessel 1992); mature lesions display fully formed bone surrounded by a fibrous capsule. MOT is isolated within the traumatized region of the muscle and may regress without treatment in as many as 35% of cases (Shafritz and Kaplan 1998). MOT may be suspected when there is pain and swelling associated with limitation of movement of an adjacent joint. Within a 4-week time frame, there may be a decline in pain, with irregularities and shadows parallel to bone seen on radiographs.

Myositis Ossificans Traumatica

MOT is representative of disorders of osteogenesis that occur within muscle secondary to traumatic intramuscular hematoma (Ackerman 1958; Rothwell 1982). MOT may follow events involving repeated strain, such as may occur in overuse injury of the adductor longus muscle in jockeys. MOT may also follow blunt physical trauma to skeletal muscle, as may be experienced in contact sport injuries. Athletes participating in sports or activities of this nature may be more vulnerable due to contact with objects moving at high velocity (Booth and Westers 1989; Cvitanic and Sedlak 1995; Paterson 1970). MOT predominantly affects healthy, active young men (Paterson 1970). MOT may also form as a consequence of repeated forcible distention of previously immobilized muscle (Michelsson and Rauschning 1983). Any of these conditions may cause extensive bleeding within muscle, result-

Heterotopic Ossification

In general, the subgroup of acquired EO referred to as *heterotopic ossification* is highly associated with conditions resulting in extended immobility such as coma, multiple limb fractures, and burns (Hurvitz et al. 1992).

Burns

EO may develop in patients with deep burns who are immobilized for prolonged periods and in whom there is significant pain, splinting, or contracture (Elledge et al. 1988; Mielantis et al. 1975). EO develops either distal or in close proximity to a joint in patients with burns (Edlich et al. 1985; Koch et al. 1992). Delayed grafting over sites appears to contribute to EO in that increases in EO are proportional to the length of time of extremity impairment and immobilization. The development of EO in the burn population has been associated with high protein intake that results in alteration of calcium transport by the kidneys (November-Dusansky et al. 1980). A mechanical influence appears to have definite bearing in that prolonged immobilization followed by joint manipulation also is associated with EO formation in a burn population (Koch et al. 1992). In addition, it is well known that healing after a burn is associated with increased vascularization and formation of fibroblasts (from mesenchymal cells) (Crawford et al. 1986). The average time of onset for EO to ensue after a burn is 12 weeks (Crawford et al. 1986). In the burn population, both direct and indirect influences on tissues make joint ankylosis a critical problem (Koch et al. 1992; Mital et al. 1987). The most commonly reported site of EO is the posterior region of the elbow joint, which is affected in 82.5% of burn patients with upper extremity involvement (Elledge et al. 1988). The nature of the elbow joint articulation may contribute to its vulnerability to EO development as well as to its poor response to aggressive treatment (Lundon and Hampson 1997). The presence of large total body surface area and upper extremity burns, in addition to delayed definitive therapy of the involved site (excision and grafting), are considered predictive of EO development in this population.

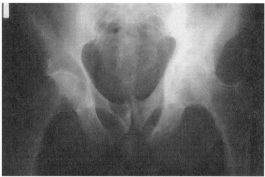

A

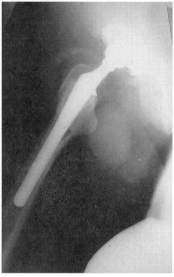

B

Figure 10-11. A. This 55-year-old man presented with marked narrowing of the left hip joint space because of osteoarthritis. **B.** Only 3 months after total hip arthroplasty, ectopic ossification is present in this same patient. (Reprinted with permission from K Lundon, D Hampson. Acquired ectopic ossification of soft tissues: implications for physical therapy. Can J Rehab 1997;10:231–246.)

Total Hip Arthroplasty

As a result of traumatic insult to the acetabular rim, bleeding and/or the reamings (which consist predominantly of bone marrow, stem cells, and fine particulate bone matter) may spill into soft tissues at the time of THA surgery, which may create a highly osteogenic environment (Elmstedt et al. 1985; Marks et al. 1988; Ritter and Vaughan 1977). A large volume of ectopic bone in the periarticular tissues around a hip replacement can be associated with impingement that is painful and adversely affects ROM (Ahrengart et al. 1988).

EO can be witnessed at 12–15 weeks post-THA (Figure 10-11). EO occurs as a complication of between 5% and 52% THA cases (Brooker 1973; Elmstedt 1985). Infected hip joints, active ankylosing spondylitis, previous incidence of EO, preoperative degenerative joint disease concentrated in the inferomedial aspect of the joint associated with osteophytes, recipients of a posterior and transtrochanteric surgical approach to the hip, and Paget's disease are conditions conducive to EO formation after hip surgery (Healy et al. 1995; Vicar and Coleman 1983). Male gender also appears to be associated with development of EO in these populations (Pedersen et al. 1989), as is trauma to the hip joint experienced with fracture and dislocation. Classification of ectopic bone formation after THA has been established in relation to the presence and degree of EO formation in the postoperative course (Brooker et al. 1973).

Neurologic Insult (Spinal Cord Injury and Traumatic Brain Injury)

The association of extent of head injury and development of EO is well documented (Anderson 1995; Garland et al. 1982; Marks et al. 1988), particularly when there is musculoskeletal trauma (Furman et al. 1999). Spasticity is considered an important neurogenic influence in the development of EO in patients with TBI and SCI (Garland 1988). Local microtrauma, disturbance of calcitonin and PTH levels, and a genetic predisposition also have been associated with the development of EO with SCI (Wittenberg et al. 1992).

The most common time frame for development of a lesion is 1 to 4 months after SCI, but it can occur as early as 18 days or as late as 1 year post-SCI (Lal et al. 1989). EO is known to selectively occur caudal to the level of the spinal cord lesion (Kewalramani 1977; Lal et al. 1989) and occurs at distinct sites of the hip (Kewalramani 1977; Wittenberg et al. 1992). The incidence of EO in the SCI population ranges from 1% to 53% (average of 20%), with 5% progressing to complete ankylosis (Garland 1988; Lal et al. 1989). Age, completeness of lesion, presence of pressure sores, and spasticity are significant contributing factors related to EO formation in the SCI population (Lal et al. 1989). A significantly higher incidence of EO was observed in a subset of 20 to 30-year-olds with SCI, in males (23%) compared to females (10%), and in patients sustaining lesions at the cervical and mid-thoracic spine compared to thoracolumbar and lumbar levels (Wittenberg et al. 1992). It is noteworthy that in SCI patients bone metabolism also is characterized by sub-lesional osteoporosis (occurring caudal to the neurologic lesion), which may be observed as early as 6 weeks after SCI (Chantraine et al. 1995).

EO is most commonly detected 2 months after incident of a TBI (Marinissen 1993). The most commonly affected sites of ectopic bone formation as studied in a pediatric and adolescent population with TBI include the hip (specifically the adductor mass) (Mital et al. 1987), the elbow, and the shoulder (Garland 1988; Hurvitz et al. 1992). The incidence of EO in the TBI population varies between 11% and 75%, with 16% progressing to ankylosis (Garland 1988). Coma and spasticity have been identified as common neurogenic factors in the development of EO in this population (Furman et al. 1999; Hurvitz et al. 1992; Mital et al. 1987).

Diagnosis of Ectopic Ossification

Physical Examination

A differential diagnosis of conditions such as hematoma, callus, muscle tumors, osteomyelitis, periostitis, and neoplasms (sarcoma) must be made to determine the identity of a hard, painful mass. The presence of EO should be suspected in any patient who presents with sudden loss of joint range with concurrent pain and loss of function (Garland 1988; Koch et al. 1992). The early diagnosis of EO is critical to minimize deformities, ankylosis, and disability associated with its development.

Imaging

The three-phase bone scan has been noted to detect EO 4–6 weeks earlier than plain film radiographs and can detect clinically silent cases that are not captured by plain film imaging (Crawford et al. 1986; Freed et al. 1982; Hurvitz et al. 1992). Because of signal characteristics inherent to different tissues, computed tomography and MRI allow the relationship between EO and bone to be clearly established (Béthoux et al. 1995). Plain film radiographs assist in the differential diagnosis of EO in that they can discriminate EO from other causes of decreased joint mobility, such as scar contracture or muscular rigidity (Elledge et al. 1988). In the case of acute MOT, however, MRI may be considered more accurate than competing imaging modalities because it can detect peripheral edema and displays signal characteristics consistent with the presence of proteinaceous fluid or myxoid stroma (Cvitanic and Sedlak 1995).

Biochemistry

The earliest indicator of EO is an elevated serum alkaline phosphatase reading, although laboratory tests for this enzyme in isolation of other evaluative tests are of limited value. Alkaline phosphatase is an enzyme secreted by osteoblasts when they are actively depositing bone matrix.

Normative adult values are 25–92 U/liter; however, in periods of active bone growth, such as fracture healing (which may complicate establishing the diagnosis of EO), levels can rise to 160 U/liter. Alkaline phosphatase levels have been recorded as high as 446 U/liter during active EO formation (Schaeffer and Sosner 1995). Hydroxyprolinuria (an increase in the urinary excretion of the nondialyzable fraction of hydroxyproline), as well as an initial peak of serum creatine phosphokinase, also have been reported (Béthoux et al. 1995).

Management Strategies for Acquired Ectopic Ossification

Regardless of cause, EO adversely affects mobility, self-care, activities of daily living, and functional independence, necessitating careful management in affected populations.

Pharmacology

Bisphosphonates. The diphosphonate ethane-1-hydroxy-1,1-diphosphonic acid (EHDP) is known to interfere with bone resorption and mineralization processes based on both in vivo and in vitro experiments. It is generally accepted that EHDP can prevent the conversion of amorphous calcium phosphate compounds to hydroxyapatite crystals, hence retarding the mineralization process. EHDP has been used to prevent ossification after myositis in the acute phase, to retard recalcification after surgical removal of existing ectopic bone, and also to prevent EO after operative intervention (Kewalramani 1977). In addition, administration of EHDP leads to the appearance of unmineralized osteoid tissue in pre-existing bone, and it may be used in an effort to resorb established EO (Garland et al. 1983; Plasmans et al 1978).

Nonsteroidal Anti-inflammatory Drugs Nonsteroidal anti-inflammatory agents such as indomethacin (Dorn et al. 1998; Ritter and Gioe 1982) and ibuprofen (Elmstedt et al. 1985; Persson et al. 1998) used after THA have proven to be effective in the prevention of EO by suppressing both the production of osteoid as well as ossification (Pedersen et al. 1989). Nonsteroidal anti-inflammatory agents

exert their effect on EO through inhibition of the synthesis of prostaglandins and related substances, which promote the initiation of inflammation and have been useful in minimizing the occurrence of EO in patients with TBI as well as preventing its recurrence once excised (Mital et al. 1987). The presence of prostaglandins is probably of importance for bone formation, because elevated levels of prostaglandins have been documented to appear in the muscle tissue surrounding a fracture site, although their source (bone or soft tissue) remains unclear. The use of anti-inflammatory medication may be associated with occasional gastrointestinal side effects and disturbed bone healing with prosthetic components (Schai et al. 1995). Thus, it is considered only as the second most effective treatment (after radiation) for the prevention of EO in this population.

Radiation Therapy

Early delivery of radiotherapy has proven to be an efficient means of preventing EO formation post-THA (Ayers et al. 1991; Schai et al. 1995), although the effectiveness of its delivery as a single event (Healy et al. 1995) rather than as a "fractionated" application (Coventry and Scanlon 1981) is controversial (Pellegrini et al. 1992). The mechanism by which early radiation therapy prevents EO development is by arresting pluripotential mesenchymal cells from proliferating and differentiating into osteoblasts (Ahrengart et al. 1988), thereby preventing the osteoblast-precursor cells from multiplying and forming active osteoblasts. It is thought by some that radiation assists in the prevention of EO but is of negligible value once the ectopic bone is visible by plain film radiography (Coventry and Scanlon 1981; Pittenger 1991). In one study, preoperative irradiation for prophylaxis of EO after THA effectively diminished the incidence of EO in this population (Vanleeuwen et al. 1998). In contrast, in a small group of multitrauma patients, radiation therapy was regarded not only to be useful in the prophylaxis of EO but also in its resolution (Schaeffer and Sosner 1995). A combination of irradiation within 16–20 hours before THA and the use of nonsteroidal anti-inflammatory drugs effected a decrease in the incidence of clinically relevant heterotopic ossification after total hip replacement (Kölbl et al. 1998).

Clinical Note

Manipulation to restore movement in the populations discussed remains a controversial management option in that there is, in both human and animal studies, some suggestion of its role in exacerbating EO formation. In one animal model study, it was determined that joints immobilized in extension and then forcibly exercised facilitated the development of EO in the extensor muscle group. Joints immobilized in flexion and subsequently subjected to forcible exercise led to the development of EO in the flexor muscles (Michelsson and Rauschning 1983). Forcible mobilization in previously immobilized muscle may lead to occasional hematomas in the muscle. Based on these findings, the prescription of exercise for a human joint after immobilization should involve only gentle active-assisted exercises within the pain-free range to decrease the chances of EO development (Michelsson and Rauschning 1983). Muscles such as the quadriceps that originate from large areas of bone and have actions that cross over an immobilized joint appear to be particularly vulnerable to EO formation.

Surgical Resection

Surgical excision of EO is recommended only after its complete maturation (6 months–2 years, depending on the population), and administration of a bisphosphonate regimen is recommended to prevent the possible recurrence of EO (Garland et al. 1985). In the case of MOT, premature removal of early lesions results in local recurrence of EO (Shafritz and Kaplan 1998).

Physical Management

Regardless of cause, deformities and limitation of motion subsequent to EO development present a serious impediment to the rehabilitative course. The classic treatment in the acute phase of MOT is *r*est, *i*ce, *c*ompression, and *e*levation (RICE), along with the application of pharmacologic agents. In the case of MOT, some recommend that passive movements should be avoided and that the affected joint rest in the early active phase of EO development. During the late phase of EO development, graduated active-assisted movements within the pain-free range should be encouraged as pain and swelling subside (Kewalramani 1977; Paterson 1970). A return to training should be avoided until a full stretch of the affected muscle group has been achieved (King 1998). In the burn population, physical therapy intervention, including active or active-assisted ROM exercises for major joints and preservation of muscle strength,

is considered important early in the treatment period. If decreased ROM and EO develop, perseverance with active-assisted exercises within the pain-free range of the patient is advocated (Elledge et al. 1988; Koch et al. 1992). In one study, before the diagnosis of EO, patients with burns were managed with an exercise program of active and active-assisted movements. In patients who persisted with passive and active-assisted ROM beyond the range of pain-free movements (thereby passively stretching periarticular structures), EO manifested and progressed to joint ankylosis. It is of interest that postoperative burn patients in whom EO developed and who continued to follow a program of active exercise within the pain-free range gained excellent ROM (Crawford et al. 1986). Although the triggering mechanisms appear similar, the clinical manifestations and the response to treatment in the TBI and SCI populations are dissimilar (Garland 1988). In those in whom a complete SCI lesion has been sustained, there is minimal to mild pain associated with EO, and musculature may be flaccid, thereby allowing joint mobilization in this population without great difficulty. The forces generated by muscle spasticity may promote EO formation (Lal et al. 1989) and, as patients with TBI frequently have increased tone about the involved joint, mobilization is rendered difficult (Garland et al. 1982). In this population, however, some consider that aggressive ROM and positioning must be initiated regardless of the possible effects of this intervention on spasticity and muscle guarding around the joint (Anderson 1995).

Avascular Necrosis (Ischemic Bone Disease)

Regional interruption of blood flow to the skeleton causes an important group of acquired disorders of cartilage and bone referred to as *avascular necrosis*. Other terms for this condition are *ischemic bone disease* (IBD), *osteonecrosis*, or *aseptic necrosis*. This condition occurs in the absence of infection in which severe and prolonged ischemia may cause regionally located osteoblasts and chondrocytes to die. Effort to repair bone occurs by resorption of necrotic areas of bone and cartilage, which ultimately compromises skeletal strength and predisposes the individual to fracture. A number of conditions lead to IBD (Table 10-2).

Etiology

Avascular necrosis occurs in the adult population, and the specific condition depends on the patient's age, the anatomic site, and the size of the area of bone where there is interruption of blood flow. Legg-Calvé-Perthes disease is an archetypical form of IBD that manifests in a pediatric population and exemplifies a version of IBD typical of this age group. Traumatic disruption of arterial blood flow or thrombosis that disrupts the microcirculation induces bony ischemia. Permanent loss of bone tissue manifesting in osteocytic necrosis may be sustained after a minimum of 2 hours of complete ischemia and anoxia (James and Steijn-Myagkaya 1986).

Pathogenesis

Several contributing causes for vascular insufficiency of bone have been identified, including traumatic rupture, obstruction, or excessive external pressure, all of which may lead to IBD. Specific bony sites, such as the femoral head, talus, scaphoid, and proximal humerus, are particularly vulnerable to ischemia. Although great variation exists in the clinical presentation of avascular necrosis that is primarily based on the affected anatomic region, the femoral head is the most

Table 10-2. Selected Conditions Associated with Ischemic Necrosis of Cartilage and Bone

---

Endocrine/Metabolic
Glucocorticoid therapy
Cushing's disease
Alcoholism
Gout
Osteomalacia
Systemic lupus erythematosus
Diabetes mellitus
Obesity
Pregnancy
Trauma
Dislocation
Fracture

---

common site of this disorder. Common characteristics of bony sites vulnerable to avascular necrosis include coverage by cartilage and restricted collateral circulation. Arteries, veins, or sinusoids may be directly affected. The pathogenesis of disrupted blood flow in IBD is not completely understood. For many types of nontraumatic ischemic necrosis, the predisposed sites of the skeleton seem to recapitulate the conversion of red marrow to fatty marrow seen during the aging process. Fat embolism, hemorrhage, and/or abnormalities in the quality of vulnerable bone tissue may also be pathogenetic factors in some types of traumatic or nontraumatic IBDs. A process of repair is initiated, but unless the lesion is small (e.g., less than 15% of the femoral head is involved), this repair process usually is ineffective. The net result is weakening of subchondral bone with subsequent collapse of the articular surface (Mont et al. 1998).

Anatomic Location

The clinical presentation of IBD may further be divided into two major anatomic categories: *diaphysometaphyseal* and *epiphysometaphyseal*. Larger infarcts typically involve the hip and femoral condyles. Large fragments of ischemic bone can collapse, thus flattening joint surfaces and destroying articular cartilage. Ultimately, this leads to the development of osteoarthritis. Extensive epiphysometaphyseal infarction results from trauma or systemic disease and frequently involves the femoral head.

Clinical Note

Considerations in Physical Rehabilitation

One must be vigilant when treating individuals who may be at risk of developing avascular necrosis. A remarkable loss in ROM, for example, in hip internal rotation, flexion, and adduction movements, in association with an acute increase in the complaints of pain, should alert the health care professional to the potential of avascular necrosis and pathologic fracture. Once IBD is diagnosed, precautions should be taken to monitor the course and progression of weightbearing and exercise.

Clinical Presentation

Symptoms

The affected individual may experience symptoms that result primarily from events associated with focal skeletal disintegration. In the case in which the femur is involved, pain is typically the presenting complaint, with specific reference to the groin, thigh, or medial knee regions. Because knee pain may be referred from the hip, the lumbar spine and hip regions should be assessed to make a differential diagnosis of pathology. Weightbearing or loading activity aggravates the symptoms. Range of motion exercises at the hip also elicit pain, particularly when the pattern involves internal rotation, flexion, and adduction. The affected individual may present with an antalgic gait.

Radiography

The radiologic manifestations of all forms of avascular necrosis depend on the variable amount of skeletal revascularization, reossification, and resorption of infarcted bone that occur subsequent to the onset of this condition. Revascularization typically occurs within 6–8 weeks of the ischemic event and may cause excessive cancellous bone resorption seen radiographically as radiolucent bands near the necrotic areas. Subsequent new bone formation ensues on dead bone surfaces. Over the course of months or even years, dead bone may or may not be slowly resorbed. Osteosclerosis occurs if new bone encases dead bone and/or if there is bony collapse, demonstrating that these processes are focal and may occur simultaneously. A change in BMD is typical of osteonecrosis; however, it may take several months for change to be visualized radiographically (Figure 10-12). Characteristic radio-logic signs of osteonecrosis include crescent-shaped radiolucency in the subchondral bone region, patchy areas of sclerosis and lucency, bony collapse, diaphyseal periostitis, and preservation of joint space despite an affected epiphyseal region. MRI is the most sensitive way to detect the presence of IBD (Figure 10-13).

Management

The treatment of IBD varies according to the location and size of the site involved, whether bony collapse has occurred, and is also influenced by the patient's age. The direction of treatment is traditionally guided by the orthopedic surgeon and may be conservative or surgical in nature. Various therapeutic options have been proposed in the treatment of femoral head necrosis, ranging from conservative management to THA. Conservative treatment includes protected weightbearing to prevent further collapse of the affected bony area. Surgical care may include hemiarthroplasty or total joint arthroplasty; however, osteotomy may be chosen in an effort to alter the weightbearing force on a joint surface. Because the results of hip arthroplasty in patients with osteonecrosis may be relatively poor, surgical intervention is aimed at femoral head preservation. The surgical alternatives include core decompression, osteotomy, and nonvascularized and vascularized bone grafting, which might be enhanced with the use of growth and differentiation factors (Mont et al. 1998). Vascularized bone grafting (e.g., vascular iliac bone graft) may be considered in an effort to intervene causally in the case of femoral head necrosis (Kern et al. 1998). Basic and clinical research has shown the efficacy of various cellular mediators (bone morphogenetic proteins, interleukins, angiogenic growth factors) in healing bone defects,

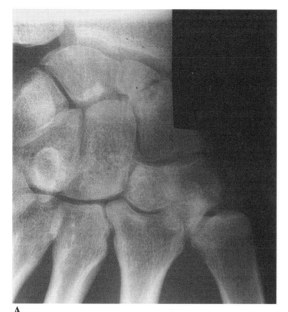

A

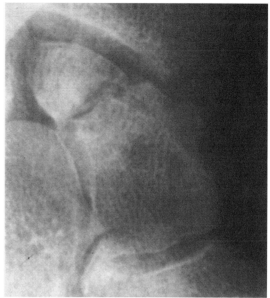

B

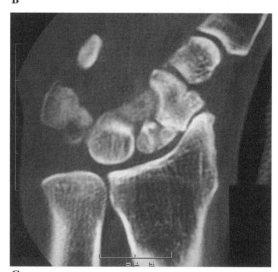

C

Figure 10-12. A. Transverse fracture of scaphoid with nonunion. **B.** Note the avascular necrosis presenting with sclerosis of the proximal pole and around the fracture site. **C.** Computed tomographic scan of a scaphoid fracture. Note signs of avascular necrosis. (Courtesy of Dr. Edna Becker, M.D., Toronto Hospital, Toronto.)

and their potential application to osteonecrosis (IBD) of the femoral head is of current interest (Mont et al. 1998).

Summary

Normal function and weightbearing is important in the maintenance of bone mass. Evidence supports that a modest reduction in function over a sufficiently long period results in significant bone loss independent of skeletal attrition caused by other factors such as aging and/or disease. Bone loss associated with immobilization may be reversed with re-ambulation; however, for some areas the rates of recovery are site-dependent and probably vary among individuals. As a general rule, bone lost under conditions of weightlessness or immobilization occurs more rapidly than it is recovered on re-ambulation.

Organ transplantation is the end-stage treatment for a number of conditions involving the renal, hepatic, cardiac, and pulmonary systems. Pharmacologic regimens to prevent rejection after organ

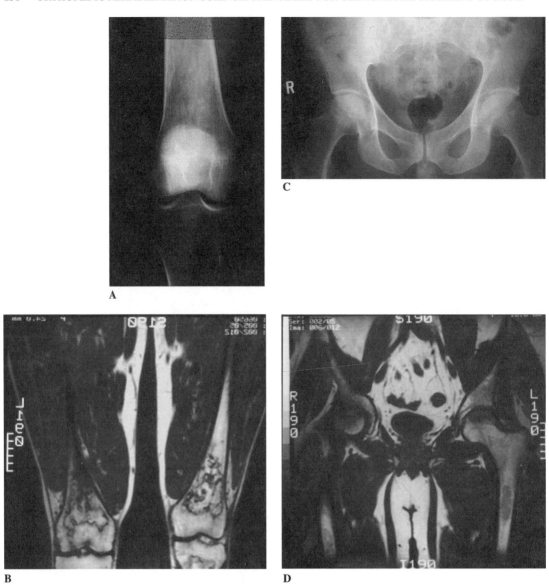

Figure 10-13. A. A bone infarct (avascular necrosis) is evident in the distal femur of this 41-year-old man who had received a short course of high-dose steroids in the past. **B.** Although changes are subtle on plain films, findings of avascular necrosis by magnetic resonance imaging (MRI) is typical and relatively dramatic. **C.** Bilateral hips as viewed on plain film imaging. Note the flattening of the right femoral head because of avascular necrosis. No clear change is evident in the left hip. **D.** MRI imaging of the sites in **C** reveals clear changes in *bilateral* femoral head regions because of avascular necrosis. This patient subsequently underwent bilateral total hip arthroplasty. (Courtesy of Dr. Edna Becker, M.D., Toronto Hospital, Toronto.)

transplantation are detrimental to bone and mineral homeostasis, because they are associated with rapid bone loss that is often superimposed on an already compromised skeleton. Routine assessment of the skeletal status of organ transplant recipients is now a consideration both before and after organ transplantation. The purpose of this assessment is twofold: first, to detect existing or pretransplantation bone disease and, second, to ensure vigilance for signs of osteopathy that may develop after organ transplantation.

Infection occurring in bone is referred to as *osteomyelitis*. Three routes exist by which an infectious organism may enter the bone: (1) hematogenous, via the bloodstream distal from the site of infection, (2) contiguous, or from an infection in the adjacent tissues, and (3) directly, from an open fracture or operative procedure. Based on the intensity of the infection, osteomyelitis may present in acute, subacute, or chronic forms. Pyogenic (pus producing) or nonpyogenic infections of the bone may occur. *S. aureus* is the most common organism of pyogenic infections, whereas nonpyogenic infections may be instigated by events associated with fungus, tuberculosis, or syphilis. Within 7–10 days after the onset of infection, a destructive lytic lesion indicated by an area of increased bone radiolucency is seen. Destruction of both cancellous and cortical bone may ensue 2–6 weeks after infection begins. Sequestra, or isolated regions of dead bone enveloped in pus, may be observed after 6 weeks. These sequestra become surrounded by a sealing zone of immature periosteal bone that also becomes infected and is referred to as the *involucrum*. The discharge of pus may occur through sinus tracts and, at this point, it is considered that chronic osteomyelitis has ensued. Aggressive and sometimes prolonged antibiotic therapy typically arrests acute osteomyelitis infection; chronic osteomyelitis carries a poor prognosis.

EO is a process whereby new bone is formed, due to metaplasia of connective tissue, in areas that normally do not ossify. Acquired EO manifests in many forms. MOT is a disorder of osteogenesis that typically occurs within skeletal muscle secondary to traumatic intramuscular hematoma. Other forms of EO include heterotopic ossification, which represents a complication of severe burns, THA, and neurologic insult (TBI and SCI). Treatment of EO includes pharmacologic intervention, radiation therapy, surgical resection, and physical management strategies. When possible, active or active-assisted exercise within the pain-free range is advocated to maintain optimal ROM in populations in whom EO has manifested. Forceful distention of periarticular structures is associated with progression to joint ankylosis.

Avascular necrosis, which is also known as *osteonecrosis* or *IBD*, is a condition that usually progresses to joint destruction, necessitating arthroplasty or other surgical intervention. The pathology of avascular necrosis involves ischemic events that are followed by necrosis of bone and marrow elements. Attempted repair of bone usually is ineffective unless the lesion is small, necessitating joint arthroplasty and surgical alternatives (e.g., core decompression, osteotomy, nonvascularized and

vascularized bone grafting) all of which may be enhanced with the application of growth and differentiation factors in the healing of this functionally impeding bone defect.

References

Ackerman LV. Extra-osseous localized non-neoplastic bone and cartilage formation (so called myositis ossificans): clinical and pathological confusion with malignant neoplasma. J Bone Joint Surg Am 1958;40:279–298.

Ahrengart L, Lindgreen V, Reinholt FH. Comparative study of the effect of radiation, indomethacin, prednisone and ethane-1-hydroxy-1,1-diphosphonate (EHDP) in the prevention of bone formation. Clin Orthop 1988;229:265–273.

Anderson D. Management of Decreased ROM from Overactive Musculature or Heterotopic Ossification. In J Montgomery (ed), Physical Therapy for Traumatic Brain Injury. New York: Churchill Livingstone, 1995;79–97.

Aringer M, Kiener HP, Koeller MD, et al. High turnover bone disease following lung transplantation. Bone 1998;23:485–488.

Ayers D, Pellegrini V, Evarts C. Prevention of heterotopic ossification in high-risk patients by radiation therapy. Clin Orthop 1991;263:87–93.

Béthoux F, Calmels P, Aigoin J, et al. Heterotopic ossification and rhabdomyolysis. Paraplegia 1995;33:164–166.

Booth DW, Westers BM. The management of athletes with myositis ossificans traumatica. Can J Sport Sci 1989;14:10.16.

Brooker AF, Bowerman JW, Robinson RA, Riley RH Jr. Ectopic ossification following total hip replacement: incidence and a method of classification. J Bone Joint Surg Am 1973;55:1629–1632.

Buring K. On the origin of cells in heterotopic bone formation. Clin Orthop 1975;110:293–302.

Burns DK, Kumar V. The Musculoskeletal System. In V Kumar, R Cotran, S Robbins (eds), Basic Pathology (6th ed). Toronto: WB Saunders, 1997;672–673.

Carmeliet G, Bouillon R. The effect of microgravity on morphology and gene expression of osteoblasts in vitro. FASEB J 1999;13:S129–S134.

Chantraine A, Minaire P. Para-osteo-arthropathies: a new theory and mode of treatment. Scand J Rehab Med 1981;13:31–37.

Chantraine A, Nusgens B, Lapiere CM. Biochemical analysis of heterotopic ossification in spinal cord injury patients. Paraplegia 1995;33:398–401.

Chen MM, Jee WSS, Ke HZ, et al. Adaptation of cancellous bone to aging and immobilization in growing rate. Anat Rec 1992;234:317–334.

Coleman P. The fate of bone after renal transplantation. Curr Opin Nephrol Hypertens 1998;7:389–395.

Compston JE. Detection of osteoporosis in patients with inflammatory bowel disease. Eur J Gastroenterol Hepatol 1997;9:931–933.

Coventry MB, Scanlon PW. The use of radiation to discourage ectopic bone: a nine year study in surgery about the hip. J Bone Joint Surg Am 1981;63:201–208.

Crawford CM, Varghese G, Mani MM, Neff JR. Heterotopic ossification: are range of motion exercises contraindicated? J Burn Care Rehab 1986;7:323–327.

Cushner FD, Morwessel RM. Myositis ossificans traumatica. Orthop Rev 1992;21:1319–1326.

Cvitanic O, Sedlak J. Acute myositis ossificans. Skeletal Radiol 1995;24:139–141.

Devos M, Dekeyse F, Mielants H, et al. Review article: bone and joint diseases in inflammatory bowel disease. Aliment Pharmacol Ther 1998;12:397–404.

Dietrick JE, Whedon GD, Shorr E. Effects of immobilization upon various metabolic and physiologic functions of normal men. Am J Med 1948;4:3–36.

Dissanayake IR, Epstein S. The fate of bone after renal transplantation. Curr Opin Nephol Hypertens 1998;7:389–395.

Dodds R, Skerry TM, Pead MJ, Lanyon LE. Proteoglycan orientation in bone; its relationship to loading disuse and clinical osteoporosis [Abstract]. Orthop Transact 1990;14:511.

Donaldson CL, Hulley SB, Vogel JM, et al. Effect of prolonged bed rest on bone mineral. Metabolism 1970;19:1071–1084.

Donohoe KJ. Selected topics in orthopaedic nuclear medicine. Orthop Clin North Am 1998;29:85–101.

Dorn U, Grethen C, Effenberger H, et al. Indomethacin for prevention of heterotopic ossification after hip arthroplasty: a randomized comparison between 4 and 8 days of treatment. Acta Orthop Scand 1998;69:107–110.

Edlich RF, Horowitz JH, Rheuban KS. Heterotopc calcification and ossification in the burn patient. J Burn Care Rehab 1985;6:363–368.

El-Khoury CU, Brandser EA, Kathol MH, et al. Imaging of muscle injuries. Skeletal Radiol 1996;25:3–11.

Elledge ES, Smith AA, McManus WF, Pruitt BA Jr. Heterotopic bone formation in burned patients. J Trauma 1988;28:584–687.

Elmstedt E, Lindholm TS, Nilsson OS, Tornkvist H. Effect of ibuprofen on heterotopic ossification after hip replacement. Acta Orthop Scand 1985;56:25–27.

Felten A, Desplaces N, Nizard R, et al. Peptostreptococcus magnus bone and joint infections after orthopedic surgery. Pathologie Biologie 1998;46:442–448.

Freed JH, Hahn H, Menter R, Dillon T. The use of the three-phase bone scan in the early diagnosis of heterotopic ossification (HO) and in the evaluation of didronel therapy. Paraplegia 1982;20:208–216.

Furman M, Ouchterlony D, Anderson R, Lundon K. Ectopic bone formation in the adult traumatic brain injury population in the acute and rehabilitation settings. Brain Cogn 1999 (in press).

Garland DE, Razza BE, Waters RL. Forceful joint manipulation in head-injured adults with heterotopic ossification. Clin Orthop 1982;169:133–138.

Garland DE, Alday B, Venos KG, Vogt JC. Diphosphonate treatment for heterotopic ossification in spinal cord injury patients. Clin Orthop 1983;176:197–200.

Garland DE, Hanscom DA, Keenan M, et al. Resection of heterotopic ossification in the adult with head trauma. J Bone Joint Surg Am 1985;67:1261.

Garland DE. Clinical observations on fracture and heterotopic ossification in the spinal cord and traumatic brain injured populations. Clin Orthop 1988;233:86–101.

Goodman TA, Merkel PA, Perlmutter G, et al. Heterotopic ossification in the setting of neuromuscular blockade. Arthritis Rheum 1997;40:1619–1627.

Grigoriadis A, Heersche J, Aubin J. Differentiation of muscle, fat, cartilage, and bone from progenitor cells present in a bone-derived clonal cell population: effect of dexamethasone. J Cell Biol 1988;106:2139–2151.

Grigoriadis A, Heersche J, Aubin J. Continuously growing bipotential and monopotential myogenic, adipogenic, and chondrogenic subclones isolated from the multipotential RCJ 3.1 clonal cell line. Dev Biol 1990;142:313–318.

Gristina A, Naylor P, Myrvik Q. Mechanisms of musculoskeletal sepsis. Orthop Clin North Am 1991;22:363–371.

Grotz W, Rump LC, Niessen A, et al. Treatment of osteopenia and osteoporosis after kidney transplantation. Transplantation 1998;66:1004–1008.

Grotz W, Rump LC, Schollmeyer P. Osteoporosis in transplant recipients: recommendations for avoidance and therapy. Biodrugs 1997;7:433–440.

Hansson TH, Roos BO, Nachemson A. Development of osteopenia in the fourth lumbar vertebra during prolonged bed rest after operation for scoliosis. Acta Orthop Scand 1975;46:621–636.

Healy WL, Lo TCM, DeSimone AA, et al. Single-dose irradiation for the prevention of heterotopic ossification after total hip arthroplasty. J Bone Joint Surg Am 1995;77:590–595.

Hinck SM. Heterotopic ossification: a review of symptoms and treatment. Rehab Nurs 1994;19:169–173.

Horlick MF. Perspective on the impact of weightlessness on calcium and bone metabolism. Bone 1998;22(Suppl 5):105–111.

Hurvitz EA, Mandac BR, Davidoff G, et al. Risk factors for heterotopic ossification in children and adolescents with severe traumatic brain injury. Arch Phys Med Rehab 1992;73:459–462.

James J, Steijn-Myagkaya GL. Death of osteocytes. Electron microscopy after in vitro ischaemia. J Bone Joint Surg Br 1986;68:620–624.

Jowsey J, Coventry MB, Robins PR. Heterotopic Ossification: Theoretical Consideration, Possible Etiologic Factors, and a Clinical Review of Total Hip Arthroplasty Patients Exhibiting This Phenomenon. The Proceedings of the Hip Society. St. Louis: Mosby, 1977;210–221.

Kaysinger KK, Ramp WK, Lang GJ, Gruber HE. Comparison of human osteoblasts and osteogenic cells from heterotopic bone. Clin Orthop 1997;342:181–191.

Kern O, Lockner C, Weber U. Long term results of joint preserving therapy of osteonecrosis of the femoral head with a vascular pedicled iliac bone graft. Orthopade 1998;27:482–490.

Kewalramani LS. Ectopic ossification. Am J Phys Med 1977;56:99–121.

King JB. Post-traumatic ectopic calcification in the muscles of athletes: a review. Br J Sports Med 1998;32:287–290.

Koch BM, Mei Wu C, Randolph J, Eng GD. Heterotopic ossification in children with burns: two case reports. Arch Phys Med Rehab 1992;73:1104–1106.

Kölbl O, Knelles D, Barthel T, et al. Preoperative irradiation versus the use of nonsteroidal anti-inflammatory drugs for prevention of heterotopic ossification following total hip replacement: the results of a randomized trial. Int J Radiation Oncol Biol Phys 1998;42:397–401.

Krolner B, Toft B. Vertebral bone loss: an unheeded side effect of therapeutic bed rest. Clin Sci 1983;4:537–540.

Lal S, Hamilton BB, Heinemann A, Betts HB. Risk factors for heterotopic ossification in spinal cord injury. Arch Phys Med Rehab 1989;70:387–390.

Leblanc AD, Schneider VS, Evans HJ, et al. Bone mineral loss and recovery after 17 weeks of bed rest. J Bone Miner Res 1990;5:843–850.

Lennkh C, de Zwaan M, Bailer U, et al. Osteopenia in anorexia nervosa: specific mechanisms of bone loss. J Psychiatr Res 1999;33:349–356.

Li XJ, Jee WSS, Chow SY, Woodbury DM. Adaptation of cancellous bone to aging and immobilization in the rat: a single photon absorptiometry and histomorphometry study. Anat Rec 1990;227:12–24.

Liedman B, Bosaeus I, Mellstrom D, Lundell L. Osteoporosis after total gastrectomy: results of a prospective clinical study. Scand J Gastroenterol 1997;32:1090–1095.

Lucas TS, Bab IA, Lian JB, et al. Stimulation of systemic bone formation induced by experimental blood loss. Clin Orthop 1997;340:267–275.

Lundon K, Hampson D. Acquired ectopic ossification of soft tissues: implications for physical therapy. Can J Rehab 1997;10:231–246.

Marinissen JC. Management of heterotopic ossification following traumatic brain or spinal cord injury. Orthop Phys Ther Clin North Am 1993;2:71.

Marks PH, Paley D, Kellam JF. Heterotopic ossification around the hip with intramedullary nailing of the femur. J Trauma 1988;28:1207–1213.

Masaki K, Shiomi S, Kuroki T, et al. Longitudinal changes of bone mineral content with age in patients with cirrhosis of the liver. J Gastroenterol 1998;33:236–240.

Mazess RB, Whedon GD. Immobilization and bone. Calcif Tissue Int 1983;35:265–267.

Michelsson J, Rauschning W. Pathogenesis of experimental heterotopic bone formation following temporary forcible exercising of immobilized limbs. Clin Orthop 1983;176:265–272.

Mielantis H, Vanhove E, De Neels J, Veys E. Clinical survey of and pathogenic approach to para-articular ossifications in long term coma. Acta Orthop Scand 1975;46:190–198.

Mital MA, Garber JE, Stinson JT. Ectopic bone formation in children and adolescents with head injuries: its management. J Pediatr Orthop 1987;7:83–90.

Mont MA, Jones LC, Einhorn TA, et al. Osteonecrosis of the femoral head: potential treatment with growth and differentiation factors. Clin Orthop 1998;355(Suppl): 314–335.

Morey ER, Baylink DJ. Inhibition of bone formation during space flight. Science 1978;201:1138–1141.

Mourad LA. Alterations of Musculoskeletal Function. In KL McCance, SE Huether (eds), Pathophysiology: The Biologic Basis for Disease in Adults and Children (2nd ed). St. Louis: Mosby–Year Book, 1994; 1434–1481.

Mulley G, Espley AJ. Hip fracture after hemiplegia. Post Grad Med J 1979;55:264–265.

November-Dusansky A, Moylan J, Linkswiler H. Calciuretic response to protein loading in burn patients. Burns 1980;6:198–201.

Ott SM, Aitken ML. Osteoporosis in patients with cystic fibrosis. Clinics Chest Med 1998;19:555.

Paterson DC. Myositis ossificans circumscripta: report of four cases without history of injury. J Bone Joint Surg Br 1970;52:296–301.

Patzakis M, Rao W, Wilkins J, et al. Analysis of 61 cases of vertebral osteomyelitis. Clin Orthop 1991;264:178–183.

Pedersen NW, Kristensen SS, Schmidt SA, et al. Factors associated with heterotopic bone formation following total hip replacement. Arch Orthop Trauma Surg 1989;108:92–95.

Pellegrini V, Konski A, Gastel J, et al. Prevention of heterotopic ossification by irradiation after total hip arthroplasty. J Bone Joint Surg Am 1992;74:186–200.

Persson PE, Sodemann B, Nilsson OS. Preventive effects of ibuprofen on periarticular heterotopic ossification after total hip arthroplasty: a randomized double-blind prospective study of treatment time. Acta Orthop Scand 1998;69:111–115.

Peszczynski M. The fractured hip in hemiplegic patients. Geriatrics 1957;12:264–265.

Pittenger DE. Heterotopic ossification. Orthop Rev 1991;20: 33–39.

Plasmans CMT, Kuypers W, Slooff TJJH. The effect of ethane-1-hydroxy-1,1-diphosphonic acid (EHDP) on matrix induced ectopic bone formation. Clin Orthop 1978;132:233–243.

Prince RL, Price RI, Ho S. Forearm bone loss in hemiplegia: a model for the study of immobilization osteoporosis. J Bone Miner Res 1988;3:305–310.

Ritter MA, Gioe T. The effect of indomethacin on para-articular ectopic ossification following total hip arthroplasty. Clin Orthop 1982;167:113–117.

Ritter MA, Vaughan RB. Ectopic ossification after total hip arthroplasty. J Bone Joint Surg 1977;59:345–351.

Roberts D, Lee W, Cuneo RC, et al. Longitudinal study of bone turnover after acute spinal cord injury. J Clin Endocrinol Metab 1998;83:415–422.

Rodino MA, Shane E. Osteoporosis after organ transplantation. Am J Med 1998;104:459–469.

Rothwell AG. Quadriceps hematoma: a prospective clinical study. Clin Orthop 1982;171:97–103.

Russell RGG, Kanis JA. Ectopic Calcification and Ossification. In BEC Nordin (ed), Metabolic Bone and Stone Disease (2nd ed). Edinburgh: Churchill Livingstone, 1984;344–365.

Schaeffer M, Sosner J. Heterotopic ossification: treatment of established bone with radiation therapy. Arch Phys Med Rehab 1995;76:284–286.

Schai P, Brunner R, Morscher E, Schubert K. Prevention of heterotopic ossification in hip arthroplasties by means of an early single-dose radiotherapy (6 Gy). Arch Orthop Trauma Surg 1995;114:153–158.

Schoon EJ, Wolffenbuttel BHR, Stockbrugger RW. Osteoporosis as a risk in inflammatory bowel disease. Drugs Today 1999;35:17–28.

Schulte C, Dignass AU, Mann K, Goebell H. Reduced BMD and unbalanced bone metabolism in patients with inflammatory bowel disease. Inflamm Bowel Dis 1998; 4:268–275.

Seibel MJ. Diagnosis and monitoring of posttransplantation osteopathies. Acta Medica (Austriaca) 1997;24:1–4.

Shafritz AB, Kaplan FS. Differential expression of bone and cartilage related genes in fibrodysplasia ossificans progressiva, myositis ossificans traumatica and osteogenic sarcoma. Clin Orthop 1998;346:46–52.

Smith MC, Rambaut PC, Vogel JM. Bone Mineral Measurement—Experiment M078. In RS Johnson, LF Dietlein (eds), Biomedical Results from Skylab. Washington, DC: Scientific and Technical Information Office, 1977;183 (NASA SP-377).

Smith R. Fibrodysplasia (myositis) ossificans progressiva: clinical lessons from a rare disease. Clin Orthop 1998; 346:7–14.

Sud AM, Wilson MW, Mountz JM. Unusual clinical presentation and scintigraphic pattern in myositis ossificans. Clin Nucl Med 1992;17:198–199.

Thornton WE, Rummel JA. Muscular Deconditioning and Its Prevention in Space Flight. In RS Johnson, LF Dietlein (eds), Biomedical Results from Skylab. Washington, DC: Scientific and Technical Information Office, 1977;191 (NASA SP-377).

Tilton FE, Degioanni TTC, Schneider VS. Long-term follow-up of Skylab bone mineralization. Aviat Space Environ Med 1980;51:1209–1213.

Tirpitz C, Pischulti G, Klaus J, et al. Osteoporosis in patients with inflammatory bowel disease: prevalence and risk factors. Zeitschrift Gastroenterol 1999;37:5–12.

Tsuzuku S, Ikegami Y, Yabe K. Bone mineral density differences between paraplegic and quadriplegic patients: a cross sectional study. Spinal Cord 1999;37:358–361.

Uhthoff HK, Jaworski ZFG. Bone loss in response to long-term immobilization. J Bone Joint Surg Br 1978;60: 420–429.

Urena P. Plasma biochemical markers of bone remodeling in patients with renal insufficiency. J Clin Ligand Assay 1998;21:159–170.

Vancleemput J, Daenen W, Geusens P, et al. Prevention of bone loss in cardiac transplant recipients: a comparison of bisphosphonates and vitamin D. Transplantation 1996;61:1495–1499.

Vanleeuwen WM, Deckers P, Delange WJ. Preoperative irradiation for prophylaxis of ectopic ossification after hip arthroplasty: a randomized study in 62 hips. Acta Orthop Scand 1998;69:116–118.

Vicar AJ, Coleman CR. A comparison of the anterolateral, transtrochanteric, and posterior surgical approaches in primary total hip arthroplasty. Clin Orthop 1984;188: 152–159.

Walton M, Rothwell AG. Reactions of thigh tissues of sheep to blunt trauma. Clin Orthop 1983;176:273–281.

Whedon GD. Disuse osteoporosis: physiological aspects. Calcif Tissue Int 1984;36:S146–S150.

Whedon GD, Shorr E. Metabolic studies in paralytic anterior poliomyelitis. II. Alterations in calcium and phosphorus metabolism. J Clin Invest 1957;36: 966–981.

Wittenberg RH, Peschke U, Botel U. Heterotopic ossification after spinal cord injury: epidemiology and risk factors. J Bone Joint Surg Br 1992;74:215–218.

Woo SLY, Akeson WH, Coutts RD, et al. A comparison of cortical bone atrophy secondary to fixation with plates with large differences in bending stiffness. J Bone Joint Surg Am 1976;58:190–195.

Yamamoto M, Tabata Y, Ikada Y. Ectopic bone formation induced by biodegradable hydrogels incorporating bone morphogenetic protein. J Biomater Sci Polym Ed 1998;9:439–458.

Yamauchi M, Young DR, Chandler GS, Mechanic GL. Cross-linking and new bone collagen synthesis in immobilized and recovering primate osteoporosis. Bone 1988;9:415–418.

Zittel TT, Maier GW, Starlinger M, Becker HD. Calcium and bone metabolism after gastrectomy. Chirurg 1997a;68: 784–788.

Zittel TT, Zeeb B, Maier GW, et al. High prevalence of bone disorders after gastrectomy. Am J Surgery 1997b;174: 431–438.

Chapter 11
Bone Neoplasms

Aileen M. Davis

A neoplasm is the growth of new tissue that serves no physiologic function, such as a bone tumor. Primary bone tumors may be benign, with no risk of metastasis, or they may be malignant, with the potential to metastasize from the site of the primary bone of origin. Metastatic bone tumors are malignancies that develop in bone secondary to a primary cancerous tumor at another anatomic site.

The three most common types of primary cancer that can metastasize to bone are breast, prostate, and lung carcinoma (National Cancer Institute of Canada 1998). In females, breast, lung, and colorectal cancers account for 50% of the new cases of cancer annually; prostate, lung, and colorectal cancers account for at least 50% of new cancers in males (National Cancer Institute of Canada 1998). Breast, prostate, and lung cancer most frequently metastasize to bone with rates of 50–85%, 50–70%, and 30–50%, respectively (Fisher et al. 1997; Orr et al. 1995; Mundy 1997a). Mundy (1997a) reported that of approximately 500,000 cancer deaths per year in the United States, two-thirds to three-quarters of patients have bone metastases at the time of death. Common sites of bone metastases include the rib cage, spine, pelvis, long bones of the extremities, and skull (Galasko 1986). Bone metastases contribute significant morbidity (manifested as pain, hypercalcemia, anemia, fracture, neurologic deficit, and reduced activity), resulting in decreased quality of life for patients with cancer (Frassica et al. 1992; Kanis 1995; Mercandante 1997).

In contrast to this relatively high rate of metastatic bone tumors, primary bone tumors are rare, occurring with an incidence of 2–3 per million (Malawar et al. 1997). Although the frequency of primary bone tumors is low, the morbidity imparted by surgically removing tumor from the involved bone and reconstructing the skeletal defect may be significant (Bell et al. 1997; McGoveran et al. 1999; Roberts et al. 1991; Probyn et al. 1998; Abudu 1996; Unwin et al. 1996; Kawar et al. 1998).

Pathophysiology of Neoplastic Bone Disease

The normal structure and function of bone were reviewed in Chapters 1–4. The three major functions of bone are (1) to provide structural support with attachments for muscle, ligaments, and tendons; (2) to provide hematopoiesis; and (3) to maintain mineral homeostasis. Any or all of these functions of bone can be impaired by primary, and especially metastatic, involvement of the skeleton (Guise and Mundy 1998).

Metastatic Bone Disease

The mechanism of development of metastatic bone disease is not completely understood. The development of metastases involves multiple steps that depend on features and interactions of both the

Clinical Note

Many of the associated morbidities of metastatic bone disease are amenable to rehabilitation interventions. Patients treated for primary bone neoplasms also require rehabilitation to achieve their optimal level of function. However, the rehabilitation specialist requires an understanding of the pathophysiology of neoplastic bone disease, the rationale and process of diagnosis, and the rationale and process of medical and surgical treatment to develop an informed approach to rehabilitation of the patient with neoplastic bone disease.

malignant tumor cells and normal host cells (Orr et al. 1995; Kanis 1995; Mundy and Yoneda 1995; Mundy 1997b). The process of metastatic tumor development includes tumor cells shedding from the primary site, invasion of adjacent tissues, entry of cells into tumor capillaries, and then entry into the general circulation via the tumor capillaries (Mundy 1997b). The circulating tumor cells then adhere to host cells (specifically to the basement membrane of the host cells), disrupt it, and then migrate through the basement membrane to seed in the host organ (Mundy 1997b). Production of proteolytic enzymes, expression or loss of cell adhesion molecules, and the presence of growth factors mediate these processes (Orr et al. 1995; Kanis 1995; Mundy and Yoneda 1995; Mundy 1997b; Miyasaka 1995).

Bone provides a particularly amenable host environment for tumor cells owing to its marrow structure, the haversian canal system, and its abundance of growth factors (Orr et al. 1995; Kanis 1995; Mundy and Yoneda 1995; Mundy 1997b). The vertebral column is particularly amenable, because the venous blood from the vena cava and prostate flow directly into the venous vertebral plexus (Batson 1940). The vertebral venous plexus is a valveless system allowing cephalad and caudad blood flow under low pressure (Batson 1940), conditions favorable for adhesion of tumor cells in the vertebrae and extradural tissues.

Once tumor cells have seeded in the bone, the bone is destroyed by a variety of osteoblast- and osteoclast-related factors. In normal tissue, bone formation (osteoblastic activity) and resorption (osteoclast activity) are balanced (Smith 1990). However, in the presence of tumor, this balance is destroyed, resulting in increased resorption and lysis (Orr et al. 1995; Kanis 1995; Mundy 1997b; Mundy and Guise 1997). Osteoclastic bone resorption is the primary cause of hyper-

calcemia in patients with metastatic cancer (Kanis 1995; Mundy and Guise 1997; Walls 1995).

Pain is common in patients with osteolytic or osteoblastic lesions of bone. Bone resorption compromises the structural and mechanical integrity of the bone and, if sufficiently weakened, the bone may fracture. Metastatic tumor growth in the vertebrae may result in collapse of the vertebrae; thus, pathologic fracture of the vertebrae, in addition to tumor growth, may result in cord compression and neurologic deficits. These complications of metastatic bone tumors are indications for medical, surgical, and rehabilitation intervention.

Primary Bone Tumors

Primary bone tumors may be benign or malignant. Benign tumors grow at the local site, whereas malignant tumors have metastatic potential. Primary malignant tumors may be derived from mesenchymal cells (e.g., chondrosarcoma, osteosarcoma) or marrow elements (e.g., lymphoma, myeloma). Primary malignant tumors are graded based on their degree of cytologic atypia. (Atypia refers to the extent of cellular abnormality on histologic examination.) Low-grade tumors have less atypia than high-grade tumors, slower growth and destruction of bone at the local site, and a small risk of metastasizing. In contrast, high-grade tumors are locally aggressive, rapidly destroy bone, and have a high risk of metastatic spread.

Primary tumors of bone are classified according to their histologic deviation from normal bone tissue (Bertoni and Bacchini 1998). Chondrogenic tumors are the most common primary bone tumors; their histologic pattern has features of hyaline cartilage. Approximately one-third of all cartilage tumors are benign *osteochondromas* or *exostoses* (bony outgrowth) on long bones (Bertoni and Bacchini 1998). *Chondromas* occur centrally or subperiosteally and frequently contain calcification or ossification. *Chondroblastoma* and *chondromyxoid fibroma* are also benign cartilage tumors. In contrast to benign cartilage tumors, *chondrosarcomas* are malignant tumors whose cells produce malignant chondroid matrix. Primary chondrosarcomas tend to occur in previously normal bone. Secondary chondrosarcomas result from malignant transformation of a benign cartilage tumor (e.g., osteochondroma developing into a chondrosarcoma).

Osteogenic tumors are the second largest group of primary bone tumors. *Osteosarcomas* are the most frequent type of osteogenic tumors (Bertoni and Bacchini 1998; Spina et al. 1998). Osteosarcomas may arise in normal bone or secondarily to preexisting conditions and tumors (e.g., Paget's disease, bone infarct, fibrous dysplasia, giant cell tumor). Benign tumors of osteogenic origin include *osteoid osteoma* and *osteoblastoma*.

Giant cell tumor (a benign lesion) and *Ewing's sarcoma* (a malignant tumor) are primary bone tumors that do not resemble any normal cell of origin on histologic examination. Giant cell tumors are characterized by a histologic pattern in which round and oval cells produce giant cells (Bertoni and Bacchini 1998). The histologic diagnosis of Ewing's sarcoma is made by demonstrating positivity of cellular elements with special immunohistochemic stains.

The process of primary bone tumor development is not understood; however, certain genetic abnormalities are associated with increased frequency of tumor occurrence (Bell and Wunder 1997). For example, the tumor cells of patients with primary sarcoma have abnormalities in the *p53* gene (a tumor suppressor gene) in approximately 30% of patients (Toguchida et al. 1992). Ongoing evaluation of genetic abnormalities is required to determine their clinical relevance in diagnosis, treatment, and prognosis of primary bone tumors.

Diagnosis of Bone Tumors

History and physical examination, radiographic imaging, and tissue histology are the methods used for bone tumor diagnosis.

Metastatic Bone Tumors

Signs and Symptoms

In patients with a known history of cancer, pain is the primary presenting feature (Kanis 1995; Levesque et al. 1998; Phillips 1998). Pain is often present at rest as well as with activity and may impair mobility. Neurologic deficits may be present with spinal metastases (Bunting 1995). The patient may present with a pathologic fracture through a metastatic lesion.

Imaging

Plain radiographs are the first test ordered when a metastatic bone lesion is suspected, because it allows evaluation of the overall bone structure, mechanical properties, and risk of fracture (Healey 1997). Metastatic bone lesions usually have a "moth-eaten" appearance, with ill-defined edges (Figure 11-1). Three radiographic patterns may occur: osteolytic, osteoblastic, and mixed (Wilner 1982). *Osteolysis* represents tumor destruction of the host bone, whereas *osteoblastic* areas within the lesion represent the host bone's reaction to the tumor. This reactive bone often lacks mechanical strength. Rapidly growing metastatic lesions often have mixed osteolytic and osteoblastic patterns, because the reparative reaction cannot keep up with the rate of tumor growth.

A total body bone scan measures metabolic bone activity and also is useful because it allows identifi-

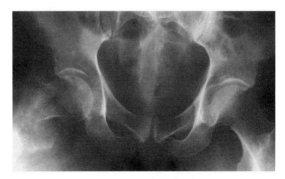

Figure 11-1. Plain x-ray demonstrating a metastatic lesion in the proximal femur. Note the "blown out" appearance of the bone and the ill-defined edges of tumor.

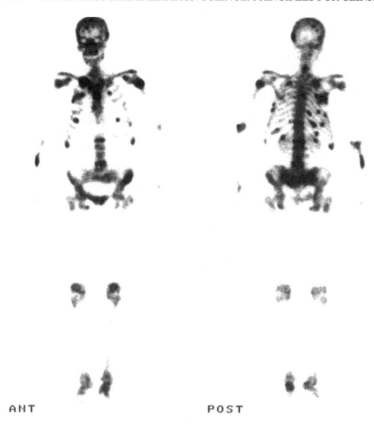

Figure 11-2. Total body bone scan demonstrating multiple metastatic sites throughout the bony skeleton.

ANT   POST

cation of multiple sites of disease (Figure 11-2), some of which may be asymptomatic (Healey 1997). Computed tomography (CT) and magnetic resonance imaging (MRI) provide three dimensional images of the lesion (Healey 1997). CT demonstrates the mineral content of the bone and delineates the structural integrity of the bony cortex. MRI defines the disease in the bone marrow and the extent of any soft tissue tumor extension. These studies are particularly helpful in planning treatment, be it with radiotherapy or surgery. They also provide a method of evaluating response to treatment with chemotherapy or radiotherapy.

Laboratory Biochemistry

Certain blood tests are helpful in diagnosing metastatic tumors. Elevated levels of prostate-specific antigen are highly suggestive of prostate cancer (Lorente et al. 1996; Wolff et al. 1996) and elevated calcium levels are also common in diffuse metastatic disease (Kanis 1995).

Pathologic Diagnosis

Tissue biopsy sometimes is required to confirm that the tumor is a metastatic lesion. However, most patients presenting with metastatic disease have a history of primary malignancy elsewhere and biopsy is often unnecessary.

Primary Bone Tumor

Signs and Symptoms

When a primary bone tumor is suspected, the history and physical examination supply important information that leads the physician to suspect a benign or malignant lesion. Patients with benign lesions report minimal pain unless there has been a pathologic fracture or aggressive bone destruction (Levesque et al. 1998). Consequently, reports of pain associated with the lesion are usually a sign of a more aggressive, and potentially malignant, tumor.

This pain is probably related to bone destruction by the tumor and pressure on the soft tissues by the rapid growth of the tumor (Levesque et al. 1998).

Imaging

Plain radiographs are again important, because they provide information about not only the mechanical integrity of the bone, but also about the possible histologic diagnosis (Campanacci et al. 1998; Levesque et al. 1998). The radiographic appearance varies by histologic diagnosis. For example, bone forming primary malignancies (osteosarcoma) usually show evidence of bone formation (osteoblastic changes) on x-ray (Seeger et al. 1998). A chondrosarcoma is characterized by lytic areas and calcification throughout the lesion (Masciocchi et al. 1998).

As with metastatic lesions, CT and MRI scans of the local region provide detail about the bony architecture and extent of disease (Figure 11-3), including bone marrow involvement or soft tissue extension in the case of MRI (Levesque et al. 1998). CT of the thorax is an important addition in evaluating primary malignant tumors of bone, because the lung is the most common site of metastatic disease spread (Peabody et al. 1998).

Histologic diagnosis or confirmation of the type of tumor is obtained by tissue biopsy. Bone tumor histologic diagnosis is extremely important, because patients with osteosarcoma and Ewing's sarcoma are assumed to have micrometastases at the time of diagnosis. Without chemotherapy, the 5-year survival rate for these patients is less than 20%, whereas chemotherapy in conjunction with surgery results in a 5-year survival rate of more than 50% (Jaffe et al. 1974; Link et al. 1991; Rosen et al. 1974; Glasser et al. 1992; Goorin and Anderson 1991; Ferrari et al. 1997).

Anatomic location, histologic type of tumor, extent of tumor, and presence or absence of metastatic disease are critical factors in determining the course of treatment for the patient.

Medical and Surgical Treatment

Metastatic Bone Tumors

The goal of treatment in patients with metastatic bone disease is to relieve pain (Phillips 1998) and

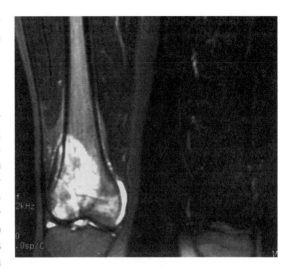

Figure 11-3. Magnetic resonance image of the distal femur demonstrating tumor replacement of the bone and marrow canal. Note the extension of the bright signal beyond the bone indicating a soft tissue mass.

to optimize patient function as quickly as possible. Treatment decisions require consideration of both the patient (i.e., general health, level of activity, expected survival time) and the disease (i.e., previous treatment, response to previous treatment, other sites of disease).

Treatment for each patient should be individualized. Radiotherapy is often the first treatment for a painful metastasis that is not a fracture risk (Hoskin 1995; Levesque et al. 1998; Twycross 1995). Certain tumors, such as breast, prostate, and thyroid tumors, are responsive to chemotherapy or hormonal therapy. Bisphosphonate compounds (Body et al. 1991), such as pamidronate or clodronate, inhibit osteoclast activity and can improve pain control in patients with metastatic bone pain. Salicylic acids and nonsteroidal anti-inflammatory drugs (NSAIDs) are also effective in reducing bone pain (Eisenberg et al. 1994). Opioids may be used in conjunction with NSAIDs in cases of severe pain (Phillips 1998).

Surgery is indicated if no response to medical management of pain occurs, if pathologic fracture of the bone exists, or in some cases of impending pathologic fracture (Levesque et al. 1998). Surgical interventions most often include excision of the involved bone and replacement with a prosthetic device (e.g., at the hip), or curettage of the lesion

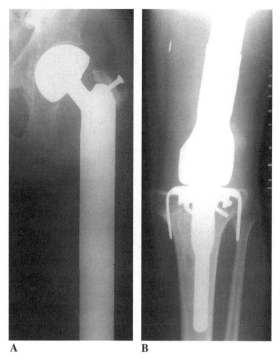

Figure 11-4. A,B. Endoprosthetic replacement of the entire femur, including the knee joint.

and packing of the bony defect with bone cement supported by internal fixation with pins, plates, and screws (Harrington 1995).

Primary Bone Tumors

If a tumor is benign and asymptomatic and the history does not indicate growth of the lesion, no intervention beyond follow-up with plain radiographs is required (Levesque et al. 1998). Serial follow-up is required over a 2-year period to document that the lesion does not progress. If a benign tumor is symptomatic, the patient should be treated for the condition, which most frequently involves excision of the tumor and bone grafting if there is a central bony defect.

Primary malignant tumors of bone may be treated by surgery alone or in combination with chemotherapy and surgery. The treatment protocol is determined by the tumor histology. For example, the survival rate of patients with osteosarcoma or Ewing's sarcoma has been dramatically improved by the use of adjuvant chemotherapy (Ferrari et al. 1997; Glasser et al. 1992; Goorin and Anderson

1991; Jaffe et al. 1974; Link et al. 1991; Rosen et al. 1974). Other bone tumors (e.g., chondrosarcoma) have not proven to be responsive to chemotherapy.

Surgery involves complete removal of the tumor with reconstruction of the bony defect. In selecting a reconstruction technique appropriate to the bony anatomic defect, the surgeon chooses from several options, including autogenous bone graft, bone transplant, and prosthetic reconstruction (Enneking 1987). When a tumor is malignant, it must be completely removed, along with a cuff of normal tissue surrounding the tumor. This limits the potential for tumor regrowth at the local site and the potential for metastatic spread of the tumor. In contrast, benign tumors may be curetted from the bone, leaving microscopic tumor behind. Benign microscopic tumor has minimal to no risk of recurrence.

In treating benign tumors such as giant cell tumor or chondromyxoid fibroma, the tumor would be curetted from bone, and the bony cavity, depending on its size, would be packed with autologous bone graft, morselized allograft bone, or bone cement (Blackley et al. 1998).

In treating a malignant tumor, the reconstructive technique chosen depends on the anatomic structure and the bone that must be removed. For example, a patient may have an osteosarcoma of the distal one-third of the femur, with soft tissue extension into the quadriceps muscle. If the tumor extends into the femoral condyles and involves the knee joint, an extra-articular excision is performed (the knee joint is removed in its entirety, as part of the tumor specimen), and the skeletal defect is reconstructed with an endoprosthesis that replaces the resected portions of the femur and tibia and provides an artificial knee joint (Abudu 1996; Kawar et al. 1998). If the tumor in the distal femur does not extend below the epiphyseal scar, the surgeon may opt to reconstruct the bony defect with a bone transplant. The tumor would be resected en bloc (in one specimen) such that the bone at either end is free of tumor and a cuff of normal soft tissue exists around the specimen. Cadaveric allograft bone from the bone bank would be fashioned to fit the defect in the femur; it would be filled with antibiotic impregnated bone cement and fixed to the proximal and distal ends of the remaining host femur (Wunder et al. 1995). The advantage of this technique is that it allows young patients to retain their own joint and articular cartilage (Figures 11-4 and 11-5).

The surgical reconstructive options are guided by (1) the amount of tissue that must be removed to obtain a sufficient margin of normal tissue around the tumor, (2) the remaining functional anatomic tissue, and (3) the potential function afforded the patient after surgery. The longevity of the reconstructive procedures (Unwin et al. 1996; Kawar et al. 1998; Horowitz 1993) has become a major consideration in the development of new reconstructive technologies.

Rehabilitation

The purpose of rehabilitation is to enhance quality of life by assisting patients in achieving their maximum function within the limits imposed by their cancer and its treatment. The specific goals of rehabilitation of the cancer patient depend on the disease site(s), the prognosis, the treatment or combination of treatments (type of tumor resection and reconstruction and use of chemotherapy and radiotherapy), the age and medical condition of the patient, and the patient's wishes.

Unless working in a specialized facility that treats patients with primary bone tumors, most rehabilitation specialists interact with patients who have metastatic bone disease. Although patients with metastatic disease may have a limited life expectancy, a significant proportion of patients are successfully rehabilitated after stabilization of a pathologic fracture, as demonstrated by work by Bunting et al. (1992). Fifty-eight patients who had been admitted to a rehabilitation hospital after stabilization were evaluated. On admission, none of the 58 patients could ambulate independently; assistance was required for bed mobility and transfers. Thirty-four patients were discharged home after their rehabilitation and seven patients were transferred to another care facility. Seventeen patients died of their disease. Overall, independent ambulation and activities of daily living were significantly improved. Hypercalcemia was a poor prognostic indicator for successful rehabilitation.

Allan et al. (1995) reported the results of periacetabular reconstruction in 25 patients with metastatic disease. Only 50% were alive 6 months after surgery. Of the surviving patients, however, at a mean of 14 months postsurgery all patients had progressed from wheelchair or nonweightbearing sta-

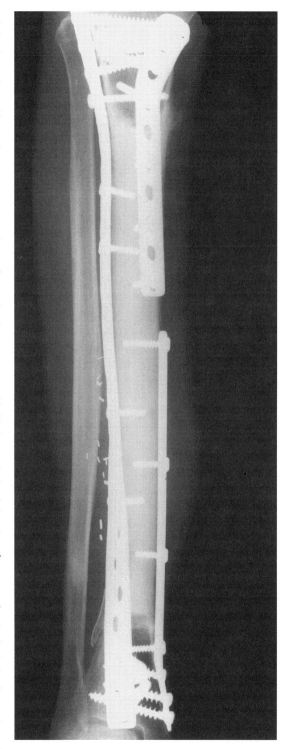

Figure 11-5. A cement-impregnated intercalary allograft used to reconstruct the tibia. Note the screws used distally and proximally to fix the bone transplant to the patient's own bone.

tus to ambulating partial weightbearing. Sixty-two percent of the patients were discharged home. Seven of the 25 patients died within 6 weeks of surgery and, in retrospect, were poor surgical candidates. Three patients had diffuse lung metastases, one patient had multiple bone metastases, one had liver metastases, and one had cerebral metastases. As emphasized by this study, patient selection is important when surgical intervention for metastatic bone cancer is considered.

The role of the treatment team in the rehabilitation process is to educate individuals about their disease and its treatment and to assist in setting and achieving realistic rehabilitation goals. Multidisciplinary team members may include the surgeon, nurse, physical therapist, occupational therapist, speech pathologist, prosthetist, chaplain, clinical dietitian, social worker, psychiatrist, psychologist, medical oncologist, radiation oncologist, and palliative care physician. Communication among team members is essential for each to understand the disease process, prognosis, and the proposed continuum of care for the patient.

Assessment and Goal Setting

Although many rehabilitation problems associated with cancer and its treatment exist, a study of 805 patients with cancers of varying sites identified that psychological and physical problems are most common (Lehman et al. 1978). Clinicians have general expectations about the nature of psychological and physical problems and likely rehabilitation outcomes, based on knowledge of the disease site and the treatment plan. However, each patient needs to be assessed individually to identify specific problems and treatment goals.

The initial assessment consists of a patient interview and objective evaluation to establish a problem list. The interview records information from the individual's history including symptoms, home situation, work, leisure, and potential goals for rehabilitation. In assessing psychological functioning, knowledge of the individual's goals, values, needs, and lifestyle are critical. Objective tests (e.g., joint range of motion, strength, sensation) are then performed. Analysis of both subjective and objective information identifies problems to be addressed by the rehabilitation program. Together, the clinician

and the patient establish treatment goals that correspond to the problem list. Both short- and long-term goals are identified. The proposed treatment plan varies, depending on whether the patient is being treated with curative or palliative intent.

The physical examination depends on the disease site. The patient is assessed for impairments such as abnormal sensation, reduced motion at a joint, or loss of muscle strength. For many patients with bone tumors, the whole extremity is involved, such that the joints and muscles proximal and distal to the surgical site must also be assessed. In determining whether assessment findings are abnormal, the functional limitations imposed by the tumor excision and reconstruction need to be considered. For example, an endoprosthesis used to reconstruct the knee joint may have a flexion stop on the prosthesis, such that greater than 100 degrees of flexion is not possible.

The patient's ability to perform activities of daily living such as personal hygiene, domestic chores, and work also merit assessment. Frequently, fatigue and lack of endurance impair these functions.

Regardless of whether treatment is curative or palliative, family members need to be included in the rehabilitation process. Unless family members are involved, they will not understand the patient's limitations and the impact of these limitations on the functioning of the family unit. Due to persistent posttreatment fatigue, a patient may be unable to assume his or her usual role within the family unit; other members may need to assume more responsibilities.

The first assessment and treatment plan forms the basis of the rehabilitation program; however, ongoing assessment and re-establishment of short-term treatment goals needs to occur throughout the rehabilitation process.

Precautions and Contraindications

Rehabilitation interventions are based on an understanding of the disease and the treatment, underlying physiology of tissue healing, muscle function, biomechanics, and the component functions necessary to perform various activities and tasks. Rehabilitation interventions include education, counseling, identification of compensatory strategies using intact mechanisms, exercise, physical modalities, and access to resources (e.g., technology, support groups, financial assistance, job retraining). However, these rehabilitation interventions need to be applied with an understanding of the precautions and contraindications imposed by the surgery, chemotherapy, or radiotherapy used to treat the cancer patient.

In surgical cases, the rehabilitation clinician must know what tissues have been resected and the reconstructive procedure done. During musculoskeletal surgery, muscles and tendons are separated and reattached to new sites, whereas bones and joints may be reconstructed with an endoprosthesis or allograft. The clinician's knowledge of the surgical procedure allows the development of treatment programs that provide protected weightbearing and avoid premature stretching of reconstructed soft tissues.

Different treatment modalities (radiotherapy, chemotherapy, and surgery) require different precautions and contraindications. Radiotherapy delays soft tissue healing and frequently results in abnormal sensation in the acute post-treatment period. Thus, the risk of burns from electrodes or thermal or cold modalities is significantly increased.

Radiotherapy can produce devascularization of bone, osteoporosis, or osteoradionecrosis. The rehabilitation specialist needs to understand the extent of mechanical instability present in the skeleton. This is particularly important in the lower extremity in which protected weightbearing may be required to protect against fracture. The rehabilitation specialist may also design and manufacture orthotic devices to prevent fracture in the upper extremity.

Chemotherapy delays bone healing after fracture or after primary tumor skeletal reconstruction. Allograft bone (i.e., cadaveric bone transplants used to reconstruct skeletal defects after tumor resection) does not have the same healing properties as normal bone. When allograft bone has been used to reconstruct the lower limb, the physical therapist must be guided in instituting a weight-training program and in progressing the patient's weightbearing status by the surgeon's interpretation of serial x-rays.

Although hydrotherapy provides an ideal exercise environment when protected weightbearing is required, it may be contraindicated in patients receiving chemotherapy, because the immunosuppression imparted by chemotherapeutic drugs increases the risk of infection. The medical oncologist usually advises chemotherapy patients against hydrotherapy and use of public whirlpools or swimming facilities.

Common Rehabilitation Problems and Their Management

Patient and family education are important for the success of the rehabilitation program. Unless the disease, recovery potential, and need for post-treatment adaptation is understood, it is unlikely that the patient will be successfully rehabilitated. Preoperative teaching allows the clinician to establish what the patient knows about the disease and treatment, to reinforce that understanding, and to correct any misapprehensions. Educational aids, such as videotapes, anatomic models, and diagrams, are useful. Meetings with carefully selected patients who have similar deficits provide peer support and complement the interventions of the multidisciplinary team.

Post-treatment education includes techniques of energy conservation and pacing of activities. Specific tasks may be taught to the patient or family members. For example, patients with spinal cord tumors who experience bowel and bladder dysfunction require routine use of enemas and intermittent catheterization; the patient or a family member may be taught such procedures.

Physical function is significantly impacted by general fatigue and lack of endurance. Patients who experience severe pain, weakness, or immobilization before treatment have increased difficulty mobilizing and regaining their physical function after treatment. An exercise program instituted during hospitalization begins strengthening and improving cardiovascular function and mobility. Postoperative pain and shortening of soft tissues may limit range of motion at specific joints. Once soft tissues are healed, gentle stretching improves joint mobility. Range of motion exercises in conjunction with elevation and compression will also decrease edema. With excision of an extremity tumor involving bone and resection or undermining of muscle, selective strengthening of various muscle groups may be required. The potential for regaining strength depends on the remaining volume of functioning tissue. When a lower extremity tumor has been resected, assistive devices may be required for ambulation. These may be temporary, with the patient progressing from crutches to cane to no assistive devices as bone heals.

Limb amputation occurs infrequently, owing partly to modern imaging techniques that allow the surgeon to determine tumor extent more accurately.

For those patients who undergo amputation, however, special consideration needs to be given to extended wound healing times that may delay the fitting of prostheses. Early postoperative prosthetic fitting is encouraged; however, patients continuing on chemotherapy are slow to heal and may have significant, ongoing weight loss. A prosthesis may not fit in the months after completion of treatment, and periodic adjustment may be required.

For patients with terminal disease, supportive care is directed towards symptom control using heat and cold modalities and pain medications. For those with metastatic bone disease, walkers, crutches, canes, and orthoses redirect weightbearing from the limbs and spine. Exercise maintains strength and cardiovascular status, decreasing fatigue. In the face of metastatic disease, the ultimate goal is to maximize the patient's function as quickly as possible. Assistive devices and personal care may be required in the home. As the patient's level of function and independence improves, the need for home assistance may diminish. Alternatively, for those receiving supportive care for terminal illness, the needs may increase significantly. Constant reassessment is necessary to re-evaluate treatment plans and goals.

Return to work after treatment for cancer depends on many factors, including the degree of residual disability, employer concerns about work performance, provision of modified work, and coworker and employer attitudes (or the patient's perceptions of their attitudes) toward the cancer patient (Malone et al. 1994). The role of the rehabilitation team is to assess the patient's capacity to return to their premorbid employment. If modified duties are required, the adaptations and limitations must be defined to assist the patient and employer in accommodating the changes. When further education and job retraining are necessary, the team should assist in identifying vocational goals and in accessing retraining programs.

Many patients experience fear and anxiety after their cancer diagnosis; appropriate resources for psychosocial support must be accessed. Psychological problems may also include a sense of disfigurement, altered body image, and concerns about sexuality. Imagery, relaxation therapy, biofeedback, and supportive counseling are frequently used psychological techniques (Body et al. 1997). Support groups provide a peer experience and help patients to understand how others have adapted to their disease and treatment sequelae.

For individuals who were active socially in volunteer work or recreational sports, the limitations imposed by fatigue, immobility, or prolonged lack of exercise, can manifest psychologically. The rehabilitation team needs to promote participation in important activities by helping the patient to adopt alternate social activities and energy-conserving strategies.

Ongoing exercise has been shown to be beneficial to both the psychological and physical well-being of cancer patients. Friedenreich and Courneya (1996) published a structured literature review of ten studies on the impact of exercise on the quality of life of cancer patients. Although the review was qualitative due to heterogeneous study samples and variable study designs, the authors concluded that exercise improved the psychological and physiological function of cancer patients.

Summary

Bone tumors are most frequently metastatic from breast or prostate carcinoma. Although incompletely understood, it is thought that metastatic tumor spread occurs via the circulatory system. Primary bone tumors are most frequently benign. Chondrosarcoma and osteosarcoma are the most common primary malignant bone tumors. Primary bone tumors are thought to develop when abnormalities occur during the process of cell division. This process may be mediated by genetic abnormalities.

The diagnosis and treatment of bone neoplasms is a challenging task that relies on the skills of a multidisciplinary medical team including medical, radiation, and surgical oncologists; pathologists; radiologists; therapists; and social workers. The history, physical examination, radiologic imaging, and tissue pathology provide the necessary information for determining the diagnosis. Once diagnosis has been made, treatment may include any or all of chemotherapy, radiotherapy, and surgery.

The rehabilitation specialist is an integral member of the treatment team whose contribution facilitates maximization of function of the cancer patient. The physical, psychological, and social problems faced by cancer patients vary, depending on the disease site, individual personality and coping style, and the point along the trajectory of treatment and recovery. Early in the recovery process, it may be necessary to work on improving range of motion of a joint, whereas further into recovery more functional activities and teaching adaptations to the broader contexts of daily life are more appropriate. The rehabilitation process is one of ongoing education, assessment, problem delineation, and treatment.

To assist cancer patients in achieving maximum outcomes for physical, psychological, and social health, members of the multidisciplinary team and the patient must work toward mutually defined goals reflecting the disease, its treatment, and the patient's needs. The ultimate result of successful rehabilitation is the enhancement of the patient's quality of life. The future challenge for rehabilitation is the evaluation of interventions under controlled conditions such that clinical decision making reflects evidence-based care.

References

Abudu A, Carter SR, Grimer RJ. The outcome and functional results of diaphyseal endoprostheses after tumour excision. J Bone Joint Surg Br 1996;78:652–657.

Allan DG, Bell RS, Davis A, Langer F. Complex acetabular reconstruction for metastatic tumor. J Arthroplasty 1995;10:301–306.

Batson OV. The function of the vertebral veins and their role in the spread of metastases. Arch Surg 1940;112:138–149.

Bell RS, Davis AM, Wunder JS, et al. Allograft reconstruction of the acetabulum after resection of stage-IIB sarcoma. J Bone Joint Surg Am 1997;79:1663–1674.

Bell RS, Wunder JS. Molecular alterations in sarcoma management. Curr Opin Orthop 1997;8:66–70.

Bertoni F, Bacchini P. Classification of bone tumors. Eur J Radiol 1998;27:S74–S76.

Blackley HR, Wunder JS, Davis AM, et al. Treatment of giant cell tumors of long bones with curettage and bone grafting. J Bone Joint Surg Am 1999;81:811–820.

Body JJ, Coleman RE, Piccart M. Use of bisphophonates in cancer patients. Cancer Treat Rev 1996;22:265–287.

Body JJ, Lossignol D, Ronson A. The concept of rehabilitation of cancer patients. Curr Opin Oncol 1997;9:332–340.

Bunting RW. Rehabilitation of cancer patients with skeletal metastases. Clin Orthop 1995;312:197–200.

Bunting RW, Boublik M, Blevins FT, et al. Functional outcome of pathologic fracture secondary to malignant disease in a rehabilitation hospital. Cancer 1992;69:98–102.

Campanacci M, Mercuri M, Gasbarrini A, Campanacci L. The value of imaging in the diagnosis and treatment of bone tumors. Eur J Radiol 1998;27:S116–S122.

Eisenberg E, Berkey CS, Carr DB, et al. Efficacy and safety of nonsteroidal antiinflammatory drugs for cancer pain: a meta-analysis. J Clin Oncol 1994;12:2756–2765.

Enneking WF. Limb Salvage in Musculoskeletal Oncology. New York: Churchill Livingstone, 1987.

Ferrari S, Bacci G, Picci P, et al. Long-term follow-up and post-relapse survival in patients with non-metastatic osteosarcoma of the extremity treated with neoadjuvant chemotherapy. Ann Oncol 1997;8:765–771.

Fisher G, Mayer D, Struthers C. Bone metastases. Part I—Pathophysiology. Clin J Oncol Nurs 1997;2:29–35.

Frassica F, Gitelis S, Slim F. Metastatic bone disease: general principles, patho-physiology, evaluation, and biopsy. Amer Acad Orthop Surg 1992;41:293–300.

Friedenreich CM, Courneya KS. Exercise as rehabilitation for cancer patients. Clin J Sport Med 1996;6:237–244.

Galasko CS. Skeletal metastases. Clin Orthop 1986;210:18–30.

Glasser DB, Lane JM, Huvos AG, et al. Survival, prognosis, and therapeutic response in osteogenic sarcoma. The Memorial Hospital experience. Cancer 1992;69:698–708.

Goorin AM, Andersen JW. Experience with multiagent chemotherapy for osteosarcoma. Improved outcome. Clin Orthop 1991;270:22–28.

Guise TA, Mundy GR. Cancer and bone. Endocrine Rev 1998;19:18–54.

Harrington KD. Orthopaedic management of extremity and pelvic lesions. Clin Orthop 1995;312:136–147.

Healey JH. Metastatic Cancer to the Bone. In VT Devita, SH Hellman, ST Rosenberg (eds), Cancer Principles and Practice of Oncology (5th ed). Philadelphia: Lippincott–Raven, 1997;2573.

Horowitz SM, Glasser DB, Lane JM, Healey JH. Prosthetic and extremity survivorship after limb salvage for sarcoma. How long do the reconstructions last? Clin Orthop 1993;293:280–286.

Hoskin PJ. Radiotherapy in the management of bone pain. Clin Orthop 1995;312:105–119.

Jaffe N, Frei E, Traggis D. Adjuvant methotrexate and citrovorum-factor treatment of osteogenic sarcoma. N Engl J Med 1974;291:59–74.

Kanis JA. Bone and cancer: pathophysiology and treatment of metastases. Bone 1995;17:101S–105S.

Kawar A, Muschler GF, Lane JM, et al. Prosthetic knee replacement after resection of a malignant tumor of the distal part of the femur. Medium to long-term results. J Bone Joint Surg Am 1998;80:636–647.

Lehman JF, DeLisa JA, Warren CG, et al. Cancer rehabilitation: assessment of need, development and evaluation of a model of care. Arch Phys Med Rehab 1978;59:410–419.

Levesque J, Marx RG, Bell RS, et al. A Clinical Guide to Primary Bone Tumors. Baltimore: Williams & Wilkins, 1998.

Link MP, Goorin AM, Horowitz M, et al. Adjuvant chemotherapy of high-grade osteosarcoma of the extremity. Updated results of the Multi-Institutional Osteosarcoma Study. Clin Orthop 1991;270:8–14.

Lorente JA, Morote J, Raventos C, et al. Clinical efficacy of bone alkaline phosphatase and prostate specific antigen in the diagnosis of bone metastasis in prostate cancer. J Urol 1996;155:1348–1351.

Malawar MM, Link MP, Donalson SS. Sarcomas of the Soft Tissues and Bone. In VT Devita, SH Hellman, ST Rosenberg (eds), Cancer Principles and Practice of Oncology (5th ed). Philadelphia: Lippincott–Raven, 1997;1789.

Malone M, Harris AL, Luscombe DK. Assessment of the impact of cancer on work recreation, home management and sleep using a general health status measure. J R Soc Med 1994;87:386–389.

Masciocchi C, Sparvoli L, Barile A. Diagnostic imaging of malignant cartilage tumors. Eur J Radiol 1998;27: S86–S90.

McGoveran BM, Davis AM, Bell RS, Gross AE. Allograft-prosthesis composite technique and functional outcomes in proximal femoral reconstruction following sarcoma resection. Can J Surg 1999;42:37–45.

Mercadante S. Malignant bone pain: pathophysiology and treatment. Pain 1997;69:1–18.

Miyasaka M. Cancer metastasis and adhesion molecules. Clin Orthop 1995;312:10–18.

Mundy GR. Malignancy and the skeleton. Horm Metab Res 1997a;29:120–125.

Mundy GR. Malignancy of bone metastasis. Cancer 1997b; 80:S1546–S1553.

Mundy GR, Guise TA. Hypercalcemia of malignancy. Am J Med 1997;103:134–143.

Mundy GR, Yoneda T. Facilitation and suppression of bone metastasis. Clin Orthop 1995;312:34–44.

National Cancer Institute of Canada, Canadian Cancer Statistics 1998. Toronto: National Cancer Institute of Canada, 1998.

Orr FW, Sanchez-Sweatman OH, Kostenuik P, Singh G. Tumor-bone interactions in skeletal metastasis. Clin Orthop 1995;312:19–33.

Peabody TD, Gibbs CP, Simon MA. Evaluation and staging of musculoskeletal neoplasms. J Bone Joint Surg Am 1998;80:1204–1218.

Phillips LL. Managing the pain of bone metastases in the home environment. Am J Hospice Palliative Care 1998;8:32–42.

Probyn LJ, Wunder JS, Bell RS, et al. A comparison of outcome of osteoarticular allograft reconstruction and shoulder arthrodesis following resection of primary tumours of the proximal humerus. Sarcoma 1998;2: 151–157.

Roberts P, Chan D, Grimer RJ, et al. Prosthetic replacement of the distal femur for primary bone tumours. J Bone Joint Surg Br 1991;73:762–769.

Rosen G, Suwansirikul S, Kwon C. High-dose methotrexate with citrovorum factor rescue and Adriamycin in osteogenic sarcoma. Cancer 1974;33:1151–1163.

Seeger LL, Yao L, Eckardt JJ. Surface lesions of bone. Radiology 1998;206:17–32.

Smith L. Normal Physiology of Bone and Bone Minerals. In T Andreoli, C Carpenter, F Plum, L Smith (eds), Cecil Essentials of Medicine (2nd ed). Philadelphia: WB Saunders, 1990;512–519.

Spina V, Montanari N, Romagnoli R. Malignant tumors of the osteogenic matrix. Eur J Radiol 1998;27:S98–S109.

Toguchida J, Yamaguchi T, Dayton S, et al. Prevalence and spectrum of germline mutations of the *p53* gene among patients with sarcoma. N Engl J Med 1992;326: 1301–1308.

Twycross RG. Management of pain in skeletal metastases. Clin Orthop 1995;312:187–196.

Unwin PS, Cannon SR, Grimer RJ, et al. Aseptic loosening in cemented custom-made prosthetic replacements for bone tumours of the lower limb. J Bone Joint Surg Br 1996;78:5–13.

Walls J, Bundred N, Howell A. Hypercalcemia and bone resorption in malignancy. Clin Orthop 1995;312: 51–63.

Wilner D. Cancer Metastases to Bone. In D Wilner (ed), Radiology of Bone Tumors and Allied Disorders. Philadelphia: WB Saunders, 1982;3611.

Wolff JM, Bares R, Jung PK, et al. Prostate-specific antigen as a marker of bone metastasis in patients with prostate cancer. Urologia Int 1996;56:169–173.

Wunder JS, Davis AM, Hummel JS, et al. The effect of intramedullary cement on intercallary allograft reconstruction of bone defects after tumour resection: a pilot study. Can J Sur 1995;38:521–527.

Chapter 12
Metabolic Bone Diseases

Metabolic bone disease manifests as a diverse collection of disorders generally associated with an alteration in homeostasis of calcium and phosphorus. Metabolic bone disease may often be silent, resulting in a progressive reduction of bone mass until the patient sustains a fracture, the ultimate complication of many metabolic disorders (Lenchik and Sartoris 1998). Osteoporosis (OP), osteomalacia (rickets), hyperparathyroidism, hypoparathyroidism, renal osteodystrophy, and Paget's disease all represent or manifest in metabolic bone disorders. OP, osteomalacia, and Paget's disease are reviewed in this chapter because the conditions themselves and their sequelae have a great impact on the field of physical rehabilitation.

Osteoporosis

OP is one of the most prevalent age-associated diseases affecting the skeleton and is currently a major public health problem affecting the geriatric population. In fact, OP is the most common form of metabolic bone disease. OP is a disease characterized by a low bone mass and the development of nontraumatic or atraumatic fractures as a direct result of the low bone mass (Johnell 1995). The following is a definition of OP: "a disease characterized by low bone mass and microarchitectural deterioration of bone tissue, leading to enhanced bone fragility and a consequent increase in fracture risk" (Consensus Development Conference 1991).

A nontraumatic fracture has been arbitrarily defined as one occurring from trauma equal to, or less than, a fall from a standing height. The absolute diagnosis of OP is made in the occurrence of a traumatic or nontraumatic fracture, whereas the previously asymptomatic state (before the fracture) is referred to as *osteopenia*. In true OP, bone fragility increases to such an extent that normal physical activity causes spontaneous fractures, bone pain syndrome, or both, mainly affecting the spine. In physiologic osteopenia, reduced bone strength and mass fits correspondingly reduced physical activities and muscle strength so well that fractures do not happen without falls or other injuries (Frost 1997).

OP and osteopenia are the most common metabolic bone diseases in the developed countries of the world. The World Health Organization classifies bone mineral density (BMD) into four levels: (1) normal, a value for BMD higher than 1 standard deviation (SD) below the young adult mean; (2) low bone mass (osteopenia), a value for BMD more than 1 SD below the young adult mean, but not more than 2.5 SD below this mean; (3) OP, a value for BMD more than 2.5 SD below the young adult mean; (4) severe OP (established OP), a value for BMD more than 2.5 SD below the young adult mean, accompanied by one or more fragility fractures (Melton 1996).

Age-related bone loss is a universal phenomenon in humans. Peak bone mass is believed to be attained typically in the third to fourth decade of life; bone mass is the difference between peak adult

Table 12-1. Risk Factors Associated
with the Development of Osteoporosis

Genetic
    White/Asian ethnicity
    Positive family history (maternal history of hip fracture)
    Small body frame (<127 lb)
Lifestyle
    Smoking
    Inactivity
    Nulliparity
    Excessive exercise (amenorrhea)
    Early natural menopause
    Late menarche
    Immobilization
Nutrition
    Milk intolerance
    Low dietary calcium intake
    Vegetarian dieting
    Excessive alcohol intake
    Consistently high protein intake
Medical disorders
    Anorexia nervosa
    Thyroid disease (hyperthyroidism)
    Primary hyperparathyroidism
    Cushing's syndrome
    Type 1 diabetes
    Gastrointestinal and hepatobiliary dysfunction
    Osteogenesis imperfecta
    Organ transplantation
Drugs
    Corticosteroid therapy
Clinical risk factors
    Radiographic: Evidence of osteopenia/vertebral deformity
    Previous fragility fracture (e.g., of the hip, spine, or wrist)
    Loss of height, thoracic kyphosis

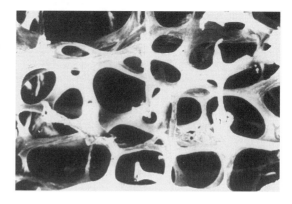

Figure 12-1. Type I osteoporosis. Note the thinning and loss of connecting trabeculae in cancellous bone.

In an effort to develop a predictive model for osteoporotic fracture, it has been determined that the strongest risk factors for osteoporotic fracture include age, race, low body mass index, and inactivity (Turner et al. 1998). BMD, body sway related to postural stability, and muscle strength also were identified as independent and powerful synergistic predictors of osteoporotic fracture incidence (Nguyen et al. 1993).

The incidence of osteoporotic fracture increases with age, and the incidence is higher in women than in men. The female to male ratio for vertebral fractures is 7 to 1 and is 2 to 1 for hip fractures. The lifetime risk of a 50-year-old woman to sustain an osteoporotic fracture during her remaining life is approximately 30–40% (Delmas 1995). In fact, for females, the risk of an osteoporotic fracture is higher than the combined risk of breast, endometrial, and ovarian cancer (Rozenberg et al. 1997). Some of the most common fractures occur in the thoracic and lumbar vertebrae of the spine and proximal femur (hip fracture). Thinning and actual loss of horizontal connecting trabeculae within cancellous bone (Figure 12-1) leads to characteristic weakness of the cancellous regions of bone, increasing the patient's susceptibility to vertebral compression fractures, distal radial fractures, and intertrochanteric femoral fractures (Silver and Einhorn 1995). The spine is the most frequent site of fracture, but fractures of the hip are responsible for the greatest morbidity and mortality (Riggs and Melton 1992; Kanis et al. 1997). Almost without exception, a hip fracture requires admission to a hospital. A 15–20% mortality rate exists after a hip

bone mass and the loss of bone mass that has since occurred. From long-term prospective studies, it can be concluded that peak bone density and bone loss are important predictors of subsequent fracture and that fracture can be predicted over a long period (Jergas and Gluer 1997; Kudlacek et al. 1998). Although OP is multifactorial, genetic factors play an important role in the pathogenesis of OP; up to 75% of the variance in bone mass may be genetically determined (Table 12-1). In fact, segregation analysis of bone mass in families has suggested a model in which bone mass is controlled by a large number of genes with small effect, rather than a few genes with large effect (Grant and Ralston 1997).

fracture caused by OP. Perhaps more important, it is estimated that fewer than one-third of patients are restored to their previous level of function within 12 months after the fracture. High morbidity rates and lengthy hospital stays associated with fractures resulting from this condition are, and will become, an increasingly significant drain on health care resources.

Vertebral Changes

In the thoracic spine, wedging progresses from the premenopausal through early postmenopausal to late postmenopausal years. The degree of change between the premenopausal and early postmenopausal period is as marked as that found in later life (Evans et al. 1993). Evidence exists, however, that changes in vertebral shape do not necessarily equate with osteoporotic collapse (Kleerekoper and Nelson 1992). Increasing age may be associated with an increase of the anteroposterior (AP) dimension of all vertebrae, which could act to increase loadbearing in older subjects. It is theorized that the apparent decline in bone density increases as a declining bone mineral content occupies a larger volume (Evans et al. 1993).

Vertebral fractures are usually described as central (biconcave), wedge, or crush, which may variously involve a part, or the whole, of the vertebrae (Figure 12-2). Wedging is more common at the anterior than the posterior aspect of the vertebrae, and these fractures often occur with minimal trauma, such as might be experienced with coughing or lifting (Kanis and McCloskey 1992). In fact, wedge deformities appear to be the most frequent deformity, clustering at the midthoracic and thoracolumbar regions of the spine in both men and women (Ismail et al. 1999). Trabecular abnormality, which is significantly correlated with aging, may be the necessary and sufficient condition for vertebral deformities in involutional OP (Oda et al. 1998). All deformity types are linked with adverse outcomes although crush deformities may show greater height loss than other deformity types (Ismail et al. 1999). The failure load of any vertebral body depends on the density and architecture of the trabecular bone and on the shape, size, and organization of the vertebral body. The magnitude of a load applied to the spine depends on the specific activity; for example, bending and lifting activ-

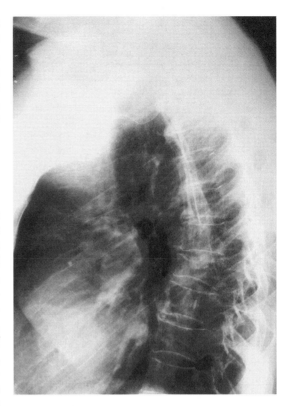

Figure 12-2. Thoracic kyphosis. Note the wedge fracture involving the anterior portion of a thoracic vertebral body.

ities generate loads on the spine that exceed the failure load of vertebrae with very low BMD (Myers and Wilson 1997).

Epidemiology of Osteoporosis-Related Fractures

It has been estimated that future worldwide incidence of hip fracture will approximately double to 2.6 million by the year 2025 and to 4.5 million by the year 2050 (Gullberg et al. 1997). Major demographic changes are projected to occur in Asia; however, the socioeconomic impact of hip fractures are projected to increase markedly throughout the world (Gullberg et al. 1997). As many as 40% of women in the United States experience a fracture in association with OP by the age of 70 years, and 15% of these women sustain a hip fracture by the age of 80 years (Bilezikian and Silverberg 1992). The estimated lifetime risk of sustaining a proximal femoral fracture in women and men at the age of 50 years is 17.5% and 6.0%, respectively (Melton 1991).

Pathogenesis

The excessive bone loss that characterizes the pathogenesis of OP results from abnormalities in the bone remodeling cycle. OP is considered a heterogeneous condition characterized by different patterns of osteoclast and osteoblast dysfunction. In health, the bone turnover cycle is initiated by resorption of old bone, recruitment of osteoblasts, deposition of new matrix, and mineralization of that newly deposited matrix. In postmenopausal OP, the normal balance of bone removal and replacement cycles is disrupted in favor of resorption, after which a weak effort at replacement of bone tissue occurs. In age-related OP, in which both males and females are affected more equally, an osteoblast insufficiency is the likely cause of aberrant bone remodeling effort.

Classification

Two categories of OP have been identified: primary and secondary. Primary OP is further divided into two types (type I and type II). Type I OP occurs in menopausal women (both surgical and natural), manifests with diminished levels of associated sex steroid hormones, and affects predominantly cancellous and endocortical bone (Arlot et al. 1990). Type II OP results as a consequence of aging in both men and women and affects both the cortical and cancellous bone compartments. Type II OP encompasses the composite influences of long-term remodeling inefficiency, as well as age-related systemic changes in calcium and vitamin D metabolism, intestinal and renal system decline, and aberration in parathyroid hormone secretion (Marcus 1996). The hip fracture is the clinical hallmark of type II OP.

Low Turnover versus High Turnover

With both age and menopause, the ultimate decrease in bone mass appears to come from a decline in bone formation (Heersche et al. 1998).

Low Turnover (Type II, Age-Related). With the normal aging process, there appears to be a progressive impairment of the signaling between bone resorption and bone formation so that with every cycle of remodeling the deficit between resorption and formation is increased because osteoblast activity, osteoblast recruitment, or both is insufficient. In the case of type II OP, excessive bone loss occurs when activation of the skeleton is not increased. Results of histomorphometric analyses of osteoblastic function in cancellous bone in which there is established OP confirm a reduction in total osteoblast number, percentage of active osteoblasts (those engaged in making osteoid), and especially in the efficiency of those active osteoblasts (Byers et al. 1997). Age-related changes in bone are discussed in greater detail in Chapter 5.

High Turnover (Type I, Postmenopausal). Bone turnover is a function of the number of cycles in progress at any one time. Conditions that increase the rate of activation of the bone remodeling process increase, in turn, the proportion of the skeleton undergoing remodeling at any one time, with the overall result of an increased rate of bone loss. This type of bone loss relates predominantly to that incurred at menopause or with surgical ovariectomy (Figure 12-3). The lack of follicular development that characterizes menopause leads to a marked reduction in serum levels of estradiol and progesterone. Knowledge of the role that estrogen and progesterone deficiency plays in the pathogenesis of postmenopausal OP and the mechanism of their actions has grown considerably (Heersche et al. 1998; Pacifici 1996). A close look at estrogen deficiency in human beings reveals that the major effect of estrogen deficiency is an increase in the rate of bone remodeling unit activation (Heersche et al. 1998). This may occur via the effect of estrogen in modulating the production of cytokines and growth factors from bone marrow and bone cells (Ershler et al. 1997; Pacifici 1996). Type I OP is characterized by accelerated cancellous bone resorption related to this estrogen and progesterone deficiency; it is identified by a fracture pattern that predominantly involves the bodies of the vertebrae and distal radius in which there is a large representation of cancellous bone tissue.

Figure 12-3. A. Dual energy x-ray absorptiometry (DEXA) scan of the lumbar spine region in a surgically ovariectomized female. Note the dramatic loss in bone mineral density relative to age-matched females. **B.** DEXA scan of the femoral neck region in a surgically ovariectomized female. Note the loss in bone mineral density relative to age-matched females. This loss is less dramatic than that seen in the lumbar spine region.

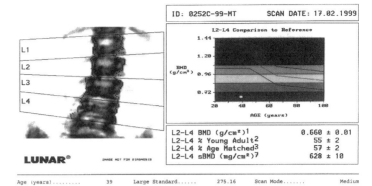

```
ID: 0252C-99-MT          SCAN DATE: 17.02.1999

            L2-L4 Comparison to Reference
```

L2-L4 BMD (g/cm²)[1]		0.660 ± 0.01
L2-L4 % Young Adult[2]		55 ± 2
L2-L4 % Age Matched[3]		57 ± 2
L2-L4 sBMD (mg/cm²)[7]		628 ± 10

Age (years)........	39	Large Standard......	275.16	Scan Mode......	Medium
Sex...............	Female	Medium Standard.....	203.79	Scan Type...........	DPXIQ
Weight (Kg)........	55.0	Small Standard.....	146.08	Collimation (mm)...	1.68
Height (cm)........	161	Low keV Air (cps)...	709340	Sample Size (mm).....	1.2x 1.2
Ethnic.............	White	High keV Air (cps)..	424420	Current (µA)........	750
System.............	5037	Rvalue (%Fat)....... 1.375(8.3)			

Region	BMD[1] g/cm²	Young Adult[2] %	T	Age Matched[3] %	Z
L1	0.574	51	-4.6	53	-4.3
L2	0.654	54	-4.6	56	-4.2
L3	0.676	56	-4.4	58	-4.0
L4	0.650	54	-4.6	56	-4.3
L1-L2	0.616	54	-4.5	55	-4.1
L1-L3	0.640	55	-4.4	57	-4.1
L1-L4	0.643	54	-4.5	56	-4.1
L2-L3	0.666	56	-4.4	57	-4.1
L2-L4	0.660	55	-4.5	57	-4.2
L3-L4	0.662	55	-4.5	57	-4.2

1 - See appendix on precision and accuracy.
    Statistically 68% of repeat scans will fall within 1 SD. (±0.01 g/cm²)
2 - USA AP Spine Reference Population, Ages 20-45.
3 - Matched for Age, Weight(25-100kg), Ethnic.
7 - Lunar BMD for L2-L4 is 0.660 g/cm². See J Bone Miner Res 1994; 9:1503-1514

A

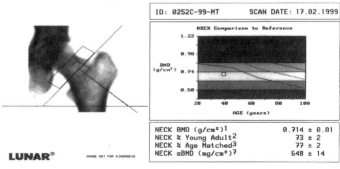

```
ID: 0252C-99-MT          SCAN DATE: 17.02.1999

            NECK Comparison to Reference
```

NECK BMD (g/cm²)[1]		0.714 ± 0.01
NECK % Young Adult[2]		73 ± 2
NECK % Age Matched[3]		77 ± 2
NECK sBMD (mg/cm²)[7]		648 ± 14

Age (years)........	39	Large Standard......	275.16	Scan Mode......	Medium
Sex...............	Female	Medium Standard.....	203.79	Scan Type...........	DPXIQ
Weight (Kg)........	55.0	Small Standard.....	146.08	Collimation (mm)....	1.68
Height (cm)........	161	Low keV Air (cps)...	709340	Sample Size (mm).....	1.2x 1.2
Ethnic.............	White	High keV Air (cps)..	424420	Region height (mm)...	60.0
System.............	5037	Rvalue (%Fat)....... 1.348(22.1)		Region width (mm)....	15.0
Side...............	Left	Current (µA)........	750	Region angle (deg)...	54

Region	BMD[1] g/cm²	Young Adult[2] %	T	Age Matched[3] %	Z
NECK	0.714	73	-2.2	77	-1.8
WARDS	0.629	69	-2.2	74	-1.7
TROCH	0.502	64	-2.6	66	-2.3
SHAFT	0.730	-	-	-	-
TOTAL	0.642	64	-3.0	67	-2.7

1 - See appendix on precision and accuracy.
    Statistically 68% of repeat scans will fall within 1 SD. (±0.01 g/cm²)
2 - USA Femur Reference Population, Ages 20-45.
3 - Matched for Age, Weight(25-100kg), Ethnic.
7 - Lunar BMD for NECK is 0.714 g/cm². See J Bone Miner Res 1994; 9:1503-1514

B

Secondary Osteoporosis

In secondary OP, a clear etiologic mechanism causes OP. Up to 20% of women who otherwise appear to have postmenopausal OP can be shown to have additional etiologic factors above and beyond their age, gender, and ethnic background. Glucocorticoid excess carries the risk of inducing secondary OP (Wolinsky-Friedland 1995; Ziegler and Kasperk 1998). The most significant adverse effects of glucocorticoid drugs on the skeleton include a direct inhibition of matrix synthesis by the osteoblast, reductions in calcium absorption in both the gut and renal tubule, and the production of hypogonadism, especially in men (Reid 1997). OP induced by glucocorticoid excess appears to be caused by changes in the birth and death of bone cells, in particular a decrease in osteoblastogenesis in the bone marrow, and an increased rate of osteoblast and osteocyte apoptosis (Manolagas 1998). A 10–40% reversible reduction in bone density may result with glucocorticoid use, with the loss more marked in cancellous bone and in those individuals in whom a high cumulative dose of the steroid exists. Fractures are common, affecting approximately 30% of individuals who take glucocorticoids for a period of 5 years or more. Because of the predilection of glucocorticoid bone loss for cancellous bone, osteopenia typically occurs in the vertebrae and ribs and is less striking in the long bones (Wolinsky-Friedland 1995).

Osteoporosis in Men

No abrupt cessation of testicular function or "andropause" occurs in males comparable with menopause in females. However, both total and free testosterone levels do decline with age. Testosterone deficiency is associated with heightened bone turnover and is a major risk factor for osteoporosis in men (Francis 1999; Katznelson 1998). The most important factors in the development of OP in males are hypoandrogenism, hypoestrogenism, an association with alcohol consumption and smoking, malnutrition, lack of sun exposure, and chronic liver disease (Treves et al. 1998). It is well recognized that estrogens are important in skeletal maintenance in men and women (Anderson 1998). A positive association between BMD and greater serum estradiol levels at all skeletal sites, and a negative association between BMD and testosterone at some sites, was reported in males older than 65 years (Ebeling 1998).

Osteoporotic fractures, especially hip fractures, are a leading cause of morbidity and mortality among elderly men (Boonen et al. 1997). However, the female to male ratio of femoral neck fractures is still approximately 2.8 (Treves et al. 1998). Age-associated endocrine deficiencies encompass a decline in circulating androgen levels and decreased activity of the growth hormone insulin-like growth factor I axis, which may also contribute to femoral bone loss and hip fracture occurrence in elderly men (Boonen et al. 1997).

Establishing a Diagnosis

Imaging

Plain Film Radiography. Cancellous bone resorption in the axial skeleton is a dominant process in type I OP and results in marked thinning and dissolution of transverse trabeculae with relative preservation of the primary trabeculae or those aligned along lines of stress. In areas in which cancellous bone predominates, such as in the spine and pelvis, the combination of osteopenia and reinforcement of primary trabeculae may produce a striated bony appearance. The reinforced primary trabeculae have a sharp appearance in osteoporotic bones. The loss of cancellous bone mass also accentuates the cortical outline, producing the so-called picture framing or empty box phenomenon seen in OP of the vertebral bodies (see Figure 12-2). The vertebral bodies become weakened and the intervertebral disk may protrude into the adjacent vertebral body. The degree of protrusion varies, ranging from bending and buckling of the endplates (biconcave appearance) to herniation of disk material into the vertebral body. In more advanced cases, complete compression fractures of the vertebral bodies occur.

Because no gold standard for the definition of vertebral fracture exists, controversy has centered on whether mild vertebral deformities are truly fractures or simply normal variation in vertebral size and shape. A lack of consensus regarding the radiographic definition of vertebral fracture makes it difficult to determine the frequency with which vertebral fractures occur in postmenopausal women. BMD and height ratios as determined by lateral radiographs of nonfractured vertebrae have been shown to be independent predictors of vertebral fracture risk; even mild deformities may represent real consequences of OP because they are more pronounced among women with obvious fracture (Tomomitsu et al. 1997). When findings suggest vertebral fracture, AP and lateral radiographs of the thoracolumbar spine should be obtained. A decrease of 15–25% in the anterior, central, or posterior height of a vertebral body compared with either adjacent normal vertebrae or a population reference is consistent with vertebral fracture (Melton et al. 1989). However, the use of a fixed percentage reduction in vertebral height identified that a 20–25% reduction in vertebral height minimizes the sample size required for clinical trials and epidemiologic studies (Black et al. 1999).

Dual-Energy X-Ray Absorptiometry. Bone densitometry, in its various applications, has become an established tool to confirm the presence of OP, to assess the severity of bone loss before treatment, and to monitor efficacy of therapy. Dual-energy x-ray absorptiometry (DEXA) is the preferred method to capture bone density, because it has the lowest precision error (Rozenberg et al. 1995). Identification of individuals at risk of OP can be achieved through DEXA (Figure 12-4). Bone density has been shown to be significantly associated with the risk of fracture. In fact, a decrease in each SD of BMD below mean values predicts a doubling of the fracture risk (Rozenberg et al. 1997). An interesting interpretation by Kanis et al. (1997) of the value of BMD is as follows:

"The performance of bone mineral density in predicting fracture is regarded to be at least as good as that of blood pressure in predicting stroke, and considerably better than the use of serum cholesterol to predict coronary artery disease."

Bone density measurements at the site of fracture appear to perform better than measurements at other sites in predicting future osteoporotic fracture of any type (Melton et al. 1996). However, fractures at other sites also may predict vertebral fractures; for example, the presence of wrist fractures increases the risk of vertebral fractures and the presence of vertebral fractures increases

the risk of hip fractures (Kotowicz and Melton 1994). Simple geometric measures of bones, such as hip axis length and vertebral depth, may be derived from images of bone densitometry scans and also are predictive of hip fracture or vertebral fracture independent of bone density (Jergas and Gluer 1997).

A lack of a significant age-related decrease of bone mass has been reported using the conventional AP view of the lumbar spine by DEXA in women older than 65 years of age (Duboeuf et al. 1991; Liu et al. 1997). This contrasts with a large (15–20%) decrease of bone density between the ages of 65 and 85 years at other skeletal sites, such as the radius, the hip, and the calcaneus (Delmas 1995). This phenomenon was partly attributable to the fact that lumbar spine osteophytes affect most subjects older than 60 years of age and contribute substantially to lumbar spine BMD measured in the AP position by DEXA. Some investigators assert that diagnosis of OP and assessment of osteoporotic fracture risk in the elderly should be based on hip BMD and not that from the AP lumbar spine, unless spinal osteoarthritis has been excluded (Liu et al. 1997). Alternatively, if qualitative computed tomography is available for BMD assessment, it might be the preferred technique to investigate the spine in women with expected artifactual images (osteophytes, scoliosis) at the spine (Rozenberg et al. 1995).

Quantitative Ultrasound. Quantitative ultrasonic measures of bone quality have been shown to have a predictive capability of fracture that is comparable to that of bone density (Gluer et al. 1997); however, some studies suggest a relationship between quantitative ultrasound (QUS) and bone strength beyond that which can be explained by BMD (Rossini et al. 1998).

Peripheral Assessment of Skeletal Status in Osteoporosis. Single photon absorptiometry and radiographic absorptiometry are traditional approaches in the peripheral measurement of bone mass (e.g., at the distal radius or os calcis). New peripheral approaches include single x-ray absorptiometry, peripheral dual x-ray absorptiometry, peripheral quantitative computed tomography, QUS, and magnetic resonance imaging.

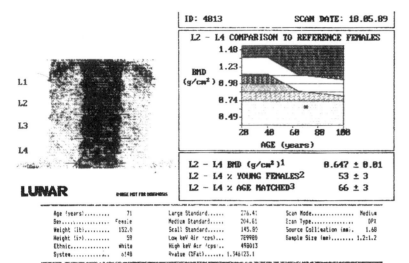

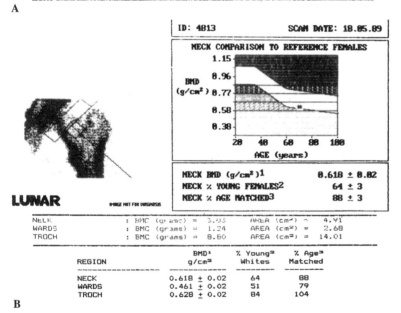

Figure 12-4. A. Dual energy x-ray absorptiometry (DEXA) scan of the lumbar spine region in a 71-year-old woman. Note the dramatic loss in bone mineral density relative to age-matched women. **B.** DEXA scan of the femoral neck region in a 71-year-old woman. Note the lack of an equally substantial loss in bone mineral density at this site, relative to the lumbar spine region.

Laboratory: Biochemistry

Screening for renal and hepatic function, primary hyperparathyroidism, and malnutrition is useful for establishing a definitive diagnosis of OP. The calciotropic hormones (parathyroid hormone, calcitriol [vitamin D], or calcitonin) are generally not considered useful measurements for establishing a diagnosis of OP. Accurate assessment of bone turnover can, however, be made with the more useful bone biochemical markers including serum levels of bone alkaline phosphatase and osteocalcin (formation) and with urine deoxypyridinoline and pyridinoline cross-links (resorption) (Riggs and Khosla 1995; Takahashi et al. 1999).

A bone mass measurement (DEXA) and a biochemical index of bone turnover provide different but complementary information that, together, aid in predicting risk of bone loss and osteoporotic fracture (Eyre 1997).

Clinical Assessment of Osteoporosis

The risk factors for, and prevalence of, skeletal deformities that occur in women with OP is presented in Table 12-2.

Axial Skeleton: Vertebral Osteoporosis

The clinical manifestation of sustaining vertebral fracture(s) include kyphosis, back pain, and loss of height. New crush fractures may give rise to severe back pain that characteristically decreases in severity over several weeks or months (Kanis and McCloskey 1992). Among symptomatic patients, pain is most commonly experienced while standing

Table 12-2. Skeletal Deformities in Women with Osteoporosis: Associated Risk Factors and Prevalence

Skeletal Deformities	Risk Factors for Skeletal Deformities	Prevalence of Skeletal Deformities and Fractures
Vertebral compression fractures (anterior wedging of the vertebral bodies): Kyphosis Reduced height Altered lumbar lordosis	Back flexion and heavy lifting (Sinaki 1982) Gonadal steroid hormone deprivation (DeSmet et al. 1988; Nguyen et al. 1995) Weak back extensor muscles (Sinaki et al. 1993)	Studies of women with post-menopausal or senile spinal osteoporosis aged 48–89 revealed a 78% (Satoh et al. 1988) and an 82% (Itoi 1991) prevalence of spinal deformity. Based on a study of 27,000 women with osteoporosis (Santavirta et al. 1992), thoracic spine fractures were as follows: Age 55–64: 5.1 per 1,000 Age 65–74: 15 per 1,000 Age 75+: 29 per 1,000
Hip fracture Femoral neck Intratrochanteric Subcapital	Height (Nevitt and Cummings 1993) Weak triceps (Nevitt and Cummings 1993) Landing on a hard floor (Nevitt and Cummings 1993) Postmenopausal status (Millar and Hill 1994)	Hospital admissions (in Canada) attributed to femoral neck fractures in 1990 (Millar and Hill 1994) were as follows: Age 55–60: 6.6 per 10,000 Age 60–64: 13 per 10,000 Age 65–69: 23 per 10,000 Age 70–74: 45 per 10,000 Age 75–79: 83 per 10,000 Age 80–84: 223 per 10,000 Age 85+: 332 per 10,000 Mortality rate attributed to femoral neck fractures in women aged 55 and older in 1990 (in Canada): 16.2 per 100,000 (Millar and Hill 1994). Women 60 years of age, with a residual life expectancy of more than 21 years, have a 14% risk of sustaining a hip fracture (Lauritzen et al. 1993).
Wrist fracture	Height (Nevitt and Cummings 1993) Weak grip strength (Nevitt and Cummings 1993)	Women 60 years of age, with a residual life expectancy of more than 21 years, have a 17% risk of sustaining a wrist (radial) fracture (Lauritzen et al. 1993).

Source: Reprinted with permission from D Grant, K Lundon. The Canadian Model of Occupational Performance applied to females with osteoporosis. Can J Occup Ther 1999;66:3–13.

and during physical stress such as bending (Leidig et al. 1990).

Some vertebral (insufficiency) fractures may occur in the absence of acute symptoms; however, in one study 13% of patients reported a sudden onset of back pain, 13% of whom had a fall, 24% lifted a heavy load, 44% had no apparent reason, and 19% reported a more gradual onset of complaints (Leidig-Bruckner et al. 1997). Fractures are most typical in the anterior portion of the vertebral bodies of the thoracic spine, ranging from T7 to L1. Acute symptoms may include sudden onset of mild to severe middle to low back pain and limitation of motion. Once an acute vertebral fracture has been sustained, the individual may report that physical activity exacerbates pain and may be willing to perform only protected movement (e.g., splints with coughing). The nature of the pain of vertebral fractures has been reported to be localized, deep-seated, and interspersed with episodes of stabbing pain, with pain rarely extending to the legs (Leidig et al. 1990). Some pain relief may be accomplished by lying down; however, some individuals report exacerbation of symptoms when changing positions in bed (Leidig et al. 1990). Within 4–6 weeks, acute skeletal pain should dissipate; however, it may persist for several weeks. The reappearance of pain may signal a new fracture. Involvement of spinal tract symptoms is rare.

The purpose of spinal x-rays is to provide evidence of vertebral fractures and gross tissue alteration. A compressed vertebra may be revealed on plain film radiographs; however, the fractured vertebra may collapse gradually and only may be observed 2 or more months later (Millard et al. 1997). If a number of vertebrae are involved, the severity of individual vertebral deformities progresses, and simultaneous weakening of the postural muscles occur with a strong tendency toward an increased degree of kyphosis.

The diagnosis of existing vertebral fractures is critical because the probability of sustaining new spine and hip fractures is increased in women with one vertebral fracture; the presence of multiple fractures may place the individual at risk for a chronic state of debilitation. However, vertebral fractures may never come to medical attention due to the fact that symptoms may not be severe enough to prompt the individual to seek medical care (Ettinger et al. 1992). In fact, surveys of spine radiographs in older subjects suggest that many vertebral fractures have occurred in the absence of acute symptoms.

The gravity of the situation is underlined by the fact that once a vertebral body has fractured, the restoration of its normal anatomy is not possible. In fact, refractures of the same vertebrae with further abnormalities of shape and size is common. These vertebral fractures give rise to chronic pain, disability, and obvious spinal deformity known as *kyphosis*. All vertebral fractures are associated with loss of stature. In the thoracic spine, loss of stature is associated with a progressive increase in the degree of kyphosis because of both morphological adaptation of both the vertebral bodies and intervertebral disks (Goh et al. 1999). In the lumbar spine, loss of stature is associated with progressive flattening of the lordotic curve (Figure 12-5). Biomechanical indications for prevention of vertebral fractures point to the need to strengthen bone by maintaining or increasing density and the need to lower the magnitude of forces applied to the spine in the elderly or other susceptible people by avoiding such risk activities as lifting. The strength of bone and the load-bearing capacity should be considered in relation to the forces applied to the spine (Myers and Wilson 1997).

Clinical Measurement of Spinal Kyphosis. As the number of vertebrae involved increases and the severity of individual vertebral deformities progresses, these anatomic deformities become more pronounced. Therefore, if postural correction is not addressed at this point, the condition progresses. There is gradual loss of the waistline contour and protuberance of the abdomen and, in severe cases, the lower ribs may approximate the pelvic rim and ultimately lie within the pelvis. Severe vertebral deformity has been associated with significantly increased risk of general disability, impaired bending in men, and impaired rising from a chair in women (Burger et al. 1997). In the same study, moderate vertebral deformity was more frequent among men, whereas the prevalence of severe deformity was considerably higher in women. In addition, vertebral deformities with age may be only slightly less common in men than in women. It appears that severe progression with age occurs in women only; severe vertebral deformity is highly related to functional

Figure 12-5. Classification of spinal kyphosis. (Reprinted with permission from E Itoi. Roentgenographic analysis of posture in spinal osteoporotics. Spine 1991;16:750–756.)

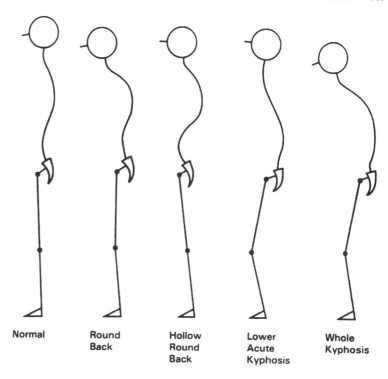

Normal   Round Back   Hollow Round Back   Lower Acute Kyphosis   Whole Kyphosis

impairment, especially in men (Burger et al. 1997; Matthis et al. 1999).

All patients suspected of having OP, with or without fracture, should have an evaluation of spinal bone mass. Measurement of kyphosis by noninvasive instruments, such as the DeBrunner's kyphometer (Figure 12-6) and the flexicurve ruler (Figure 12-7), should be applied in the evaluation of spinal deformities to evaluate a baseline and subsequent progression of the disease (Lundon et al.

Clinical Note

It is apparent that impairment of general well-being, functional disability, pain, and altered body shape in patients with OP extends beyond the measurement of fractures but additionally is influenced by the presence of microfractures, muscle imbalances, irritation of joints, periarticular structures, and the status of intervertebral disks (Ettinger et al. 1992; Ettinger et al. 1994). One point of view is that OP is one of the nonfatal conditions that leads more to changes in the quality of life rather than to changes in the quantity of life (Rudberg et al. 1992). Common physical and social outcomes of OP, such as loss of height, kyphosis, decreased mobility, pain, loss of independence, and depression, contribute to a diminished quality of life for the individual with this condition (Grant and Lundon 1999; Zimmerman et al. 1995).

The loss of stature results in progressive changes in length of the paraspinal muscles, resulting in considerable discomfort and muscle fatigue. Back pain is a major complaint in the osteoporotic patient. It is thought that a great deal of chronic back pain from spinal OP is derived from the fatigued paraspinal muscles as well as structural bone changes inherent to spinal kyphosis. After multiple fractures and subsequent spinal deformity ensue, chronic back pain may develop as a result of muscle spasms caused by altered spinal biomechanics. Affected individuals often report the pain to be located in the paraspinal regions and that the spine region itself is not tender. Pain is often reported to be worse with prolonged standing and is relieved by walking.

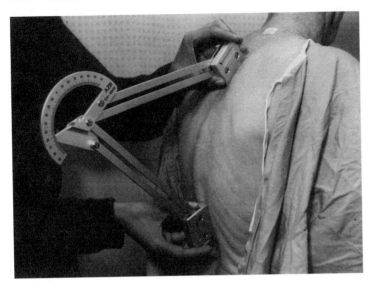

Figure 12-6. DeBrunner's kyphometer for noninvasive measurement of spinal kyphosis. (Reprinted with permission from K Lundon, A Li, S Bibershtein. Interrater and intrarater reliability in the measurement of kyphosis in postmenopausal women with osteoporosis. Spine 1998;23:1978–1985.)

1998). In addition, height reduction (HR), distance from occiput to wall (DOW), and the distance from the iliac crest to the ribs (DIR) are easily obtained physical measurements and are useful for monitoring disease progression.

Management Strategies

The general goal in the care of the skeleton in which a fracture has been sustained because of OP is to restore, as closely as possible, the anatomic and functional prefracture state of the affected individual. The clinical paradox is that immobilization should be limited in the primary fracture healing phase, because longer immobilization has the potential to lead to accelerated bone loss. There does not appear to be anything about an osteoporotic fracture that would result in severely delayed fracture union.

Psychosocial Impact of Osteoporosis

A distorted body image, which results from the loss of height as well as the protuberant abdomen, can contribute to debilitating psychosocial issues

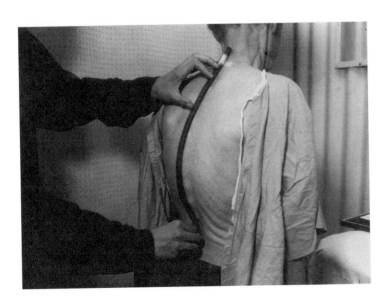

Figure 12-7. The flexicurve ruler for noninvasive measurement of spinal kyphosis. (Reprinted with permission from K Lundon, A Li, S Bibershtein. Interrater and intrarater reliability in the measurement of kyphosis in postmenopausal women with osteoporosis. Spine 1998;23:1978–1985.)

> **Clinical Note**
>
> *Summary of Issues of Concern in the Management of the Individual with Osteoporosis*
>
> **Relief of pain**
> **Restoration of function**
> **Maintain quality of life**
> **Prevention of further fractures**

in these individuals. Fears, adaptations because of physical changes and limitations, as well as concerns about self-image all warrant consideration to best target disease management and intervention strategies. Some of the clinical consequences of osteoporotic vertebral fractures are back pain, functional limitations, and impairment of well-being and mood, warranting a multidisciplinary therapeutic approach to intervention. Although parameters of quality of life were not observed to be linearly related to the degree of radiologically assessed vertebral deformity, osteoporotic patients with two or more vertebral fractures tended to have more functional limitations than those with only one fracture (Leidig-Bruckner et al. 1997). In other words, spinal deformation and the clinical course of OP appears to be insufficiently reflected by radiologic indices of vertebral deformity alone.

Ettinger et al. (1992) found a relationship between vertebral fractures and pain and functional limitations only among patients with severe vertebral fractures. In this study, a significant relationship was observed between components of quality of life (disability score, pain) and clinical measures of spinal deformation (HR, DOW, and DIR). The overall clinical consequences of OP are decreased mobility; increased fear of falling and fractures; dissatisfaction with body image; and respiratory and gastrointestinal problems associated with severe kyphosis, height loss, or both (Lydick et al. 1997). Other associated age-related conditions, such as impaired vision and hearing, decreased strength and coordination, neurologic dysfunction, arthritis, and diabetes mellitus, increase the risk of falling and consequently the risk of fractures.

It appears that with respect to quality of life components, functional limitation is most specific to spinal OP and is related to clinical measures of spinal deformation. Kyphosis, by both clinical and quantitative assessment, is associated with diminished function, especially performance of mobility tasks (Ryan and Fried 1997). In another study, Cook et al. (1993) identified that emotional dysfunction is a serious problem in a significant proportion of patients with spinal OP and is highly associated with functional disabilities.

A number of instruments exist for measuring health-related quality of life for women with OP and back pain caused by OP-related vertebral fractures (Guyatt and Cook 1994; Lydick et al. 1997). The OP targeted quality of life questionnaire (OPTQoL) is a validated measure to help in understanding the natural history of OP, to aid in screening individuals for disease-related problems, and to provide information regarding prevention and treatment programs (Lydick et al. 1997). The Osteoporosis Quality of Life Questionnaire (OQLQ) addresses five domains: symptoms, physical function, activities of daily living, emotional function, and leisure (Guyatt and Cook 1994). A summary of the functional limitations, related skeletal deformities, and subsequent impact of OP on occupation is presented in Table 12-3.

Physical Rehabilitation

All efforts must be made to reduce the number of OP-related fractures in an individual at risk. In some regions, practice guidelines have been developed for primary care clinicians (Kanis et al. 1997). It is therefore necessary to emphasize various interventions and attitudes that act to lessen

Table 12-3. Mechanisms of Development of Skeletal Deformities and Their Functional Limitations: Impact on Occupation

Skeletal Deformities	Mechanisms of Development	Functional Limitations	Impact on Occupation (Self-care, Productivity, and Leisure)
Vertebral compression fractures (anterior wedging of the vertebral bodies): Kyphosis Reduced height Altered lumbar lordosis	Gradual compression of reduced mineralized mid-thoracic and thoracolumbar vertebrae leads to anterior wedging and the development of hyperkyphosis (DeSmet et al. 1988). To compensate for hyperkyphosis, the following may eventually develop: Altered lumbar lordosis Posterior tilt of the sacrum and pelvis Knee flexion However, such compensation only seems to promote back pain (Itoi 1991). Demineralization of vertebrae, combined with traumatic event(s) or regular activity that normally does not result in fractures, can induce both compression fractures and anterior wedging of the vertebral body. Back flexion promotes vertebral compression fractures and may increase kyphosis (Sinaki 1982).	Musculoskeletal Back pain (Itoi 1991; Ryan et al. 1994; Satoh et al. 1998). Reduced range of lumbar extension (Satoh et al. 1998). Respiratory Reduced inspiratory function due to severe kyphosis (Culham et al. 1994; Lisboa et al. 1985). Back pain (Galindo Ciocon et al. 1995; Helmes et al. 1995). Limited movement patterns: The individual should avoid stooping, bending, and heavy lifting (Sinaki 1982).	Self-care Difficulty finding suitable clothing (Ryan et al. 1994). Difficulty bathing and washing (Ryan et al. 1994). May have difficulty with toileting, dressing, transfers, and continence (Galindo-Ciocon et al. 1995). Sleep disturbance (Ryan et al. 1994). The individual should avoid sleeping in the fetal position (Sinaki 1982). Productivity Fatigue. Reduced functional reach (Lyles et al. 1993). Heavy lifting or strenuous activity may result in back pain (Sinaki 1982). May need lower back support (Sinaki 1982). Reduced sitting and standing tolerance (Cirullo 1989). Fear of falling and fractures (Cook et al. 1993). Overall, the effect of kyphosis on the ability to perform daily activities is not considered significant (Ryan et al. 1994).
Hip fracture: Femoral neck Intratrochanteric Subcapital	Hip fractures often occur before a fall. Fall mechanism: People who experience hip fractures tend to fall sideways or straight down, land near or on their hip, and are unlikely to break a fall by grasping or hitting an object (Nevitt and Cummings 1993).	Reduced mobility and possible nursing home admission (Melton 1993).	Self-care and productivity Increased dependency on others (Roberts and McGraw 1991).
Wrist fracture	Fall mechanism: There is a tendency to fall backward, land on one hand, and be unable to break the fall (Nevitt and Cummings 1993).	Wrist range of motion and strength are limited for 8–12 months (Ware 1993).	Patients remain independent in self-care.

Source: Reprinted with permission from D Grant, K Lundon. The Canadian Model of Occupational Performance applied to females with osteoporosis. Can J Occup Ther 1999;66:3–13.

Clinical Note

In addition to postural correction, education, and attention to modification of activities of daily living, specific exercise regimes in the management of OP should

1. Be weightbearing in nature (essential for normal development and maintenance of a healthy skeleton)
2. Include cyclic, resistance, site-specific muscle strengthening exercises (antigravity)
3. Promote strengthening of paraspinal back extensor muscles

---

the risk of falling or initiating fractures in vulnerable regions. It is never too late to start preventive and curative treatment for OP, even in those in whom a fracture has occurred, because all individuals with OP are at risk of further fractures (Dequeker 1997).

Education.   It is important to educate for lifting techniques and avoidance of activities involving stooping and bending that promote spinal flexion. Physical therapy intervention is requisite to decrease paraspinal muscle spasm, to specifically strengthen back extensors (when appropriate to prevent future vertebral fractures; see Exercise), and to evaluate posture and gait.

Exercise.   There is evidence to suggest that a degree of skeletal spinal deformity may result in different body shapes, depending on the patient's ability to counter the skeletal deformity by the use of muscles and ligaments (Sinaki et al. 1988; Sinaki et al. 1996). De Smet et al. (1988) reported that although the Cobb's angle (one measure of kyphosis) was highly correlated with anterior wedge fracturing of the vertebrae, significant kyphosis can also be present in those without any vertebral height deformation or fracturing. Reduced back extensor strength in individuals with OP has been documented by Sinaki et al (1988), whereas increasing back extensor strength by specific exercise in healthy postmenopausal women has been shown to decrease thoracic kyphosis (Itoi et al. 1994).

Significant positive correlation between back extensor strength and level of physical activity suggests that levels of physical activity and back muscle strength may be important contributors to the BMD of lumbar vertebral bodies (Sinaki and Offord

1988). Postmenopausal bone loss was unaffected by a modest exercise program despite an increase in muscle strength. Nonloading muscle exercise was ineffective in retarding vertebral bone loss in these same ambulatory, healthy postmenopausal women (Sinaki et al. 1989).

A meta-analysis of the effectiveness of physical activity for the prevention of bone loss in postmenopausal women pointed to its general effectiveness for preventing spinal BMD loss at the L2-L4 level, but not on the forearm or femoral neck regions (Berard et al. 1997). However, a randomized controlled study demonstrated that strength training exercises can increase or stabilize bone density of the hip and spine, while improving muscle mass, strength, and balance in postmenopausal women (Nelson et al. 1994). In a nonrandomized longitudinal study of 59 postmenopausal women with vertebral fractures, early extension exercises were determined to be more beneficial than flexion exercise in preventing future vertebral fractures; subsequent vertebral fractures occurred in fewer women performing extension exercises (Sinaki and Mikkelsen 1984).

In general, the skeleton responds in a site-specific manner to mechanical loading (Hughes et al. 1995). For example, continuous 1 year psoas training prevented lumbar bone loss in postmenopausal women (Revel et al. 1993). Bone responds favorably to select forms of mechanical loading (Lanyon 1996). Load magnitude appears to be the salient factor in determining the magnitude of the skeletal response. The general goal of physical activity in the management of OP is to positively influence bone mass by preventing or attenuating the loss of bone during the aging process. A greater effect through peak load and strength training (magnitude and low repetition)

Clinical Note

Management of Acute Compression Fractures (Frost 1998)

General Management

The acute stage lasts approximately 3 weeks, with pain located in the fracture regions. In the 3-week long acute stage after vertebral compression fracture, the patient should remain on bed rest for the initial 4–8 days until able to turn easily from side to side. After this period, a back support should be provided. In the subsequent 10-week healing stage the patient should lie down for 20 minutes every 2 hours (referred to as the *intermittent horizontal rest regimen* [IHRR]). If lordotic low back pain develops, IHRR may be advocated for a further 10 weeks.

Specific Management

According to Frost (1998), recovery from acute symptomatic vertebral compression fractures in OP occurs in the following three stages, each with its specific management strategy:

1. *Acute stage*: The acute stage lasts approximately 3 weeks. Pain may present in the fracture regions. Bed rest, without bathroom trips, is prescribed until the individual can turn side to side (4–8 days). On getting up, a thoracolumbar back support is indicated. After a week postfracture, the individual may begin sitting and walking while wearing the back support, for approximately 10 minutes at a time, 10 times a day. Between times, the individual should lie down and avoid sitting. The number of times the individual may be up during the next week is then doubled. The back support is not needed while sleeping. The individual may be encouraged in the use of thin head pillows, lying in a supine position with supported flexed hips and knees. Lying on one's side with a pillow between the knees is an alternative sleep position.
2. *Bone healing stage*: The bone healing stage lasts approximately 10 weeks. After 3 weeks postfracture, the IHRR is to lie down 20 minutes every 2 hours during the day, continuing for 10 weeks. Sitting is contraindicated. By the ninth postfracture week (6 weeks into IHRR), the back support may become unnecessary. Use of the support is discontinued gradually by removing it 3 hours before bedtime during the first week, 6 hours before that during the second week, and 9 hours before bedtime during the third week (ninth week of IHRR). At 13 weeks postfracture, the patient may resume normal activities. Frost (1998) reports that more than 50% of the patients enter the third recovery stage.
3. *Lordotic low back pain stage*: The lordotic low back pain stage lasts approximately 10 weeks if managed appropriately. These patients begin to feel low lumbar back pain in the latter part of the day even though the fracture typically affects T5-L1. The IHRR is reinstituted. For lasting relief, doing the IHRR for another 10 weeks may be required.

versus number of loading cycles (repetition only → endurance training) in positively affecting BMD has been demonstrated in humans (Kerr et al. 1996).

No evidence supports the idea that exercise alone can prevent the rapid decrease in bone mass in the peri-postmenopausal years or replace the bone loss associated with the low level of repro-ductive hormones that accompanies menopause. Nevertheless, healthy women should be encouraged to exercise, regardless of whether the activity has a marked osteogenic component (American College of Sports Medicine [ACSM] Position Stand on Osteoporosis and Exercise 1995; Ernst 1998). The additive effects of weightbearing exercise and hormone replacement therapy (HRT) on bone mineral accretion, coupled with other adaptations to the exercise (such as increased strength and functional capacity) could effectively reduce the incidence of falls and osteoporotic fractures (Kohrt et al. 1995). An additional benefit of exercise is to reduce the risk of falls and to lessen the likelihood of sustaining trauma from falls leading to fracture. The optimal program for older persons should include activities that improve strength, flexibility, and coordination to possibly indirectly, but effectively, decrease the incidence of osteoporotic fractures by lessening the likelihood of falling (ACSM Position Stand on Osteoporosis and Exercise 1995).

The majority of evidence supporting application of exercise to benefit the adult osteoporotic skeleton stems from longitudinal studies, the vast majority of which identify its role in the conservation and not the increase in bone mass (Ernst 1998). Physical activity has been related to optimal bone mass and improved physical function and inherently carries the benefit of reducing the risk for fracture. Among older, community-dwelling women, however, physical activity was associated only with a reduced risk for hip fracture but not wrist or vertebral fracture (Gregg et al. 1998). Therefore, although vigorous physical activity is associated with increased BMD, this advantage does not necessarily always translate into lower fracture rates when all fractures are considered together (Fries 1996).

Pharmacologic Management

Clinical decisions concerning pharmacologic intervention depend not only on the level of bone mass, but also on age-associated risk factors, the existence of previous fractures, and the risk to benefit ratio of particular therapeutic regimens (Delmas 1997). Nearly all of the pharmacologic treatments available are antiresorptive agents that act to prevent bone loss and, in some cases, have been shown to reduce fracture risk. HRT and possibly the bisphosphonates appear to be non–site specific and may reduce fracture risk at both the spine and hip. It is important to be aware, however, that changes in bone mass induced by pharmacologic treatment do not always predict the corresponding changes in fracture rate (Compston 1997).

Hormone Replacement Therapy

ESTROGEN AND PROGESTIN THERAPY.   Estrogen supplementation has been most successful in the prevention and attenuation of early (peri-menopausal) postmenopausal bone loss. The estrogens commonly used are estradiol-17β, estrone sulphate, and conjugated equine estrogens. If the postmenopausal woman still has an intact uterus, then estrogen also stimulates growth of the uterine endothelium, which can lead to erratic bleeding, endometrial hyperplasia, and neoplasia (Sarrel 1997). This unwanted effect is prevented by the addition of a progestogen, usually in a cyclical fashion. Therefore, HRT for menopausal women comprises treatment with continuous estrogens, and cyclic or continuous progestogens in women who have not been hysterectomized to regularize or abolish uterine bleeding (Stevenson 1997; Witt and Lonsberg 1997). Although the benefits of estrogen replacement therapy in preventing bone loss and reducing the incidence of fractures are well established, such therapy is contraindicated in some women and continues to not be an acceptable option for others (Castelobranco 1998).

Much controversy exists regarding the use of estrogen in postmenopausal women. The link between breast cancer and HRT continues to be controversial (Burke et al. 1997). Postmenopausal estrogen deficiency, however, may result in an array of physiologic disorders including vasomotor symptoms, urogenital atrophy, an increase in the risk of coronary heart disease, osteoporotic fractures, and Alzheimer's disease (Alsina 1996). The decision to use HRT is made on an individual basis, taking into consideration all benefits (e.g., diminished climacteric symptoms and decreased cardiovascular risk) and potential risks (e.g., possible enhanced breast cancer risk and appearance of side effects). HRT is of greatest benefit when initiated at the cessation of menses; however, delayed HRT initiated as late as 65 years of age can still be effective. A decrease in the incidence of osteoporotic fracture is remarkable when the duration of estrogen replacement therapy exceeds 7 years (Roux 1997). Finally, postural balance function may be better preserved in long-term estrogen users than in nonusers (Naessen et al. 1997). Effects of loss of estrogen on postural balance function may be one mechanism underlying the rapid increase in distal forearm fractures seen early after menopause.

ANDROGENS.   A decrease in blood androgen levels is well documented in women who experience natural or surgical menopause (Abraham and Carpenter 1997). Anabolic steroids can be broadly divided according to structural additions at the carbon-17 position. Stanozolol and oxymetholone are 17β-alkylated agents. Testosterone and nandrolone are 17β-esterified derivatives. The anabolic steroids most commonly used in the treatment of OP are stanozolol and nandrolone; however, their use is not universally approved. The anabolic steroids prevent bone loss, probably by their preferential effect on endocortical bone (Kanis et al. 1997).

Other Medications

CALCITONIN.   Synthetic salmon calcitonin is available as a subcutaneous injection, but it also can be delivered nasally. Calcitonin stabilizes bone turnover by inhibiting bone resorption and slowing down the rate of bone loss. Some individuals develop a resistance to calcitonin therapy; however, this may be alleviated by reductions in dosages, use of intranasal administration, and interrupted administration.

BISPHOSPHONATES.   Bisphosphonates, previously referred to as *diphosphonates*, are potent inhibitors of bone resorption. Bisphosphonates are used therapeutically in humans to decrease bone resorption in conditions such as Paget's disease, tumor bone disease, and OP (Francis 1997; Johansen et al. 1996; Reginster et al. 1997). The class of drugs known as the *geminal bisphosphonates* are groups of synthetic compounds characterized by a P-C-P bond, each with its own physicochemical and biological characteristics. Many of the bisphosphonates are powerful inhibitors of bone resorption; however, they not only prevent bone loss, but may increase bone mass and improve the biomechanical properties of the skeleton (Fleisch 1997). The bisphosphonates have a complex mechanism of action involving the three following events:

1. A direct effect on osteoclast activity.
2. Both direct and indirect effect on osteoclast recruitment. The indirect effect is mediated by cells of the osteoblastic lineage and involves their production of an inhibitor of osteoclastic recruitment.
3. A shortening of osteoclast survival by apoptosis.

Large amounts of bisphosphonates can also inhibit mineralization through a physicochemical inhibition of crystal growth (Fleisch 1997).

Etidronate is a member of the group of bisphosphonates that stabilize, or may even increase, bone mass and possibly reduce the rate of vertebral fractures. Given cyclically, it is antiresorptive in nature (Fleisch 1997). A 4-year randomized study demonstrated an additive effect of etidronate and HRT on hip and spine BMD in postmenopausal women with established OP (Wimalawansa 1998). In this study, patients who received combined therapy had significantly higher BMD in both the vertebrae and in the femora in comparison with patients who were treated with HRT or etidronate alone after 4 years. Alendronate (Fosamax) is currently used for the treatment of postmenopausal and glucocorticoid-induced OP (Saag et al. 1998; Ragsdale et al. 1998; Lin et al. 1999; Hosking et al 1999). In women with low BMD but without vertebral fracture, long-term (more than 3 years) alendronate therapy appears to safely increase BMD and decrease the risk of sustaining the first vertebral deformity (Minne et al. 1999; Black and Thompson 1999). Alendronate appeared to significantly reduce the risk of clinical fractures among women with OP but not among women with higher BMD (Cummings et al. 1998). After critical analysis of randomized clinical trials for different therapies, alendronate appeared to demonstrate the greatest fracture benefit (Meunier 1999).

SODIUM FLUORIDE.   Sodium fluoride is one pharmacologic agent that acts to increase bone mass; however, little evidence exists showing that this increase in bone mass translates to any reduction in vertebral fractures. Although fluoride salts have been shown to be capable of linearly increasing spinal BMD in postmenopausal OP, the effects of this gain in density on the vertebral fracture rate remain controversial. A large prospective clinical trial involving osteoporotic women with vertebral fractures determined that a combined fluoride, calcium, and vitamin D regimen was no more effective than calcium and vitamin D supplements alone in the prevention of new vertebral fractures (Meunier et al. 1998). However, early treatment of idiopathic OP in men with no previous vertebral fractures using a fluoride-calcium regimen appeared to improve cancellous and cortical bone density, reduce the incidence of vertebral fractures, and attenuate back pain (Ringe et al. 1998).

Surgery

The presence of OP in patients who are candidates for spinal surgery can impact surgical management. If use of instrumentation is indicated because of instability or deformity, certain principles must be applied. These include using multiple sites of fixation, accepting lesser degrees of deformity correction, and avoiding ending the instrumentation within kyphotic segments (Hu 1997).

Paget's Disease of Bone

Paget's disease is a chronic age-related skeletal disorder characterized by focal areas of elevated and abnormal bone remodeling activity. Although a viral infection of osteoclasts has been suggested, it is considered to be a metabolic bone disorder (Singer and Mills 1983). Paget's disease (osteitis deformans) is a common bone disorder with incidence and presentation affecting men more than women typically in those older than 40 years of age. Paget's disease is an asymmetric, monostotic (single bone site affected) or polyostotic (multiple bone sites affected) bone disease featuring increased osteoclast-mediated bone resorption and subsequent compensatory increases in bone formation. The overall result is a disorganized mosaic of woven and lamellar bone at focal sites. This structural change produces hypertrophic bone that is more vascular, mechanically weaker, and ultimately more susceptible to deformity or fracture than normal bone (Ooi and Fraser 1997). Complications of Paget's disease also may involve joints (osteoarthritis) and the nervous system.

Paget's disease occurs in geographic and ethnic clusters predominating in people of northern European ancestry, from the United Kingdom, as well as western Europe, Australia, and New Zealand. It is rare in Scandinavia, Asia, and Africa. In Europe and North America, Paget's disease is predominantly a disease of the elderly, affecting 1–3% of adults older than 40 years of age.

Etiology

The etiology of Paget's disease remains speculative. It has been proposed that the changes in bone remodeling occur as the result of a viral infection of osteoclasts in pagetic bone. Osteoclasts at pagetic sites contain characteristic intranuclear and intracytoplasmic inclusion bodies, strongly supporting the role of infection with members of the paramyxovirus family. Despite the morphologic findings suggestive of viral infection (measles, respiratory syncytial virus, and canine distemper virus) the specific role remains inconclusive (Harinck et al. 1986; Delmas and Meunier 1997). It is theorized that a common viral infection, perhaps acquired early in life, in a genetically susceptible host may predispose the individual to an osteoclast lesion that manifests in late adulthood (Papapoulos 1997).

Pathophysiology

The pathophysiology of Paget's disease will remain speculative until a specific etiologic agent is determined. Major disorganization in both the architecture and the lamellar texture of bone characterizes Pagetic bone. The focal event of Paget's disease is increased resorption followed by increased bone formation, with rates of skeletal remodeling enhanced up to 20-fold (Mundy 1995). The primary abnormality appears to reside in the osteoclast. Pagetic osteoclasts are more numerous than normal and contain substantially more nuclei than do normal osteoclasts (up to 100 nuclei per cell). In addition, the number of osteoblasts is increased, causing excessive formation of a mixture of immature woven collagen matrix and lamellar bone. The corresponding hypertrophy and osteosclerosis that characterizes Paget's disease is caused by this overproduction of poor quality bone (Delmas and Meunier 1997). Although bone formation processes appear to be altered, the osteoblasts and fibroblasts that are recruited to pagetic sites are morphologically normal, and this response is considered a consequence of prior increases in bone resorption. The new bone that is formed, however, is abnormal, with the newly deposited collagen fibers laid down in a haphazard rather than linear fashion, creating more primitive woven bone. Bone matrix at pagetic sites is

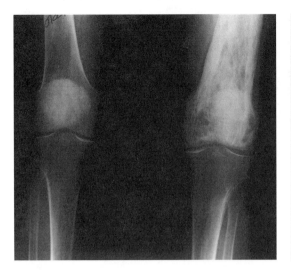

Figure 12-8. Paget's disease affecting the long bones (femora). Note the sclerotic mosaic of bone. (Courtesy of Dr. E. Becker, M.D., The Toronto Hospital, Toronto.)

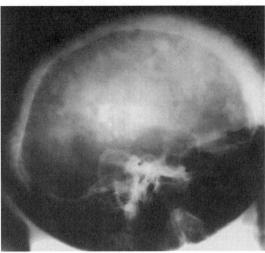

Figure 12-9. Fifty-five-year-old man with Paget's disease affecting the cranium. (Courtesy of Dr. E. Becker, M.D., The Toronto Hospital, Toronto.)

usually normally mineralized. The disease front may proceed through bone, particularly the axial skeleton, the long bones (Figure 12-8), and skull (Figure 12-9) at a steady state rate of approximately 1 cm per year. Vascular fibrous tissue increases in the marrow cavity. In time, the hypercellularity at a locus of affected bone may diminish, leaving the end product as a sclerotic mosaic of bone without evidence of active bone turnover. This phenomenon may be referred to as *burned out Paget's disease.*

Biochemistry

Urinary hydroxyproline and serum alkaline phosphatase measurements are useful markers of bone pathology in Paget's disease. A typical rise occurs in markers of bone resorption such as urine (total) hydroxyproline excretion and deoxypyridinoline cross-links. An increase in the levels of serum alkaline phosphatase may be noted, reflecting new bone formation. In patients with Paget's disease, serum calcium and phosphate levels typically are normal.

Histologic Features

The bone that becomes enclosed in individual packets consists of true woven bone and lamellar bone, giv-

ing a mosaic-pattern appearance. Marked net bone formation occurs, the bone of which is essentially normal. Differential diagnosis of malignancy from pagetic bone is achieved most easily by bone biopsy.

Bone Vascularization Changes and Paget's Disease

The increase in vascularity of pagetic bone is associated with increased arteriovenous shunting and increased local blood flow through the bone, inducing the typical increase in warmth reported over affected bones. Because of arteriovenous shunting through bone, a high cardiac-output state may be induced which, in the most extreme cases of patients with underlying cardiac disease, may precipitate cardiac failure.

Clinical Presentation

Paget's disease affects local sites in an asymmetric fashion, often involving only a single bone or portion of a bone (monostotic) or two or more bones (polyostotic). Approximately 90% of individuals affected by Paget's disease are initially asymptomatic. The bones most commonly involved in Paget's disease include the vertebrae, cranium, pelvis, sternum, and proximal ends of the long bones (e.g., the tibia), although any bony site may be affected. The lumbar and sacral regions may be affected; however, they are often asymptomatic. Twenty or thirty bones may be simultaneously targeted by Paget's disease; however, the number of bones involved does not always reflect the severity with which an individual bone may be affected. Although progression of disease within a given bone may occur, the sudden appearance of new sites of involvement years after the initial diagnosis is uncommon. Diagnosis usually is made by reports of bone pain or deformity, by x-ray, or by inadvertent detection of elevated serum alkaline phosphatase levels found through routine biochemical testing.

The most common reported complaints are pain, skeletal deformity, and change in skin temperature. Joint dysfunction related to Paget's disease may result from damage to cartilage and osteoarthritis consequent to the associated bone hypertrophy in subchondral bone (Altman 1994; Delmas and Meunier 1997). The most commonly involved joints in osteoarthritis associated with Paget's disease are the knees, hips, and spine. Some pagetic lesions are not painful, but pain can occur in varying degrees of severity, is usually constant and nagging in nature, and is most commonly experienced at the site of the lesion (Hamdy et al. 1995). Bone pain is often nocturnal and is thought to be a result of increased pressure on the periosteum or associated hyperemia.

Other clinical manifestations include diminished mobility and unsteady gait. A variety of neurologic complications are due largely to nerve root compression or nerve entrapment in which these structures are adjacent to pagetic bone near a nerve foramen or canal. Paget's disease of the skull often is associated with cranial nerve involvement, high cervical pain, and headache that radiates to the occiput and the back of the skull (Altman 1994). Mixed sensorineural and conductive hearing loss is a common clinical manifestation of Paget's disease. Low back pain may present in Paget's disease of bone because of vertebral body and facet enlargement, loss of lumbar lordosis, dorsal kyphosis (Figure 12-10), spinal impingement, and altered gait dynamics (Altman 1994). The deep-rooted bone pain of Paget's disease often is unalleviated with the use of simple analgesics

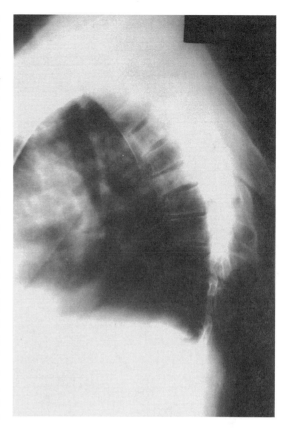

Figure 12-10. Fifty-five-year-old man with Paget's disease affecting the thoracic spine. Note the dorsal kyphosis. (Courtesy of Dr. E. Becker, M.D., The Toronto Hospital, Toronto.)

and is more marked at rest than on movement. The efficacy of physical modalities in treating pagetic pain is unclear and is best applied on an individual basis. Pagetic bone has an increased vascularity leading to perceived warmth of the bone, which affected individuals consider an unpleasant sensation. Because of abnormal bone remodeling processes inherent to the Paget's disease process, bone architecture becomes distorted, resulting in the slow and progressive development of bowing deformity, depending on the bony site. It appears that weightbearing exacerbates the development of deformity, and pathologic fractures occur most commonly in the long weightbearing bones of the lower extremities in the femoral neck, subtrochanteric, and tibial regions (Figure 12-11).

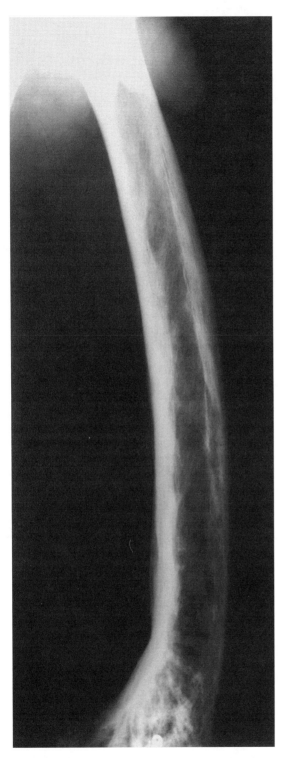

Figure 12-11. Paget's disease. Note the long bone "bowing" deformity. (Courtesy of Dr. E. Becker, M.D., The Toronto Hospital, Toronto.)

Radiographic Signs

Radionuclide bone scanning is considered the most reliable modality for identifying the distribution, extent, and activity of pagetic lesions (Delmas and Meunier 1997). The typically focal asymmetric nature of Paget's disease and the extent of spread in individual bones makes the bone scan useful in differentiating Paget's disease from that of other bone diseases, including metastatic carcinoma. A bone scan demonstrates an increased uptake of isotope at sites of disease activity and generally correlates well with the pathophysiologic activity of the disease (Klein and Norman 1995). The localized enlargement of a bone is characteristic of Paget's disease as identified radiographically. A typical presentation includes radiolucent areas of patchy arrangement indicating increased bone resorption, evidence of regional bone formation processes represented by cortical and cancellous thickening and sclerosis, and uneven widths of affected bones (see Figure 12-11). Patchy areas of resorption typical of Paget's disease are referred to as *osteoporosis circumscripta* in the skull. In the pelvis, there may be evidence of sclerosis along the iliopectineal line. Cortical bone thickening, sclerotic changes, and osteolytic areas are radiographic hallmarks of Paget's disease (Figure 12-12).

Management

The short-term objective for the treatment of Paget's disease is to alleviate the associated bone pain. Long-term objectives include the prevention of the progression of the disease. Because the primary abnormality lies in the osteoclast, inhibitors of bone resorption are used for its therapy. Pharmacologic therapy includes calcitonin, plicamycin and gallium nitrate, and the bisphosphonates. The goal of these pharmacologic therapies is to control the disease activity, to normalize biochemical parameters, and to ameliorate the symptoms. Pharmacologic efforts are critical, given that relief of bone pain, immobilization, hypercalcemia, and high-output cardiac failure associated with Paget's disease are related to the extent with which biochemical control is regained. Other symptomatic treatment

Clinical Note

Paget's Disease and Functional Mobility

Bowed lower extremities result in altered biodynamics and pressures within the joint (Altman 1994). When compared with age- and gender-matched controls, patients who have Paget's disease of bone involving the tibia, femur, or acetabular portion of the ilium demonstrated clinically and statistically significant functional and mobility impairments, as measured by a mobility skills protocol, 10-foot walk time, number of steps to complete a 360-degree turn, and 6-minute walk distance (Lyles et al. 1995). Pain, deformity, leg length discrepancy, and secondary arthritis in joints proximate to the areas of Paget's disease contribute to the functional status and mobility impairments. Furthermore, gait analysis in patients with Paget's disease identified that involvement of the femur and tibia is associated with significant reductions in gait velocity, cadence, and increased stride time (Gainey et al. 1989).

for Paget's disease includes analgesics and anti-inflammatory medication.

Surgery and Joint Arthroplasty

The conservative treatment of fractures in patients with Paget's disease is associated with a high risk of delayed union in spite of the extensive blood supply to bone in Paget's disease (Delmas and Meunier 1997). In fact, the increased vascularity of actively remodeling pagetic bone may lead to substantial blood loss in the presence of fractures due to trauma. Elective joint replacement can be successful in relieving refractory pain and for severe osteoarthritis of the hip or knee. Metabolic activity of Paget's disease subsequent to total hip arthroplasty (THA) surgery was observed to have no effect, regardless of location of disease, on the clin-

ical outcome in a 7.8-year follow-up study. For the femur, failure rates were similar for prostheses implanted in pagetic or nonpagetic bone, with cemented THA being the most viable option for these patients (Ludkowski and Wilson-MacDonald 1990). Neurosurgical intervention may be required in cases in which neurologic syndromes are present.

Osteomalacia

Osteomalacia is a generalized metabolic bone disorder manifesting in impaired mineralization of newly formed or remodeling bone. In the adult skeleton, this disorder leads to an accumulation or relative excess of unmineralized matrix or osteoid ("prebone," or immature bone). Osteomalacia occurs after the cessation of skeletal growth and

Clinical Note

Orthopedic Rehabilitation and Paget's Disease

Goals of treatment in Paget's disease are to reduce pain and encourage maintenance of, or an appropriate increase in, mobility. The use of assistive devices for ambulation must be prescribed on an individual basis that takes into consideration issues such as degree of pain, deformity, leg length discrepancies, and secondary arthritis in joints near active disease sites. Many of the problems, such as the development of bony deformity, are difficult to treat once established, but with early diagnosis and attention to prophylactic (pharmacologic and physical) therapies the progression of deformity may be somewhat attenuated.

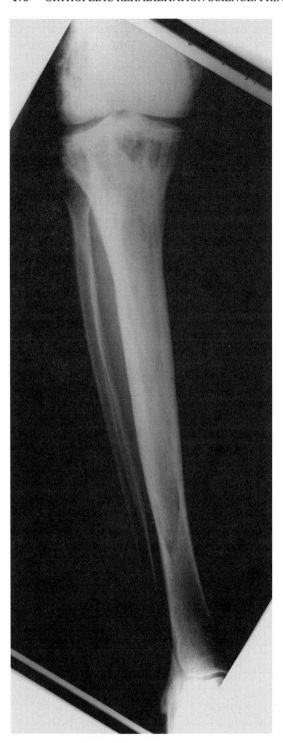

Figure 12-12. Sixty-six-year-old man presenting with Paget's disease in the tibia. Note the characteristic "flame" or "blade of grass" margin in the distal third of the tibia. (Courtesy of Dr. E. Becker, M.D., The Toronto Hospital, Toronto.)

involves only bone, not the growth plate. *Rickets* is the equivalent disease affecting the pediatric population; however, additional involvement of the epiphysis in the growing skeleton occurs in this state. Regardless of their cause, these syndromes display remarkably similar histologic and radiographic features (Pitt 1991).

Osteomalacia results when mineralization of mature cortical and cancellous bone is inadequate or delayed due to altered intake, loss, or metabolism of 1,25-dihydroxyvitamin D_3 (vitamin D) and phosphate. Although the precise role of the vitamin D metabolites in the mineralization process remains uncertain, they are generally recognized for their role in the regulation of calcium and phosphate homeostasis (Table 12-4). Adequate amounts of calcium and phosphate are essential for the normal mineralization of osteoid. Osteomalacia may develop in any condition interfering with the mineralization of bone matrix. These conditions include reduced calcium absorption (e.g., gastrointestinal disorders), reduced formation of active vitamin D (e.g., renal osteodystrophy), disorders leading to a decrease of the calcium-phosphate product (e.g., hypophosphatemia), or interference by other substances with the mineralization process (e.g., fluorosis) (Eriksen and Langdahl 1995).

The gross, histopathologic, and radiologic abnormalities of osteomalacia are the common result of a number of different diseases (Table 12-5). In general, osteomalacia is considered to be most frequently caused by altered vitamin D_3 or phosphate metabolism, both being conditions to which the elderly population is at particular risk. Because housebound or institutionalized individuals may represent a significant sector of the elderly population, this group is at risk for the development of this disorder. A deficiency in vitamin D is typical in the institutionalized elderly probably due to diminished epidemic production of its precursors and to scant exposure to sunlight (Plantalech et al. 1997).

Causes of Vitamin D Deficiency

The two causes of vitamin D deficiency are a decreased intake and a defective metabolism.

1. *Decreased intake*: In general, vitamin D deficiency occurs in those whose vitamin D intake is

Table 12-4. Sources and Action of Vitamin D

Sources

Cutaneous production: The major source of vitamin D production that is stimulated by exposure to UV radiation (sunlight).

Diet: A more minor but essential source of vitamin D, especially when cutaneous production is limited. The main natural sources of vitamin D are found in the fish-liver foods. In North America, fortification of foods such as milk and eggs has been necessary to prevent vitamin D deficiency.

Actions

Vitamin D itself has little biological activity and is initially metabolized in the liver to 25-hydroxycholecalciferol (25-OHD), the major circulating form of vitamin D. This undergoes further hydroxylation in the kidneys to form vitamin D_3 (1,25[OH]$_2D_3$), the hormonally active metabolite of vitamin D. This form acts to (1) regulate calcium absorption from the bowel, (2) influence bone remodeling, and (3) affect muscle function.

low and who, in addition, have minimal or no exposure to UV radiation. Vitamin D deficiency may be caused by an inadequate dietary intake; defective intestinal absorption of vitamin D may also occur, as observed in malabsorption syndromes (e.g., jejunoileal bypass for obesity). In addition, an age-related diminished response of the intestine to vitamin D may exist. Age-related decline in the dermal synthesis of 7-dehydrocholesterol (a precursor of vitamin D) is also known to exist (Hutchison and Bell 1992).

2. *Decreased metabolism*: Vitamin D metabolism is defective. Most diseases are not caused by simple vitamin D deficiency but involve abnormal production or regulation of its synthesis in the liver, the kidney, or both.

Causes of Phosphate Deficiency

The main cause of altered phosphate metabolism in the adult are disorders of the renal system, which often induce a condition known as *renal osteodystrophy*. Very low plasma phosphate levels are common in osteomalacic patients. Alimentary phosphate deficiency may be additionally aggravated by vitamin D deficiencies. Vitamin D promotes jejunal phosphate absorption and renal phosphate reabsorption. Disorders which affect phosphate absorption in the intestine and reabsorption in the kidney include certain malabsorption states and conditions in which large amounts of phosphate-binding antacids have been administered.

Pathophysiology

Osteomalacia is associated with many clinical, radiographic, and biochemical abnormalities, none of which are entirely pathognomonic of the disorder. In fact, osteomalacia may present with a variety of clinical and radiographic manifestations mimicking other musculoskeletal disorders (Reginato et al. 1999). Histologic examination of a bone biopsy is often essential to establish a definitive diagnosis.

Table 12-5. Classification of the Major Causes of Osteomalacia

Deficiency	Cause	Clinical Form
Vitamin D	Decreased sunlight exposure	Housebound elderly
	Malabsorption	Small bowel disease
	Decreased dietary intake	Poor nutrition
25-hydroxycholecalciferol (25-OHD)	Abnormal vitamin D metabolism	Anticonvulsant therapy
1,25(OH)$_2D_3$	Decreased 1α-hydroxylase activity	Renal failure
		Reduction in renal function
Phosphate	Decreased tubular reabsorption	Familial
	Dialysis therapy	Tumoral
	Phosphate depletion	Sporadic
	Chronic antacid therapy	Use of phosphate binders
Calcium	Inadequate calcium in diet	Poor nutrition

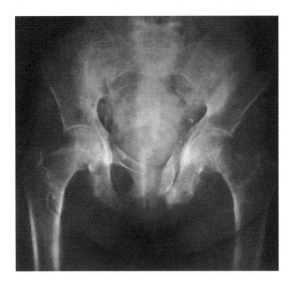

Figure 12-13. Osteomalacia resulting from chronic renal failure and associated secondary hyperparathyroidism. Note the pelvic pseudofracture. (Courtesy of Dr. E. Becker, M.D., The Toronto Hospital, Toronto.)

Histologic Features

Both static and dynamic histomorphometric measurements of bone are useful to identify high bone turnover and excessive amounts of inadequately mineralized osteoid (unmineralized bone tissue), which are the histologic hallmarks of osteomalacia. Specifically, this increase in nonmineralized bone is associated with a prolonged mineralization lag time in which large seams of osteoid coat the trabeculae of cancellous bone and contribute to an overall preserved bone volume. In cortical bone, intracortical bone resorption or "tunneling" and increased amounts of osteoid lining the haversian canals may be observed.

Biochemical

Mineralization of newly formed bone requires the deposition of adequate concentrations of calcium and phosphate. In general, the combination of moderate hypocalcemia and clear hypophosphatemia are hallmarks of adult osteomalacia (Anderson and Richardson 1992). If vitamin D deficiency exists because of dietary restrictions or malabsorption, the serum calcium and its urinary excretion may be low; serum phosphorus may be low because of

decreased intestinal phosphate absorption and increased renal phosphate clearance caused by secondary hyperparathyroidism induced by the low serum calcium levels. Levels of alkaline phosphatase and osteocalcin (bone Gla protein) may also be elevated.

Radiographic Findings

The most common radiographic change in osteomalacia is a reduction in skeletal density, a nonspecific finding of little diagnostic value (Hutchison and Bell 1992). Other disease states that share the findings of osteopenia include senile or postmenopausal OP, hyperparathyroidism, hyperthyroidism, and multiple myeloma (Doppelt 1984). Intervertebral disks may balloon out and deform the adjacent vertebrae to give them a uniformly biconcave "codfish" appearance. A similar deformity may be observed in spinal OP, but the biconcavity is more regular in osteomalacia than in OP, when the extent of vertebral deformity is variable. Radiologic evidence of gross deformity of the rib cage, pelvis, and long bones may be found. *Looser-Milkman pseudofractures* or *Looser's transformation zones* are characteristic of osteomalacia (although they may also be seen in Paget's disease); they consist of a large area of osteoid and represent a type of insufficiency fracture (Figure 12-13). These areas appear as narrow lines of radiolucency that characteristically lie either perpendicular or oblique to the bone surface at the site where the nutrient arteries enter bone. The pubic rami and femoral neck, ribs, metatarsals, border of the scapula, pelvic brim, or medial aspect of the humeral head are typical sites of activity. Looser's zones or pseudofractures, consisting of focal accumulations of osteoid, can proceed to full lateral fractures that ultimately cause skeletal deformity.

Clinical Presentation

Although the presentation of osteomalacia may vary from one individual to another, a common complaint is of vague, generalized bone pain. The soft elastic bone deforms easily and may lead to multiple vertebral compression fractures, deformity of the rib cage and pelvis, and loss in height. Deformity of the lower limbs due to malunion and bowing (varus deformity) may also be associated with pseudofractures. The patient may report generalized bone pain of a dull, aching nature. Muscle weakness, particularly in the proximal muscle groups of the lower extremities (also referred to as *pelvic girdle* or *proximal myopathy*) and back is common. This diffuse skeletal pain is typically exacerbated by physical activity, and tenderness may be elicited by palpation. Muscle weakness and hypotonia is a common accompaniment of prolonged vitamin D deficiency, although the mechanism is unknown. This condition can affect bone turnover to the extent that fractures occur in situations that otherwise might constitute only minimal to moderate impact stress. A scoliosis of the spine also may develop because of the altered biconcave shape of affected vertebral bodies. A characteristic waddling gait may manifest with this condition, and the combination of proximal myopathy and limb bowing may contribute to great difficulty in rising from a chair or climbing stairs. Functional activities (e.g., climbing stairs and ambulation) may become difficult, making requisite the use of gait aids for support. In the extreme case, the composite presentation of weakness and muscle atrophy, skeletal deformities, and fracture incidence may even lead the affected individual to become wheelchair-bound or bedridden.

Management

The goals of treatment of osteomalacia are to (1) correct hypocalcemia and resulting symptoms and prevent the consequences of hypocalcemia; (2) correct and prevent skeletal deformities and changes caused by secondary hyperparathyroidism; and (3) prevent hypercalcemia, hypercalciuria, and renal damage (Hutchison and Bell 1992). In most cases, the stereotypic presentation of osteomalacia may be cured, or at least improved, with appropriate therapy for the specific underlying abnormality. Although different underlying causes of this skeletal disorder may exist, most signs and symptoms resolve with supplementation of vitamin D, which aims to restore plasma calcium and phosphate levels to normal. Bone pain should disappear promptly. UV irradiation therapy may also be beneficial.

Physical management strategies should address postural and peripheral muscle strengthening exercise and gait retraining to achieve maximal functional status. Because of the vulnerability to fracture, care should be taken to prevent falls in this population. Sound clinical judgment and precaution should always be used when treating the osteomalacia patient with ultrasound, electric stimulation, and heat or cold. Graduated loading of the skeleton with weightbearing and resistive exercises should be closely supervised and guided by the patient's tolerance to activity.

Summary

Metabolic bone disorders are common but are often difficult to distinguish on the basis of radiologic and clinical findings. Quantitative assessment of bone mass may assist in early diagnosis because many of the conditions present with a reduction of bone mass.

OP is a condition of generalized skeletal fragility in which bone presents with sufficient weakness that fractures occur with minimal trauma. OP is a disease associated with menopause and aging. The two major determinants of risk for developing OP are peak bone mass and the rate of bone loss thereafter. Postmenopausal OP (type I) and age-related OP (type II) are the most common primary forms of bone loss seen in clinical practice. Accelerated loss of cancellous bone in type I OP results from the combination of increased bone resorption and inadequate compensation by bone formation. Disproportionate loss of cancellous bone from the axial skeleton is seen in type I OP. Vertebral fractures form an integral component of this osteoporotic syndrome. Decreased connectivity contributes largely to the fragility seen in vertebral OP, in concert with reduced bone mass. In type II OP, bone loss is global, affecting both cortical and cancellous bone. The femoral neck region is thus vulnerable to fracture with this age-related condition. In secondary OP, specific etiologic agents are responsible for bone loss. Such agents include chronic corticosteroid use and certain endocrine disorders such as thyroid disease and primary hyperthyroidism.

Osteoporotic fractures are likely caused by skeletal changes, including low bone mass, altered spatial orientation of bone, altered turnover properties, and deterioration in quality of bone tissue. Low bone mass is by far the most important risk factor for the development of osteoporotic fractures. However, other contributing causes of fractures may include extraskeletal factors such as falls, poor neuromuscular coordination and postural instability, amount of soft tissue, and physical environment.

Several important approaches exist for the long-term management of patients with chronic deformities associated with spinal OP. Of particular importance is educating patients to understand the nature of the deformity so that they can have realistic expectations concerning body image and the anticipated goals of therapy. The goals of rehabilitation should ideally include relief of pain, restoration of function, maintenance of a reasonable quality of life through encouragement to remain active, and prevention of further fractures.

Paget's disease is an age-related disorder of excessive but disordered bone remodeling. It is an asymmetric, monostotic or polyostotic bone disease featuring increased osteoclastic resorptive activity. Bone formation is irregular and chaotic, and a mixture of both woven and lamellar bone ensues. The areas of increased bone remodeling associated with Paget's disease may cause pain and deformities of the axial skeleton, the long bones, and the skull. Fracture and nerve entrapment may accompany this condition, if chronic. Although many individuals with Paget's disease of bone may be asymptomatic, many have pain and impaired function. With the development of potent bisphosphonates that behave as specific inhibitors of osteoclast-mediated bone resorption, the disease process may be controlled. Significant functional impairment may accompany Paget's disease as a result of pain and deformity associated with this condition.

Osteomalacia is a bone disease in which the mineralization of newly formed bone is impaired. Histologically, nonmineralized osteoid tissue characteristically increases and is associated with decreased mineralization rates. Osteomalacia represents gross, histologic, and radiologic abnormalities common to a number of different diseases; however, it typically manifests when a vitamin D or phosphate deficiency exists. Elderly, housebound, or institutionalized individuals are at risk for developing this disorder. Osteopenia is a nonspecific radiographic finding associated with osteomalacia which, in concert with a prolonged and relative increase in nonmineralized osteoid tissue, contributes to the likelihood of skeletal deformity and fracture. Generalized bone pain of a dull, aching nature and muscle weakness (proximal myopathy)

are common and may be exacerbated by physical activity. In concert with pharmacologic therapy, physical management strategies should address postural and peripheral muscle strengthening exercise and gait retraining to achieve maximal functional status.

References

Abraham D, Carpenter PC. Issues concerning androgen replacement therapy in postmenopausal women. Mayo Clin Proc 1997;72:1051–1055.

ACSM Position Stand on Osteoporosis and Exercise. Medicine and science in sports and exercise. 1995;27:i–vii.

Alsina JC. Benefits of hormone replacement therapy: overview and update. Int J Fertil Womens Med 1996;42(Suppl 2):329–346.

Altman RD. Articular complications of Paget's disease of bone. Semin Arthritis Rheum 1994;23:248–249.

Anderson FH. Osteoporosis in men. Int J Clin Pract 1998;52:176–180.

Anderson J, Richardson PC. Paget's Disease of Bone. In JC Brocklehurst, RC Tallis, HM Fillit (eds), Textbook of Geriatrics and Gerontology. New York: Churchill Livingstone, 1992;783–791.

Arlot ME, Delmas PD, Chappard D, Meunier PJ. Trabecular and endochondral bone remodeling in postmenopausal osteoporosis: comparison with normal postmenopausal women. Osteoporosis Int 1990;1:41–49.

Berard A, Bravo G, Gauthier P. Meta-analysis of the effectiveness of physical activity for the prevention of bone loss in postmenopausal women. Osteoporosis Int 1997;7:331–337.

Bilezikian JP, Silverberg SJ. Osteoporosis: a practical approach to the perimenopausal woman. J Womens Health 1992;1:21–27.

Black DM, Palermo L, Nevitt MC, et al. Defining incident vertebral deformity: a prospective comparison of several approaches. The Study of Osteoporotic Fractures Research Group. J Bone Miner Res 1999;14:90–101.

Black DM, Thompson DE. The effect of alendronate therapy on osteoporotic fracture in the vertebral fracture arm of the Fracture Intervention Trial. Int J Clin Prac 1999;April(Suppl 101):46–50.

Boonen S, Vanderschueren D, Geusens P, et al. Age-associated endocrine deficiencies as potential determinants of femoral neck (type II) osteoporotic fracture occurrence in elderly men. Int J Androl 1997;20:134–143.

Burger H, Van Daele PLA, Grashuis K, et al. Vertebral deformities and functional impairment in men and women. J Bone Miner Res 1997;12:152–157.

Burke CC, Gullatte MM, Vigliani M, et al. Hormone replacement therapy and breast cancer risk. Cancer Pract 1997;5:203–208.

Byers RJ, Hoyland JA, Freemont AJ. Differential patterns of

osteoblast dysfunction in trabecular bone in patients with established osteoporosis. J Clin Pathol 1997;50:760–764.

Castelobranco C. Management of osteoporosis: an overview. Drugs Aging 1998;12(Suppl 1):25–32.

Compston JE. Prevention and management of osteoporosis: current trends and future prospects. Drugs 1997;53:727–735.

Consensus Development Conference. Prophylaxis and treatment of osteoporosis Am J Med 1991;90:107–110.

Cook DJ, Guyatt GH, Adachi JD, et al. Quality of life issues in women with vertebral fractures due to osteoporosis. Arthritis Rheum 1993;36:750–756.

Cummings SR, Black DM, Thompson DE, et al. Effect of alendronate on risk of fracture in women with low bone density but without vertebral fractures: results from the fracture intervention trial. JAMA 1998;280:2077–2082.

De Smet AA, Robinson RG, Johnson BE, Lukert BP. Spinal compression fractures in osteoporotic women: patterns and relationship to hyperkyphosis. Radiology 1988; 166:497–500.

Delmas PD. Diagnostic procedures for osteoporosis in the elderly. Horm Res 1995;43:80–82.

Delmas PD. Hormone replacement therapy in the prevention and treatment of osteoporosis. Osteoporosis Int 1997; (Suppl 1):S3–S7.

Delmas PD, Meunier PJ. The management of Paget's disease of bone. N Engl J Med 1997;336:558–566.

Dequeker J. Overview of osteoporosis treatment. Br J Rheum 1997;36:5–9.

Doppelt SH. Vitamin D, rickets, and osteomalacia. Orthop Clin North Am 1984;15:671–686.

Duboeuf F, Braillon P, Chapuy MC, et al. Bone mineral density of the hip measured with dual-energy x-ray absorptiometry in normal elderly women and in patients with hip fracture. Osteoporosis Int 1991;1:242–249.

Ebeling PR. Osteoporosis in men: new insights into etiology, pathogenesis, prevention and management. Drugs Aging 1998;13:421–434.

Eriksen EF, Langdahl B. Bone changes in metabolic bone disease. Acta Orthop Scand 1995;66(Suppl 266):195–201.

Ernst E. Exercise for female osteoporosis. A systematic review of randomized clinical trials. Sports Med 1998;25:359–368.

Ershler WB, Harman SM, Keller ET. Immunological aspects of osteoporosis. Dev Comp Immunol 1997;21:487–499.

Ettinger B, Black DM, Nevitt MC, et al. Contribution of vertebral deformities to chronic back pain and disability. The study of osteoporotic fractures research group. J Bone Miner Res 1992;7:449–456.

Ettinger B, Black DM, Palermo L, et al. Kyphosis in older women and its relation to back pain, disability and osteopenia: the study of osteoporotic fractures. Osteoporosis Int 1994;4:55–60.

Evans SF, Nicholson PHF, Haddaway MJ, Davie MWJ. Vertebral morphometry in women aged 50–81 years. Bone Miner 1993;21:29–40.

Eyre DR. Bone biomarkers as tools in osteoporosis management. Spine 1997;22(Suppl 24):17–24.

Fleisch H. Bisphosphonates: mechanisms of action and clinical use in osteoporosis: an update. Horm Metab Res 1997;29:145–150.

Francis RM. Bisphosphonates in the treatment of osteoporosis in 1997: a review. Curr Ther Res Clin Exp 1997;58: 656–678.

Francis RM. The effects of testosterone on osteoporosis in men. Clin Endocrinol 1999;50:411–414.

Fries JF. Prevention of osteoporotic fractures: possibilities, the role of exercise, and limitations. Scand J Rheum 1996;25(Suppl 103):6–10.

Frost HM. Defining osteopenias and osteoporoses: another view (with insights from a new paradigm). Bone 1997;20:385–391.

Frost HM. Personal experience in managing acute compression fractures, their aftermath, and the bone pain syndrome, in osteoporosis. Osteoporosis Int 1998;8:13–15.

Gainey JC, Kadaba MP, Wootten ME, et al. Gait analysis of patients who have Paget disease. J Bone Joint Surg Am 1989;71:568–579.

Gluer CC, Jergas M, Hans D. Peripheral measurement techniques for the assessment of osteoporosis. Semin Nucl Med 1997;27:229–247.

Goh S, Price RI, Leedman PJ, Singer KP. The relative influence of vertebral body and intervertebral disc shape on thoracic kyphosis. Clin Biomech 1999;14:439–448.

Grant D, Lundon K. The model of occupational performance applied to females with osteoporosis. Can J Occup Ther 1999;66:3–13.

Grant SFA, Ralston SH. Genes and osteoporosis. Trends Endocrinol Metab 1997;8:232–236.

Gregg EW, Cauley JA, Seely DG, et al. Physical activity and osteoporotic fracture risk in older women. Ann Intern Med 1998;129:81–88.

Gullberg B, Johnell O, Kanis JA. World-wide projections for hip fracture. Osteoporosis Int 1997;7:407–413.

Guyatt GH, Cook DJ. Health status, quality of life, and the individual. JAMA 1994;272:630–631.

Hamdy RC. Clinical features and pharmacologic treatment of Paget's disease. Endocrinol Metab Clin North Am 1995;24:421–433.

Harinck H, Bijivioet O, Vellenga C, et al. Relation between signs and symptoms in Paget's disease of bone. Q J Med 1986;58:133–151.

Heersche JNM, Bellows CG, Yoichiro I. The decrease in bone mass associated with aging and menopause. J Prosthet Dent 1998;79:14–16.

Hosking DJ, Favus M, Yates AJ. Alendronate in the treatment of postmenopausal osteoporosis. Int J Clin Prac 1999;April(Suppl 101):27–35.

Hu SS. Internal fixation in the osteoporotic spine. Spine 1997;22(Suppl 24):43S–48S.

Hughes VA, Frontera WR, Dallal GE, et al. Muscle strength and body composition: associations with bone density in older subjects. Med Sci Sports Exerc 1995;27:967–974.

Hutchison FN, Bell NH. Osteomalacia and rickets. Semin Nephrol 1992;12:127–145.

Ismail AA, Cooper C, Felsenberg D, et al. Number and type of vertebral deformities: epidemiological characteristics and relation to back pain and height loss. Osteoporosis Int 1999;9:206–213.

Itoi E. Roentgenographic analysis of posture in spinal osteoporosis. Spine 1991;16:750–756.

Itoi E, Sinaki M. Effect of back-strengthening exercise on posture in healthy women 49 to 65 years of age. Mayo Clin Proc 1994;69:1054–1059.

Jergas M, Gluer CC. Assessment of fracture risk by bone-density measurements. Semin Nucl Med 1997;27:261–275.

Johansen A, Stone M, Rawlinson F. Bisphosphonates and the treatment of bone disease in the elderly. Drugs Aging 1996;8:113–126.

Johnell O. Prevention of fractures in the elderly. Acta Orthop Scand 1995;66:90–98.

Kanis JA, Delmas P, Burckhardt P, et al. Guidelines for diagnosis and management of osteoporosis. Osteoporosis Int 1997;7:390–406.

Kanis JA, McCloskey EV. Epidemiology of vertebral osteoporosis. Bone 1992;13:S1–S10.

Katznelson L. Therapeutic role of androgens in the treatment of osteoporosis in men. Baillieres Clin Endocrinol Metab 1998;12:453–470.

Kerr D, Morton A, Dick I, Prince R. Exercise effects on bone mass in post-menopausal women are site-specific and load dependent. J Bone Miner Res 1996;11:218–225.

Kleerekoper M, Nelson DA. Vertebral fracture or vertebral deformity? Calcif Tissue Int 1992;50:5–6.

Klein RM, Norman A. Diagnostic procedures for Paget's disease. Endocrinol Metab Clin North Am 1995;24:437–450.

Kohrt WM, Snead DB, Slatopolsky E, et al. Additive effects of weight-bearing exercise and estrogen on bone mineral density in older women. J Bone Miner Res 1995;10:1303–1311.

Kotowicz MA, Melton LJ III, Cooper G, et al. Risk of hip fracture in women with vertebral fracture. J Bone Miner Res 1994;9:599–605.

Kudlacek S, Schneider B, Reisch H, Willvonseder R. Density of lumbar vertebrae: risk-factors for vertebral fractures in women. Deutsche Med Wochenschrift 1998; 123:651–657.

Lanyon L. Using functional loading to influence bone mass and architecture: objectives, mechanisms, and relationship with estrogen of the mechanically adaptive process in bone. Bone 1996;18:S375–S435.

Leidig G, Minne HW, Sauer P, et al. A study of complaints and their relation to vertebral destruction in patients with osteoporosis. Bone Miner 1990;8:217–229.

Leidig-Bruckner G, Minne HW, Schlaich C, et al. Clinical grading of spinal osteoporosis: quality of life components and spinal deformity in women with chronic low back pain and women with vertebral osteoporosis. J Bone Miner Res 1997;12:663–675.

Lenchik L, Sartoris DJ. Orthopedic aspects of metabolic bone disease. Orthop Clin North Am 1998;29:103–134.

Lin JH, Russell G, Gertz B. Pharmacokinetics of alendronate: an overview. Int J Clin Prac 1999;April(Suppl 101):18–26.

Liu G, Peacock M, Eilam O, et al. Effect of osteoarthritis in the lumbar spine and hip on bone-mineral density and diagnosis of osteoporosis in elderly men and women. Osteoporosis Int 1997;7:564–569.

Ludkowski P, Wilson-MacDonald J. Total arthroplasty in Paget's disease of the hip. Clin Orthop 1990;255:160–167.

Lundon K. Age-Related Pathology of Dense Mineralized Connective Tissues: Osteomalacia and Paget's Disease. In T Kauffman (ed), Rehabilitation of the Geriatric Patient. New York: Churchill Livingstone, 1998.

Lydick E, Zimmerman SI, Yawn B, et al. Development and validation of a discriminative quality of life questionnaire for osteoporosis (the OPTQoL). J Bone Miner Res 1997;12:456–463.

Lyles KW, Lammers JE, Shipp, KM, et al. Functional and mobility impairments associated with Paget's disease of bone. J Am Geriatr Soc 1995;43:502–506.

Manolaga SC. Cellular and molecular mechanisms of osteoporosis. Aging Clin Exp Res 1998;10:182–190.

Marcus R. Clinical Review 76. The nature of osteoporosis. J Clin Endocrinol Metab 1996;81:1–5.

Matthis C, Weber U, O'Neill TW, Raspe H. Health impact associated with vertebral deformities: results from the European vertebral osteoporosis study (EVOS). Osteoporosis Int 1998;8:364–372.

Melton LJ III. Epidemiology of osteoporosis. Baillieres Clin Obstet Gynaecol 1991;5:785–805.

Melton LJ. Epidemiology of Osteoporosis and Fractures. In D Sartoris (ed), Osteoporosis Diagnosis and Treatment. New York: Marcel Dekker, 1996;57–79.

Melton LJ, Atkinson EJ, O'Fallon WM, et al. Long-term fracture risk prediction with bone mineral measurements made at various skeletal sites. J Bone Miner Res 1996;6(Suppl 1):S136.

Melton LJ III, Kan SH, Frye MA, et al. Epidemiology of vertebral fractures in women. Am J Epidemiol 1989;129: 1000–1011.

Meunier PJ. Evidence based medicine and osteoporosis: a comparison of fracture risk reduction data from osteoporosis randomised clinical trials. Int J Clin Pract 1999;53:122–124, 126–129.

Meunier PJ, Sebert JL, Reginster JY, et al. Fluoride salts are no better at preventing new vertebral fractures than calcium–vitamin D in postmenopausal osteoporosis. Osteoporosis Int 1998;8:4–12.

Millard PS, Rosen CJ, Johnson KH. Osteoporotic vertebral fractures in postmenopausal women. Am Fam Physician 1997;55:1315–1322.

Minne HW, Pollhane W, Karpf DB. The effects of alendronate on stature and the spine deformity index. Int J Clin Prac 1999;April(Suppl 101):36–39.

Mundy GR. Bone Remodeling and Its Disorders. London: M Dunitz, 1995;153–164.

Myers ER, Wilson SE. Biomechanics of osteoporosis and vertebral fracture. Spine 1997;22(Suppl 24):25S–31S.

Naessen T, Lindmark B, Larse HC. Better postural balance in elderly women receiving estrogen. Am J Obstet Gynecol 1997;177:412–416.

Nelson ME, Fiatarone MA, Morganit CM, et al. Effects of

high-intensity strength training on multiple risk factors for osteoporotic fractures. A randomized controlled trial. JAMA 1994;272:1909–1914.

Nguyen T, Sambrook P, Kelly P, et al. Prediction of osteoporotic fractures by postural instability and bone density. BMJ 1993;307:1111–1115.

Oda K, Shibayama V, Abe M, Onomura T. Morphogenesis of vertebral deformities in involutional osteoporosis: age-related, 3-dimensional trabecular structure. Spine 1998;23:1050–1055.

Ooi CG, Fraser WD. Paget's disease of bone. Postgrad Med J 1997;73:69–74.

Pacifici R. Estrogen, cytokines, and pathogenesis of postmenopausal osteoporosis. J Bone Miner Res 1996;11:1043–1051.

Papapoulos SE. Paget's disease of bone: clinical, pathogenetic and therapeutic aspects. Baillieres Clin Endocrinol Metab 1997;11:117–139.

Pitt MJ. Rickets and osteomalacia are still around. Radiol Clin North Am 1991;29:97–118.

Plantalech L, Knoblovits P, Cambiazzo E. Vitamin D deficiency in elderly nursing home residents of Buenos Aires. Med (B Aires) 1997;57:29–35.

Ragsdale AB, Barringer TA, Anastasio GD. Alendronate treatment to prevent osteoporotic fractures. Arch Fam Med 1998;7:583–586.

Reginato AJ, Falasca GF, Pappu R, et al. Musculoskeletal manifestations of osteomalacia: report of 26 cases and literature review. Semin Arthritis Rheum 1999;28:287–304.

Reginster JYL, Halkin V, Gosset C, Derosy R. The role of bisphosphonates in the treatment of osteoporosis. Drugs Today 1997;33:563–570.

Reid IR. Glucocorticoid osteoporosis: mechanisms and management. Eur J Endocrinol 1997;137:209–217.

Revel M, Mayoux-Benhamou A, Rabourdin JP, et al. One-year psoas training can prevent lumbar bone loss in postmenopausal women; a randomized controlled trial. Calcif Tissue Int 1993;53:307–311.

Riggs BL, Khosla S. Role of biochemical markers in assessment of osteoporosis. Acta Orthop Scand 1995;66(Suppl 266):14–18.

Riggs BL, Melton LJ. The prevention and treatment of osteoporosis. N Engl J Med 1992;327:620–627.

Ringe JD, Dorst A, Kipshoven C, et al. Avoidance of vertebral fractures in men with idiopathic osteoporosis by a 3 year therapy with calcium and low-dose intermittent monofluorophosphate. Osteoporos Int 1998;8:47–53.

Rossini M, Viapiana O, Adami S. Instrumental diagnosis of osteoporosis. Aging Clin Exper Res 1998;10:240–248.

Roux C. Estrogen therapy in postmenopausal osteoporosis: what we know and what we don't. Rev Rhum Engl Ed 1997;64:402–409.

Rozenberg S, Vandromme J, Kroll M, et al. Overview of the clinical usefulness of bone mineral measurements in the prevention of postmenopausal osteoporosis. Int J Fertil 1995;40:12–24.

Rozenberg S, Vandromme J, Kroll M, et al. The brittle bone: how to save women from osteoporosis. Int J Fertil Womens Med 1997;42:101–106.

Rudberg MA, Furner SE, Cassel CK. Measurement issues in preventive strategies: past, present, future. Am J Clin Nutr 1992;55:1253S–1256S.

Ryan SD, Fried LP. The impact of kyphosis on daily functioning. J Am Geriatr Soc 1997;45:1479–1486.

Saag KG, Emkey R, Schnitzer TJ, et al. Alendronate for the prevention and treatment of glucocorticoid induced osteoporosis. N Engl J Med 1998;339:292–299.

Sarrel PM. Hormone replacement therapy in the menopause. Int J Fertil Womens Med 1997:42:78–84.

Silver JJ, Einhorn TA. Osteoporosis and aging. Current update. Clin Orthopaed Related Res 1995;316:10–20.

Sinaki M, Itoi E, Rogers J, et al. Correlation of back extensor strength with thoracic kyphosis and lumbar lordosis in estrogen deficient women. Am J Phys Med Rehabil 1996;75:370–374.

Sinaki M, Mikkelsen BA. Postmenopausal spinal osteoporosis: flexion versus extension exercises. Arch Phys Med Rehabil 1984;65:593–596.

Sinaki M, Offord KP. Physical activity in postmenopausal women: effect on back muscle strength and bone mineral density of the spine. Arch Phys Med Rehabil 1988;69:277–280.

Sinaki M, Wahner HW, Offord KP, et al. Efficacy of nonloading exercises in prevention of vertebral bone loss in postmenopausal women: a controlled trial. Mayo Clin Proc 1989;64:762–769.

Singer FR, Mills BG. Evidence of a viral etiology of Paget's disease of bone. Clin Orthop 1983;178:245.

Stevenson JC. Gonadal hormones. Osteoporosis Int 1997;7 (Suppl 1):S58–S60.

Takahashi M, Kushida K, Hoshino H, et al. Biochemical markers of bone turnover do not decline after menopause in healthy women. Br J Obstet Gynaecol 1999;106:427–431.

Tomomitsu T, Miyake M, Takeda N, Fukunaga M. Age-related changes in vertebral heights ratios and vertebral fracture. Osteoporosis Int 1997;7:113–118.

Treves R, Louer V, Bonnet C, et al. Osteoporosis in men. Presse Med 1998;27:1647–1651.

Turner LW, Fu Q, Taylor JE, et al. Osteoporotic fracture among older women: risk factors quantified. J Aging Health 1998;10:372–391.

Wimalawansa SJ. A four-year randomized controlled trial of hormone replacement and bisphosphate, alone or in combination, in women with postmenopausal osteoporosis. Am J Med 1998;104:219–226.

Witt DM, Lousberg TR. Controversies surrounding estrogen use in postmenopausal women. Ann Pharmacother 1997;31:745–755.

Wolinsky-Friedland M. Drug-induced metabolic bone disease. Endocrinol Metabol Clin North Am 1995;24:395–420.

Ziegler R, Kasperk C. Glucocorticoid induced osteoporosis: prevention and treatment. Steroids 1998;63:344–348.

Zimmerman SI, Fox KM, Magaziner J. Psychosocial aspects of osteoporosis. Phys Med Rehabil Clin North Am 1995;6:441–453.

Chapter 13

Bone Changes in Joint Disease

Osteoarthritis

Changes in the Cartilage Endplate and Subchondral Bone

In the past, degenerative joint diseases (osteoarthritis [OA]) were considered to represent primarily a disorder of cartilage with secondary reactive changes occurring in subchondral bone. However, some suggest that the degenerative joint disease may, in fact, be primarily a subchondral bone disorder with secondary changes occurring in the articular cartilage (Imhof et al. 1997). Subchondral bone changes that occur early in the OA process include a redistribution of blood supply with marrow hypertension and edema, and it is likely that some micronecrosis is present. Some pathophysiologic events appear to parallel those seen in avascular necrosis of bone, and a vascular etiology becomes a consideration. It is believed that changes in the subchondral mineralized tissues are not required for initiation of cartilage fibrillation, but may be necessary for progression, and that only changes in bone and calcified cartilage close to the joint are significant to the disease (Burr and Schaffler 1997). Therefore, the articular cartilage and subchondral bone regions are increasingly considered as one highly interdependent functional unit in which the subchondral bone is more stress-sensitive than previously thought.

OA (also referred to as *osteoarthrosis* or *degenerative joint disease*) is the most common rheuma-tologic disease. This degenerative, noninflammatory joint disease is progressive and irreversible. OA is a condition acquired through metabolic, mechanical, genetic, or other associated influences; however, its precise etiology remains unknown. Information derived from longitudinal studies will likely facilitate valid inferences about causation and provide important new insights, particularly with respect to disease prevention (Felson and Zhang 1998).

Diagnostic evidence of OA includes loss of cartilage matrix macromolecules, increased chondrocyte metabolism, physical disruption of the tissue, and loss of joint function (Smith et al. 1992). At a gross tissue level, OA is characterized by progressive loss of articular cartilage, reactive changes at the margins of the joints, subchondral bone resulting in bony overgrowth, and increased subchondral bone density (Wu et al. 1990). Clinical OA generally consists of joint symptoms in concert with evidence of structural change.

Anatomy of the Subchondral Bone Region

In the subchondral bone region, a bone layer (the cortical end plate) is connected with the calcified cartilage layer. Together, the calcified cartilage and end plate represent the mineralization zone (see Chapter 3). Cancellous bone and fatty marrow is found beneath this zone. The subchondral region is supplied by numerous arterial and venous vessels that extend branches into the calcified cartilage

Clinical Note

Clinical Manifestations of Osteoarthritis

Slowly developing joint pain, stiffness, and enlargement
Limitation in range of motion
Rarely systemic (compared to rheumatoid arthritis [RA] and other connective tissue diseases)

area. In fact, channels that extend between the subchondral region and the uncalcified cartilage have been demonstrated (Milz and Putz 1994). An exchange of extracellular fluid between the cartilage and subchondral region through these channels has been speculated (Burr and Schaffler 1997).

In OA, subchondral bone underlying fibrillated cartilage is sclerotic and stiffer than normal subchondral bone. Once overlying articular cartilage is lost, exposed sclerotic bone becomes eburnated (extruded into the joint space). At the margins of joints some of the subchondral bone forms *osteophytes* that protrude into the joint space or along adjacent tendons or ligaments. Subchondral bone failure may develop as a result of compression and shear forces applied in impact models of overload arthrosis (Norrdin et al. 1998). Milder lesions demonstrate histologic thickening of subchondral bone and underlying trabeculae with advancing sclerosis as well as an increased amount of osteocyte necrosis.

Matrix

Degenerative joint disease results from an imbalance between enzyme production and inhibition, between proinflammatory cytokines and growth factors, and between anabolism and catabolism (Chevalier 1998). Biochemical investigations into the pathogenesis of OA have largely concentrated on the mechanisms involved in the destruction of the articular cartilage, whereas the biochemistry of collagenous matrix within osteoarthritic bone has received considerably less attention. For instance, significant increases in bone collagen metabolism occurred within osteoarthritic femoral heads at the subchondral region (Mansell and Bailey 1998). One

favored theory supports that bone cells from joints affected by OA can influence cartilage metabolism, explaining why increased subchondral bone activity can predict cartilage loss (Westacott et al. 1997). The polarization exhibited in the metabolism of bone collagen from osteoarthritic hips might exacerbate the processes involved in joint deterioration by altering joint morphology. This, in turn, may alter the distribution of mechanical forces to the various tissues, to which bone is a sensitive responder (Mansell and Bailey 1998).

Microdamage

The role of microdamage in OA is poorly understood; however, it is largely regarded as an important determinant of loss of bone quality in general. Results of one study indicate that there are factors that are associated with the increase of microdamage with age that are also independent of bone mass. In this study of patients with OA, bone mineral density (BMD) and microcrack density were the major determinants of cancellous bone strength, whereas BMD and anisotropy were major determinants of cancellous bone stiffness (Fazzalari et al. 1998). One theory suggests that repetitive loading of normal subchondral bone may result in microfractures that, in turn, lessen cartilage support, resulting in surface changes and other modifications of cartilage (Smith et al. 1990).

Classification Criteria

OA has been classified into two forms: idiopathic (primary) or secondary. An example of secondary OA in adulthood would be that associated with anatomic abnormalities experienced earlier in childhood such as congenital dislocation of the hip (CDH) or a slipped femoral epiphysis. Further classification is based on the combination of clinical, radiologic, and laboratory findings.

Clinical Findings

The objective diagnosis of OA is established by radiography; however, radiographic evidence of OA is found in asymptomatic individuals as well. Therefore, the diagnosis of OA relies on both clinical and radiographic presentation (Figure 13-1). Pain plus at least three of six criteria, including age older than 50 years, joint stiffness of less than 30 minutes, crepitus, bony tenderness, bony enlargement, and no palpable warmth, are required for establishing a diagnosis of OA. *Caution*: The value of using the classification criteria is limited. It is meant to allow for standardization of case reports and investigational studies and to foster consistency in communication among clinicians.

Influential Factors Associated with Osteoarthritis

Systemic and local factors affect the likelihood that a joint will develop OA (Dieppe 1995; Dieppe et al. 1997). Systemic factors include a person's age, gender, and inherited susceptibility to OA—among other factors—that all, or in part, make cartilage and subchondral bone more vulnerable to daily injuries and less capable of repair (Felson and Zhang 1998).

Demographics

Prevalence of OA increases with age; the disease is almost universal in people aged 65 and older. OA is more prevalent and may be more generalized in women than in men. Before the age of 50, men have a higher prevalence and incidence of OA than women, but after age 50, women have a higher prevalence and incidence—which is consistent with the role of postmenopausal estrogen deficiency in increasing the risk of OA (Felson and Zhang 1998). Between racial groups, differences exist in prevalence and distribution of affected joints, which may be related to differences in occupation, lifestyle, and predisposing genetic factors. Epidemiologic studies report that Chinese (from southern China), South

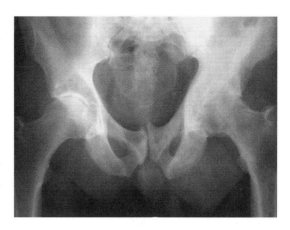

Figure 13-1. This 55-year-old man presented with marked narrowing of the left hip joint space because of osteoarthritis. Note the sclerosis of the subchondral bone regions. (Reprinted with permission from K Lundon, D Hampson. Acquired ectopic ossification of soft tissues: implications for physical therapy. Can J Rehab 1997;10:234.)

African blacks, and East Indians have a lower incidence of OA of the hip than European or American whites. In contrast, the Japanese have a high incidence of secondary OA of the hip. This appears to be related to antecedent congenital hip disease prevalent in this particular population. Congenital subluxation or dislocation of the hip and acetabular dysplasia may predispose girls and young women to premature OA of the hip (Oddis 1996). Legg-Calvé-Perthes disease (the adolescent equivalent of avascular necrosis) and slipped capital femoral epiphysis may predispose boys and young men to early hip OA (Mankin et al. 1986).

Estrogen and Osteoarthritis

In addition to the high incidence of osteoarthritis in women older than age 50, certain women develop menopausal arthritis, which presents as a rapidly progressive OA of the hand at the time of menopause. These gender and age-related prevalence patterns are consistent with the role of postmenopausal hormone deficiency in increasing the risk of OA (Felson and Zhang 1998).

Genetic Associations

Genetic factors play a role in the development of OA of the distal interphalangeal (DIP) joints of the hands (Heberden's nodes). The genetic mechanism appears to involve a single autosomal gene that is gender-influenced and dominant in females, resulting in an incidence in women 10 times greater than in men (Cicuttini and Spector 1997).

Obesity

The role of obesity in the pathogenesis of OA remains controversial. Some studies have demonstrated an increased frequency of OA in the weightbearing joints of obese patients, particularly of the knee, and in women (Anderson and Felson 1988). Longitudinal studies have proven that obesity precedes incidence of knee OA and is not a consequence of it (Felson et al. 1988). The principal reason for the association of the two is suggested to be the additional mechanical stress resulting from being overweight (mechanical theory). In obese people, a sixfold increase in force may be exerted by body weight through weightbearing joints (e.g., the knee) with simple walking; the consequences of obesity are clear. However, a second theory states that a metabolic factor, such as a hormone or biological mediator, linked with obesity induces OA. The strong relationship between the female gender and development of OA supports this theory. Excess adipose tissue may produce abnormal levels of certain hormones or growth factors that may predispose cartilage or underlying bone to OA development (Felson and Zhang 1998).

Bone Density

A general change in bone composition found in patients with OA supports the current hypothesis that the disease involves the bone in the primary pathogenesis (Li and Aspden 1997). An increase in bone mass in the subchondral bone region of the affected joints is typical of advanced OA. The loading pattern at the hip joint during gait and the BMD of the proximal femur in individuals with end-stage hip OA was examined (Hurwitz et al. 1998). Significant correlation between the hip joint movements during gait and femoral BMD indicate that hip joint loads need to be noted when explaining local variation in BMD in hip OA.

Biomechanical Factors

1. *Major injury*: In the Framingham study, men with a history of major knee injury had 5–6 times the risk of developing knee OA as those without (Zhang et al. 1996). Cruciate ligament injury and meniscal tears are strongly associated with OA of the knee. Studies indicate that elite athletes are at high risk of later development of OA especially in the weightbearing joints (Kujala et al. 1995; Roos et al. 1994).
2. *Repetitive stress*: Prolonged occupational or sports-related stress and the inception degree of OA appear to be related. For example, increased severity of OA in the right hand may exist in right hand–dominant people. Cross-sectional data have demonstrated a high risk of hip OA in persons with a high level of physical activity over their lifetime (Lane et al. 1996).

Microdamage accumulation and attempted repair by vascular invasion is considered, in select cases, to be a component of the pathogenesis of OA. The role of developing OA is not considered increased with normal joint use; however, individuals who participate in competitive sports and use structurally abnormal or injured joints while active are at increased risk (Oddis 1996). Muscle strength acts to stabilize a joint, distribute forces, or attenuate the impact of loads across a joint. If muscle contraction is not properly coordinated, the joint will exceed its normal extreme of excursion and the loading of both cartilage and subchondral bone will be excessive. It has been suggested that if the neuromuscular system cannot control the mechanical environment of the joint, the articular, periarticular, and subchondral bone tissues break down (O'Connor and Brandt 1993; Michel et al. 1992). Persons with knee OA identified radiographically, whether symptomatic or not, have weaker quadriceps muscles than those without knee OA (Slemenda et al. 1997). An extensive review of the relationship between OA and exercise can be found elsewhere (McKeag 1992). Careful review of the literature, however, indicates that the perceived association between athletic training and the development of OA appears to be due to injury and joint malalignment rather than any particular form of exercise (Smith et al. 1990).

Relationship of Osteoarthritis and Osteoporosis

An inverse relationship between OA and osteoporosis has been suggested based on the results

Clinical Note

Signs and Symptoms Associated with Osteoarthritis

- Signs and symptoms are usually local.
- Clinical signs and symptoms eventually show positive correlation with radiologic abnormalities.
- Early in the course of the disease, pain occurs after joint use and is relieved by rest. Because cartilage has no nerve supply and is insensitive to pain, pain arises from secondary effects, including other innervated intra-articular and periarticular structures affected by the disease process.
- Joint stiffness is relatively short-lived and localized. Local tenderness may be elicited, especially if synovitis (usually secondary) is present.
- Pain is evoked on passive motion of affected joints and *crepitus*, a feeling of cracking and palpable grating, may be heard as the joint is moved.
- Joint enlargement is often seen, resulting from bony swelling (e.g., proliferative change in cartilage and bone).

Sources of Pain in Osteoarthritis

Painful joints are a primary complaint in the patient with OA. Sources of pain include

- Periosteum: elevation of the innervated periosteal layer of bone because of bony proliferation
- Increased pressure on subchondral bone that is no longer covered or protected by articular cartilage
- Trabecular microfractures
- Soft tissue (ligament, capsular, synovium) distension
- Involvement of highly innervated periarticular structures, including the fascia and tendons

of several epidemiologic studies that have shown a lower incidence and prevalence of hip fractures in people with OA (Dequeker et al. 1996; Sambrook and Naganathan 1997). Because OA is a disease of cartilage and subchondral bone, the higher bone density and increased stiffness seen in the subchondral bone with OA may contribute to this occurrence. Subchondral bone taken from the femoral head of patients with OA was intermediately stiff and dense, relative to osteoporotic bone (least stiff and dense) and normal controls (most stiff and dense) (Li and Aspden 1997). In this study, osteoarthritic bone from the same regions was found to be hypomineralized but additionally displayed diminished organic and water fractions, suggesting a defect in the matrix of subchondral bone (Li and Aspden 1997). Osteoporosis is not a component of degenerative changes seen in the subchondral bone of an osteoarthritic joint. Quantitative analysis of cancellous bone structure of the femoral bone from patients with severe primary OA demonstrated increased trabecular thickness and decreased trabecular number. Increased morphometric variance indicated that severe OA, contrary to osteoporosis, is associated with heterogeneous bone structures, findings which provide some basis for understanding how OA may contribute to the prevention of osteoporotic fracture (Antonacci et al. 1997; Fazzalari and Parkinson 1998).

Pathology: Gross Histologic Changes in the Osteoarthritic Process

Structural Breakdown of Cartilage

The breakdown of articular cartilage is marked by *fissuring*, *pitting*, and *erosions*. Erosions are initially focal events (Figure 13-2). Eventually they become confluent and lead to large areas of denuded surface. Disease progression is characterized by full-thickness loss of cartilage down to the bone.

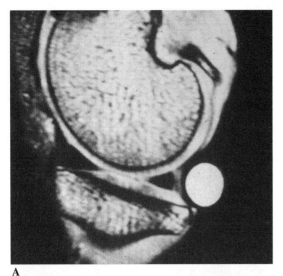

A

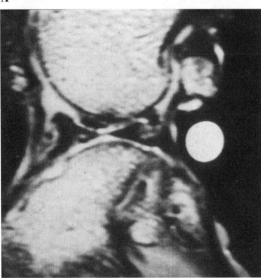

B

Figure 13-2. A. Magnetic resonance imaging (MRI) of a normal knee joint. **B.** MRI of a knee joint with moderate osteoarthritis. Note the subchondral bone sclerosis and the deterioration in the joint space and articular cartilage.

Proliferation of Cartilage and Bone

Osteophyte spur formation is seen most prominently at joint margins and represents a proliferative response of cartilage and bone inherent to the osteoarthritic process. Osteophytes form and consist of proliferating new bone capped by cartilage.

Clinical observation indicates that bone density and cartilage fibrillation are inversely related.

Thickening and Sclerosis of Subchondral Bone

A process known as *eburnation* of subchondral bone and juxta-articular bone cyst formation occurs in advanced stages of the disease.

Synovitis

Localized inflammatory changes relate to the release of inflammatory mediators or humoral and cell-mediated immune responses to damaged joint components.

Assessment of the Osteoarthritic Joint

Biochemistry

Biochemical markers for OA may serve different purposes. Markers reflect ongoing dynamic metabolic processes in the affected joint tissues including cartilage, synovium, and bone; they are of interest for the therapeutic management of OA (Lohmander 1997).

Patient-Related Measures of Joint Pain and Disability

Scoring systems such as the WOMAC OA index may be used to assess patient-related measures of joint pain and disability (Bellamy et al. 1988).

Physical Assessment

Hand.   Spurs formed at the dorsolateral and medial aspects of the DIP joints of the fingers are called *Heberden's nodes*. Flexor and lateral deviations of the distal phalanx are common. Similar changes at the proximal interphalangeal joints are known as *Bouchard's nodes* (cartilaginous). Involvement at the first carpometacarpal joint leads to tenderness at the base of the first metacarpal bone and a squared appearance of the hand. The trapezioscaphoid joint is also commonly affected.

Knee.   OA of the knee is characterized by localized tenderness over various compartments of the

Clinical Note

The individual with OA should avoid physical activities that apply excessive or abrupt forces on the affected joints because these may cause further damage to subchondral bone and cartilage and cause pain. For this reason, exercise programs must be introduced with caution and adjustments in intensity introduced in a graduated manner. In addition, participants in physical activities should avoid extreme fatigue, which is conducive to joint malalignment or injury. It is critical that programs tailored for persons with arthritis are designed and implemented with their fundamental principles supported by knowledge of disease pathophysiology, joint biomechanics, exercise science, and an appreciation of the need for adoption of physical activity into lifelong practice.

joint and pain may be elicited by both passive or active motion. Joint crepitus and associated muscle atrophy (quadriceps, especially vastus medialis) secondary to disuse are common features in OA of the knee (Marks et al. 1994).

Hip. Osteoarthritic changes in the hip lead to an insidious onset of pain often inducing an altered gait pattern of the affected individual. Pain is usually localized to the groin or along the inner aspect of the thigh although patients often complain of pain in the buttocks, sciatic region, or the knee due to pain referral along contiguous nerves. Physical examination typically demonstrates loss of joint motion with internal rotation or extension of the hip.

Foot. The first metatarsophalangeal (MTP) joint of the foot is commonly affected by OA. OA of the first MTP joint can be aggravated, for example, by shoes that are too tight. Irregularities in joint contour can be palpated. Tenderness is common when the overlying bursa at the medial aspect of this joint becomes inflamed.

Spine. OA of the spine results from involvement of the intervertebral disks, vertebral bodies, or posterior apophyseal articulations. Involvement of the lumbar spine is seen most commonly at the L3-L4 area. Associated symptoms include local pain and stiffness and radicular pain due to compression of contiguous nerve roots. Large anterior osteophytes in the cervical spine may give rise to dysphagia or respiratory tract symptoms. Compression of nerve roots or the cord itself leads to variable neurologic deficits.

Radiographic Evaluation

X-rays may appear normal if pathologic changes are mild. Characteristic and progressive changes include narrowing of the affected joint spaces (due to cartilage deterioration), subchondral bony sclerosis (eburnation), osteophyte formation at the joint margins (in the case of the knee at the tibial spines), and bony cyst formation. In more advanced OA, subluxation of the joint may result.

Management

The selection of specific therapeutic programs is tailored according to the unique presentation of the individual affected by OA. General status of health, weight, and the individual's ability to cooperate in programs designed for the therapeutic management of OA must be considered. The management of OA should also include adaptation of the surrounding environment (e.g., prescribing shoe orthotics when indicated, altering chair height, etc.).

Physical Rehabilitation

Physical activity programs should emphasize safety to avoid joint injury and malalignment, factors that likely contribute to the initial development of OA (Smith et al. 1990). When weightbearing joints are affected by OA, the protection of these joints from overuse is very important. The influence of different knee joint stresses on intra-articular oxygen partial pressure revealed that patients with OA sustained a lower increase of intra-articular oxygen partial pressure with exercise than healthy controls (Miltner et al. 1997). Joint protection and avoidance of vigorous activity may be indicated to minimize joint stress, inflammation, and tissue damage. As an example, forces transferred through the lower extremity are increased three- to fourfold when weight is shifted to each leg in walking. The use of canes, for example, can be beneficial for the purpose of joint protection.

Strengthening of the muscles surrounding the weightbearing joints affected by OA is important to optimize joint mechanics. Improvement in muscle strength around the affected joint decreases the shock to the subchondral bone and assists in reducing stress that perpetuates injury because of mechanical forces. Range-of-motion exercises are important to maintain and maximize movement. Because OA patients may be deconditioned, graduated exercise is warranted. In fact, conditioning exercise as an appropriate addition to comprehensive arthritis management has gained much support (Rogind et al. 1998), with extensive reviews of such found elsewhere (Minor et al. 1991; Panush and Brown 1987; Semble et al. 1990). The rationale of exercise for the management of OA is based on its corrective effect on disuse, atrophy, and weakness, increasing muscle and associated periarticular muscle strength, increasing intra-articular nutrient diffusion with weightbearing exercise, and effectively stimulating compression of cartilage and subchondral bone through weightbearing (McKeag 1992). A study in which 8 weeks of simple aerobic training (walking) was prescribed to subjects with OA of the knee demonstrated an outcome of increase in the amount of manageable distance on a 6-minute walking test, as compared to controls (Kovar et al. 1992). The alleviation and control of pain and muscle spasm by use of thermal agents and modalities, such as heat, and the maintenance and promotion of optimal joint range of motion is indicated on an individual basis. Application of heat to an affected joint paradoxically decreases intra-articular temperature (Oddis 1996). Weight reduction is advised for obese patients.

Pharmacology

Analgesic agents, such as acetaminophen, may be used on a continuous or as-needed (prn) basis. Aspirin is effective both as an analgesic and anti-inflammatory agent. The use of nonaspirin nonsteroidal anti-inflammatory drugs (NSAIDs) is receiving increased clinical acceptance for symptomatic relief of pain. These agents include indomethacin, ibuprofen, fenoprofen, naproxen, tolmetin, meclofenamate, piroxicam, sulindac, diflunisal, and ketoprofen. Some of these have a number of adverse side effects, particularly in the elderly population. Certain NSAIDs, including aspirin, appear to significantly reduce cartilage proteoglycan synthesis in both in vivo and in vitro studies.

Surgery

Orthopedic surgery is the most aggressive management option for OA. Surgical procedures include total or partial joint arthroplasty, osteotomy, and joint fusion. Angulation osteotomy is particularly helpful for correcting joint malalignment when significant varus or valgus deformities (e.g., of the knee) are present in unicompartmental disease. Pain is relieved by the realignment of healthy articular cartilage and its underlying bony surface within the joint space. Hip and knee replacement procedures produce striking symptomatic relief and improved range of motion. Advances in arthroscopic techniques have led to an increase in microsurgical management earlier along the course of the disease. The joint can be irrigated and débrided to remove loose bodies and to smooth out irregular joint surfaces.

Rheumatoid Arthritis and Associated Changes in Bone

Assessment and Management of the Bone Changes in the Joint Affected by Rheumatoid Arthritis

RA is associated with changes in bone and muscle mass. RA is a chronic destructive inflammatory process involving the synovial joints and ultimately destroying intra- and periarticular structures, including subchondral bone, articular cartilage, ligaments, and tendons. The damaged structures become incompetent at maintaining normal joint alignment. RA is associated with a decrease in BMD at both the lumbar spine and femoral neck regions, most marked in patients with active and severe disease and in those who take glucocorticoids (Cortet et al. 1997). The symptoms and medical management of RA puts individuals, particularly women, at risk for BMD loss and thus osteoporosis. Vertebral deformities are typical of advanced RA and seem to occur even more frequently in those treated with corticosteroids (Lems et al. 1997). Corticosteroid therapy, even in daily doses of less than 10 mg per day of prednisone equivalent, was associated with an approximately 10% decrease in bone mass after 6 months of treatment (Cortet et al. 1995). Laan et al. (1993) demonstrated that even low dose corticosteroids can, in fact, influence BMD in the vertebrae of RA patients; however, the osteopenia that results may be reversible after administration of the drugs is stopped. The bisphosphonates may have potential in the prophylaxis of osteopenia and deterring subchondral bone damage in inflammatory arthritis (Bogoch and Moran 1998; Geusens et al. 1998; Laan et al. 1999).

Stimulation of such bone loss may be induced by inflammatory arthritis, which is demonstrable in animal models. Increased bone remodeling and altered microstructure of bone occur in such inflammation-induced arthritis models, inducing a narrowed subchondral bone plate and perforation by vascular inflammatory invasion. There is also an increased femoral fracture risk in RA that may be induced by cortical bone resorption defects (Bogoch and Moran 1998). In one study, it was determined that patients with RA had a twofold increase in fracture risk, independent of their bone mass. Factors associated with this high fracture risk were corticosteroid therapy, physical inactivity, and female gender (Cortet et al. 1995).

Rheumatoid Arthritis and Arthroplasty

Osteopenia is responsible for substantial co-morbidity in patients with RA and is an important factor in the surgical management of joint disease (Bogoch and Moran 1998; Yang et al. 1997). Stiffness of subchondral bone is a factor in the stability of any prosthesis implanted in this region and it becomes an important surgical consideration in that bone from individuals with RA has significantly less stiffness than either normal or osteoarthritic bone (Yang et al. 1997).

Role of Exercise in the Management of Inflammatory Arthritis

Exercise has been shown to increase bone mineral, the potential for which becomes especially important for those treated with steroids (Zeidman and Ducker 1994). An investigation of soft tissue composition, quadriceps strength, bone quality, and bone mass revealed quadriceps strength was 20% lower in females with RA when compared to controls. In addition, significantly lower BMD existed at the femoral neck but not spine in this same group. Reduction in BMD and muscle strength in RA were not, however, accompanied by changes in soft tissue composition in this study (Madsen et al. 1998). Minimally supervised strength training resulted in significant improvements in muscle strength but not BMD over a 12-month period in patients with RA (Hakkinen et al. 1999).

Traditional treatment has included rest for the affected part, which results in a further reduction of physical condition that includes the impact of immobilization or decreased physical stress on bone. An extended abstinence from appropriate physical activity may exacerbate systemic and musculoskeletal consequences inherent to RA. Minor et al. (1991) described improvement in aerobic capacity of 120 patients with RA and OA in response to a program of aerobic activity that included walking and aquatics. When this group was compared to patients with OA and RA who performed nonaerobic range-of-motion stretching, no differences were noted in the number of inflamed joints. Aerobic exercise also appears to induce positive changes in circulating immune function, which would possibly be helpful in regulating inflammation (Shephard and Shek 1997), an influence that might extend to the bone.

However, high-impact joint loading, such as running and jumping, should be avoided so as to avoid further cartilage and subchondral bone damage. A rehabilitation or exercise regimen using cross-training principles and involving the integration of various strengthening and endurance techniques into the current exercise program can be beneficial for patients with inflammatory arthritis. By changing the pattern of joint loading on a regular basis, joint overload can be avoided (Galloway and Jokl 1993). Isometric exercise is also advised in the management of the RA joint to induce the least possible joint inflammation, intra-articular pressure, and juxta-articular bone destruction (Gerber 1990).

Summary

OA is a degenerative joint disorder with a multifactorial etiology and is the most common form of arthritis. The consensus is that OA is characterized by sclerosing of the subchondral bone region; however, whether bone changes occur concurrent with, primary to, or secondary to, cartilage deterioration is disputed. It is plausible that microdamage accumulation and repair by vascular invasion may be important components of the pathogenesis of OA. Systemic factors, such as age, gender, and inherited susceptibility to OA, may play a permissive role to the effect that local biomechanical factors play in joint breakdown. Repetitive joint injury (major and minor), joint deformity (change in angulation), obesity, and muscle weakness are biomechanical factors that likely contribute to the OA process. Current therapy of OA is largely symptomatic, and aims to decrease pain and improve function with pharmacologic agents (e.g., analgesics, NSAIDs) or joint replacement. The recognition of the role of muscle strengthening or aerobic conditioning in both alleviating disability (tertiary prevention) and as a strategy for primary prevention of OA is of utmost importance. The trend in transition from large cross-sectional epidemiologic studies to longitudinal observational studies and clinical trials should benefit knowledge of preventive strategies for OA that, to a large extent, include this physical management component.

RA is a chronic autoimmune disease characterized by the accumulation of inflammatory cells into the synovium and the destruction of joints. It is important to identify and treat individuals at risk for BMD loss due to RA and to: (1) identify those with RA and be aware of the effects of medical intervention used to treat symptoms of the disease (e.g., corticosteroids), (2) understand symptoms of the disease relating to activity levels and direct the individual in appropriate exercise, and (3) identify and correct, as able, habitual postural abnormalities (forward head posture).

References

Anderson J, Felson DT. Factors associated with osteoarthritis of the knee in the First National Health and Nutrition Examination Survey I (NHANES I): evidence for an association with overweight, race, and physical demands of work. Am J Epidemiol 1988;128:79–189.

Antonacci MD, Hanson DS, Leblanc A, Heggeness MH. Regional variation in vertebral bone-density and trabecular architecture are influenced by osteoarthritic change and osteoporosis. Spine 1997;22:2393–2401.

Bellamy N, Buchanan W, Goldsmith CH, et al. Validation study of WOMAC: a health status instrument for measuring clinically important patient relevant outcomes to antirheumatic drug therapy in patients with osteoarthritis of the hip or knee. J Rheumatol 1988;15:1833–1840.

Bogoch ER, Moran E. Abnormal bone remodeling in inflammatory arthritis. Can J Surg 1998;41:264–271.

Burr DB, Schaffler MB. The involvement of subchondral mineralized tissues in osteoarthrosis: quantitative microscopic evidence. Microsc Res Tech 1997;37:343–357.

Chevalier X. Therapeutic perspectives. Presse Med 1998;27: 88–92.

Cicuttini FM, Spector TD. What is the evidence that osteoarthritis is genetically determined? Baillieres Clin Rheumatol 1997;11:657–669.

Cortet B, Flipo RM, Blanckaert F, et al. Evaluation of bone-mineral density in patients with rheumatoid arthritis: influence of disease activity and glucocorticoid therapy. Rev Rhum 1997;64:451–458.

Cortet B, Flipo RM, Duquesnoy B, Delcambre B. Polyarthrite rhumatoide et tissu osseux (1). Densitometrie osseuse et risque fracturaire. Rev Rhum Fr Ed 1995;62: 206–213.

Dequeker J, Boonen S, Aerssens J, Westhovens R. Inverse relationship osteoarthritis-osteoporosis: what is the evidence? What are the consequences? Br J Rheumatol 1996;35:813–820.

Dieppe P. The Classification and Diagnosis of Osteoarthritis. In KE Kuettner, WM Goldberg (eds), Osteoarthritic Disorders. Rosemont, IL: American Academy of Orthopaedic Surgeons 1995;5–12.

Dieppe PA, Cushnaghan J, Shepstone L. The Bristol "OA500" Study: progression of osteoarthritis (OA) over 3 years and the relationship between clinical and radiographic changes at the knee joint. Osteoarthritis Cartilage 1997;5:87–97.

Fazzalari NL, Forwood MR, Smith K, et al. Assessment of cancellous bone quality in severe osteoarthrosis; bone mineral density, mechanics, and microdamage. Bone 1998;22:381–388.

Fazzalari NL, Parkinson IH. Femoral trabecular bone of osteoarthritic and normal subjects in an age and sex matched group. Osteoarthritis Cartilage 1998;6: 377–382.

Felson DT, Anderson JJ, Naimark A, et al. Obesity and knee osteoarthritis: the Framingham study. Ann Intern Med 1988;109:18–24.

Felson DT, Zhang Y. An update on the epidemiology of knee and hip osteoarthritis with a view to prevention. Arthritis Rheum 1998;41:1343–1355.

Galloway MT, Jokl P. The role of exercise in the treatment of inflammatory arthritis. Bull Rheum Dis 1993;42:1–4.

Gerber LH. Exercise and arthritis. Bull Rheum Dis 1990;39: 1–8.

Geusens P, Dequeker J, Vanhoof J, et al. Cyclical etidronate increases bone density in the spine and hip of postmenopausal women receiving long-term corticosteroid treatment. A double blind, randomized placebo controlled study. Ann Rheum Dis 1998;57: 724–727.

Hakkinen A, Sokka T, Kotaniemi A. Dynamic strength training in patients with early rheumatoid arthritis increases muscle strength but not bone mineral density. J Rheumatol 1999;26:1257–1263.

Hurwitz DE, Foucher KC, Sumner DR, et al. Hip motion and moments during gait relate directly to proximal femoral bone mineral density in patients with hip osteoarthritis. J Biomechan 1998;31:919–925.

Imhof H, Breitenseher M, Kainberger F, Trattnig S. Degenerative joint disease: cartilage or vascular disease? Skeletal Radiol 1997;26:398–403.

Kovar PA, Allegrante JP, Mackenzie CR, et al. Supervised fitness walking in patients with osteoarthritis of the knee. A randomized, controlled trial. Ann Intern Med 1992;116:529–534.

Kujala UM, Kettunen J, Paananen H, et al. Knee osteoarthritis in former runners, soccer players, weight lifters, and shooters. Arthritis Rheum 1995;38:539–546.

Laan RF, Buijs WC, vanErning LJ, et al. Differential effects of glucocorticoids on cortical appendicular and cortical vertebral bone mineral content. Calcif Tissue Int 1993;52:5–9.

Laan RF, Jansen TL, van Riel PL. Glucocorticosteroids in the management of rheumatoid arthritis. Rheumatology 1999;38:6–12.

Lane NE, Nevitt MC, Pressman A, et al. The relationship of physical activity and osteoarthritis of the hip in a cohort of elderly women [Abstract]. Arthritis Rheum 1996;39(Suppl 9):S309.

Lems WF, Jahangier ZN, Raymakers JA, et al. Methods to score vertebral deformities in patients with rheumatoid arthritis. Br J Rheumatol 1997;36:220–224.

Li BH, Aspden RM. Mechanical and material properties of the subchondral bone plate from the femoral head of patients with osteoarthritis or osteoporosis. Ann Rheum Dis 1997;56:247–254.

Lohmander LS. What is the current status of biochemical markers in the diagnosis, prognosis and monitoring of osteoarthritis? Baillieres Clin Rheumatol 1997;11:711–726.

Madsen OR, Egsmose C, Hansen B, Sorensen OH. Soft tissue composition, quadriceps strength, bone quality and bone mass in rheumatoid arthritis. Clin Exp Rheumatol 1998;16:27–32.

Mankin HJ, Brandt KA, Shulman LE. Workshop on etiopathogenesis of osteoarthritis: proceedings and recommendations. J Rheumatol 1986;13:1130–1160.

Mansell JP, Bailey AJ. Abnormal cancellous bone-collagen metabolism in osteoarthritis. J Clin Invest 1998;101: 1596–1603.

Marks R, Kumar S, Semple J, Percy J. Quadriceps femoris activation in healthy women with genu varum and women with osteoarthrosis and genu varum. J Electromyogr Kinesiol 1994;4:153–160.

McKeag DB. The relationship of osteoarthritis and exercise. Clin Sports Med 1992;11:471–487.

Michel BA, Fries JF, Bloch DA, et al. Osteophytosis of the knee: association with changes in weight bearing exercise. Clin Rheumatol 1992;11:235–238.

Miltner O, Schneider U, Graf J, Neithard FU. Influence of isokinetic and ergometric exercises on oxygen partial pressure measurement in the human knee joint. Adv Exp Med Biol 1997;411:183–189.

Milz S, Putz R. Luckenbildung der subchondralen Mineralisierungszone des Tibiaplateaus. Osteologie 1994;3: 110–118.

Minor MA. Physical activity and management of arthritis. Ann Behav Med 1991;13:117–124.

Norrdin RW, Kawak CE, Capwell BA, McIlwraith CW. Subchondral bone failure in an equine model of overload arthrosis. Bone 1998;22:133–139.

O'Connor BL, Brandt KD. Neurogenic factors in the etiopathogenesis of osteoarthritis. Rheum Dis Clin North Am 1993;19:581–605.

Oddis CV. New perspectives on osteoarthritis. Am J Med 1996;100(Suppl 2A):2-10S–2-15S.

Panush RS, Brown DG. Exercise and arthritis. Sports Med 1987;4:54–64.

Rogind H, Bibow-Nielsen B, Jensen B, et al. The effects of a physical training program on patients with osteoarthritis of the knees. Arch Phys Med Rehab 1998;79: 1421–1427.

Roos H, Lindberg H, Gardsell P, et al. The prevalence of gonarthrosis in former soccer players and its relation to meniscectomy. Am J Sports Med 1994;22:219–222.

Sambrook P, Naganathan V. What is the relationship between osteoarthritis and osteoporosis? Baillieres Clin Rheumatol 1997;11:695–710.

Semble EL, Loeser RF, Wise CM. Therapeutic exercise for rheumatoid arthritis and osteoarthritis. Semin Arthritis Rheum 1990;20:32–40.

Shephard RJ, Shek PN. Autoimmune disorders, physical activity, and training, with particular reference to rheumatoid arthritis. Exerc Immunol Rev 1997;3: 53–67.

Slemenda C, Brandt KD, Heilman DK, et al. Quadriceps weakness and osteoarthritis of the knee. Ann Intern Med 1997;127:97–104.

Smith EL, Smith KA, Gilligan C. Exercise, Fitness, Osteoarthritis, and Osteoporosis. In Exercise, Fitness and Health: A Consensus of Current Knowledge. Champaign, IL: Human Kinetics Books, 1990.

Smith RL, Thomas KD, Schurman DJ, et al. Rabbit knee immobilization: bone remodeling precedes cartilage degeneration. J Orthop Res 1992;10:88–95.

Westacott CI, Webb GR, Warnock MG, et al. Alteration of cartilage metabolism by cells from osteoarthritic bone. Arthritis Rheum 1997;40:1282–1291.

Wu DD, Burr DB, Boyd RD, Radin EL. Bone and cartilage changes following experimental varus or valgus tibial angulation. J Orthop Res 1990;8:572–585.

Yang JP, Bogoch ER, Woodside TD, Hearn TC. Stiffness of trabecular bone of the tibial plateau in patients with rheumatoid-arthritis of the knee. J Arthrop 1997;12: 798–803.

Zeidman SM, Ducker TB. Rheumatoid arthritis. Neuroanatomy, compression, and grading of deficits. Spine 1994;19:2259–2266.

Zhang Y, Glynn RJ, Felson DT. Musculoskeletal disease research: should we analyze the joint or the person? J Rheumatol 1996;23:1130–1134.

Index